Contents

vii   *Conference Committee*
ix   *Introduction*

KEYNOTE ADDRESS

2   **Past and future of radiologic error** [3663-06]
     P. J. Friedman, Univ. of California/San Diego Medical Ctr.

SESSION 1   DISPLAY PARAMETERS AND PERFORMANCE I

8   **Observer performance assessment of JPEG-compressed high-resolution chest images**
     [3663-01]
     W. F. Good, G. S. Maitz, J. L. King, R. C. Gennari, D. Gur, Univ. of Pittsburgh School of
     Medicine

14   **Acceptable compression ratios for CR images for PACS archives** [3663-02]
     B. M. Misra, Harvard Univ.; P. F. Judy, F. L. Jacobson, W. B. Hanlon, S. D. Davis, Brigham
     and Women's Hospital/Harvard Medical School

24   **Effect of denoising on the consistency of manually defined borders** [3663-03]
     X. Zong, GE Corporate Research and Development; E. A. Geiser, Univ. of Florida;
     D. A. Conetta, Health Sciences Ctr./Univ. of Florida

34   **Clinical validation studies on clinical workstation prototypes** [3663-04]
     B. Verdonck, K. C. Strasters, F. A. Gerritsen, Philips Medical Systems (Netherlands)

44   **Effects of radiation dose and display contrast on low-contrast phantom image visibility**
     [3663-05]
     C. C. Chamberlain, W. Huda, A. R. Wojtowycz, Health Sciences Ctr./SUNY Syracuse

SESSION 2   DISPLAY PARAMETERS AND PERFORMANCE II

56   **Radiologists' ability to use computer-aided diagnosis (CAD) to improve breast biopsy**
     recommendations [3663-07]
     Y. Jiang, R. M. Nishikawa, Univ. of Chicago Medical Ctr.

61   **Computer algorithm for automated detection and quantification of microaneurysms and**
     hemorrhages (HMAs) in color retinal images [3663-08]
     S. C. Lee, Y. Wang, Univ. of Oklahoma; E. T. Lee, Health Sciences Ctr./Univ. of Oklahoma

SESSION 3   ROC AND OTHER PERFORMANCE METHODOLOGIES

74   **Using incomplete and imprecise localization data on images to improve estimates of**
     detection accuracy [3663-09]
     R. G. Swensson, G. S. Maitz, J. L. King, D. Gur, Univ. of Pittsburgh School of Medicine

82   Differential receiver operating characteristic (DROC) method: rationale and results of recent experiments [3663-10]
D. P. Chakraborty, N. S. Howard, H. L. Kundel, Univ. of Pennsylvania School of Medicine

91   Monte Carlo validation of a multireader method for receiver operating characteristic discrete rating data: split-plot experimental design [3663-11]
D. D. Dorfman, K. S. Berbaum, R. V. Lenth, Y.-F. Chen, Univ. of Iowa

100 Gains in accuracy from averaging ratings of abnormality [3663-12]
R. G. Swensson, J. L. King, D. Gur, W. F. Good, Univ. of Pittsburgh School of Medicine

108 Dynamic viewing protocols for diagnostic image comparison [3663-13]
D. H. Foos, Eastman Kodak Co.; R. M. Slone, B. R. Whiting, Mallinckrodt Institute of Radiology/Washington Univ. School of Medicine; K. S. Kohm, S. S. Young, Eastman Kodak Co.; E. Muka, D. Hendrickson, Mallinckrodt Institute of Radiology/Washington Univ. School of Medicine

SESSION 4   PERCEPTUAL PROCESSES AND PERFORMANCE

122 Eye-position study of the effects of a verbal prompt and pictorial backgrounds on the search for lung nodules in chest radiographs [3663-14]
H. L. Kundel, C. F. Nodine, L. C. Toto, Univ. of Pennsylvania School of Medicine

129 Medical image compression using attention modeling [3663-15]
A. J. Maeder, Queensland Univ. of Technology (Australia)

136 Development of the eye-movement response in the trainee radiologist [3663-16]
D. S. Wooding, Univ. of Derby (UK); G. M. Roberts, J. Phillips-Hughes, Univ. of Wales College of Medicine (UK)

146 Chronometric analysis of mammography expertise [3663-17]
C. Mello-Thoms, C. F. Nodine, H. L. Kundel, Univ. of Pennsylvania School of Medicine

151 Influence of monitor luminance and tone scale on observers' search and dwell patterns [3663-18]
E. A. Krupinski, H. Roehrig, Health Sciences Ctr./Univ. of Arizona

157 Breast cancer screening: comparison of radiologists' performance in a self-assessment scheme and in actual breast screening [3663-19]
H. C. Cowley, A. G. Gale, Univ. of Derby (UK)

SESSION 5   TECHNOLOGY ASSESSMENT AND OBSERVER PERFORMANCE I

170 Psychophysical evaluation of the image quality of a dynamic flat-panel digital x-ray image detector using the threshold contrast detail detectability (TCDD) technique [3663-20]
A. G. Davies, A. R. Cowen, Univ. of Leeds General Infirmary (UK); T. J. Bruijns, Philips Medical Systems (Netherlands)

180 Evaluation of angiograms obtained from a laser-based x-ray source in DESA regime [3663-21]
E. M. Scalzetti, A. Krol, G. M. Gagne, T. T. Renvyle, C. C. Chamberlain, Health Science Ctr./SUNY Syracuse; J.-C. Kieffer, Z. Jiang, J. Yu, INRS/Univ. Québec (Canada)

PROCEEDINGS OF SPIE

Society for Optical Engineering

Medical Imaging 1999

Image Perception
and Performance

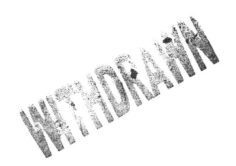

Elizabeth A. Krupinski
Chair/Editor

24–25 February 1999
San Diego, California

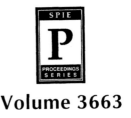

Sponsored by
SPIE—The International Society for Optical Engineering

Cooperating Organizations
AAPM—American Association of Physicists in Medicine
APS—American Physiological Society
FDA Center for Devices and Radiological Health
IS&T—The Society for Imaging Science and Technology
NEMA—National Electrical Manufacturers Association/Diagnostic Imaging
  and Therapy Systems Division
RSNA—Radiological Society of North America
SCAR—Society for Computer Applications in Radiology

Published by
SPIE—The International Society for Optical Engineering

SPIE
P
PROCEEDINGS
SERIES

Volume 3663

SPIE is an international technical society dedicated to advancing engineering and scientific
applications of optical , photonic, imaging, electronic, and optoelectronic technologies.

Please use the following format to cite material from this book:
  Author(s), "Title of paper," in *Medical Imaging 1999: Image Perception and Performance*, Elizabeth A. Krupinski, Editor, Proceedings of SPIE Vol. 3663, page numbers (1999).

ISSN 0277-786X
ISBN 0-8194-3135-4

Published by
SPIE—The International Society for Optical Engineering
P.O. Box 10, Bellingham, Washington 98227-0010 USA
Telephone 360/676-3290 (Pacific Time) • Fax 360/647-1445

187   LROC analysis of human detection performance in PET and time-of-flight PET [3663-22]
       H. C. Gifford, R. G. Wells, M. A. King, Univ. of Massachusetts Medical School

199   Diagnostic performance and image quality assessment in teledermatology [3663-23]
       E. A. Krupinski, Arizona Telemedicine/Univ. of Arizona; B. W. LeSueur, L. G. Ellsworth,
       N. Levine, R. C. Hansen, N. Silvis, P. Sarantopoulos, P. Hite, J. P. Wurzel, Univ. of Arizona
       College of Medicine; R. S. Weinstein, A. M. Lopez, Arizona Telemedicine/Univ. of Arizona

207   Classification of mammographic patterns: beyond fraction of dense tissue [3663-24]
       P. F. Judy, R. Nawfel, F. L. Jacobson, D. N. Smith, S. E. Seltzer, Brigham and Women's
       Hospital/Harvard Medical School

SESSION 6   TECHNOLOGY ASSESSMENT AND OBSERVER PERFORMANCE II

212   Effect of monitor luminance on the detection of a solitary pulmonary nodule: ROC analysis
       [3663-25]
       K.-S. Song, J. S. Lee, H. Y. Kim, T.-H. Lim, Univ. of Ulsan College of Medicine (Korea)

217   Observer performance using CRT monitors with different phosphors [3663-26]
       H. Roehrig, E. A. Krupinski, M. Sivarudrappa, Health Sciences Ctr./Univ. of Arizona

225   Web-based tool for subjective observer ranking of compressed medical images [3663-27]
       S. G. Langer, B. K. Stewart, R. K. Andrew, Univ. of Washington

SESSION 7   MODELING VISUAL SIGNAL DETECTION I

232   Evaluation of keyhole MR imaging with a human visual response model [3663-29]
       K. A. Salem, Case Western Reserve Univ.; J. L. Duerk, M. Wendt, D. L. Wilson, Case Western
       Reserve Univ. and Univ. Hospitals of Cleveland

243   Effect of image compression in model and human performance [3663-30]
       M. P. Eckstein, C. K. Abbey, F. O. Bochud, J. L. Bartroff, J. S. Whiting, Cedars-Sinai
       Medical Ctr.

253   Visual discrimination model for digital mammography [3663-31]
       J. P. Johnson, J. Lubin, Sarnoff Corp.; E. A. Krupinski, Health Sciences Ctr./Univ. of Arizona;
       H. A. Peterson, Sarnoff Corp.; H. Roehrig, A. Baysinger, Health Sciences Ctr./Univ. of Arizona

264   Signal detection in a lumpy background: effects of providing more information to the human
       than just raw data [3663-32]
       B. D. Gallas, Health Sciences Ctr./Univ. of Arizona and Univ. of Arizona; H. H. Barrett, Health
       Sciences Ctr./Univ. of Arizona, Univ. of Arizona, and Optical Sciences Ctr./Univ. of Arizona

273   Further investigation of the effect of phase spectrum on visual detection in structured
       backgrounds [3663-33]
       F. O. Bochud, C. K. Abbey, M. P. Eckstein, Cedars-Sinai Medical Ctr.

SESSION 8   MODELING VISUAL SIGNAL DETECTION II

284   Estimation of human-observer templates in two-alternative forced-choice experiments [3663-34]
C. K. Abbey, M. P. Eckstein, F. O. Bochud, Cedars-Sinai Medical Ctr.

296   Quantitative image quality of spatially filtered x-ray fluoroscopy [3663-35]
K. N. Jabri, Case Western Reserve Univ.; D. L. Wilson, Case Western Reserve Univ. and Univ. Hospitals of Cleveland

304   Detection of lesions in mammographic structure [3663-36]
A. E. Burgess, F. L. Jacobson, P. F. Judy, Brigham and Women's Hospital/Harvard Medical School

316   Producing lesions for hybrid mammograms: extracted tumors and simulated microcalcifications [3663-40]
A. E. Burgess, S. Chakraborty, Brigham and Women's Hospital/Harvard Medical School

SESSION 9   POSTER SESSION

324   Appearance matching of radiographic images using lightness index [3663-37]
E. Ogawa, K. Shimura, Fuji Photo Film Co., Ltd. (Japan)

333   Reconfigurable parallel processor for noise suppression [3663-38]
M. Cuviello, P. P. Dang, P. M. Chau, Univ. of California/San Diego

342   Image compression and feature stabilization of dynamically displayed coronary angiograms [3663-41]
J. L. Bartroff, C. A. Morioka, J. S. Whiting, M. P. Eckstein, Cedars-Sinai Medical Ctr.

347   Addendum
349   Author Index

Conference Committee

Conference Chair
> **Elizabeth A. Krupinski,** Health Sciences Center/University of Arizona

Program Committee
> **Arthur E. Burgess,** Brigham and Women's Hospital/Harvard Medical School
> **Dev P. Chakraborty,** University of Pennsylvania School of Medicine
> **Calvin F. Nodine,** University of Pennsylvania School of Medicine

Session Chairs

1   Display Parameters and Performance I
      Miguel P. Eckstein, Cedars-Sinai Medical Center

2   Display Parameters and Performance II
      Elizabeth A. Krupinski, Health Sciences Center/University of Arizona

3   ROC and Other Performance Methodologies
      Bijoy M. Misra, Brigham and Women's Hospital/Harvard Medical School

4   Perceptual Processes and Performance
      Calvin F. Nodine, University of Pennsylvania School of Medicine

5   Technology Assessment and Observer Performance I
      David S. Wooding, University of Derby (UK)

6   Technology Assessment and Observer Performance II
      Mary Pastel Anderson, FDA Center for Devices & Radiological Health

7   Modeling Visual Signal Detection I
      Dev P. Chakraborty, University of Pennsylvania School of Medicine

8   Modeling Visual Signal Detection II
      Elizabeth A. Krupinski, Health Sciences Center/University of Arizona

Introduction

The Image Perception and Performance conference has grown steadily over the past few years, as more and more people have recognized the importance of understanding how the human observer interacts with the various types of perceptual stimuli presented in the clinical environment. This year's conference was very well attended, as were the keynote address and evening workshop. The number of posters was also up somewhat from last year, although we still need to promote the use of posters as an alternative way of presenting results, or as a supplement to the 20-minute oral presentation.

The keynote address, "The Past and Future of Radiologic Error," was given by Paul Friedman, M.D., from UCSD. It was a fascinating talk that took the audience through the history of error in radiology to the influences of technology on error and error prevention. Dr. Friedman noted that with each technological advance (e.g., PACS, teleradiology) there is always the opportunity for reduction in errors, but there also seems to be just as many opportunities for new sources of error. For example, teleradiology allows the general radiologist to ship images off to the expert radiologist for interpretation, reducing the potential for error. However, the expert radiologist has to deal with viewing images (often digitized) on a CRT monitor, leading to potentially new sources of error in their interpretation. The talk was extremely well received, and afterward a number of people commented on how much they appreciated hearing about the topic through the eyes of a radiologist who deals with these critical issues on a day-to-day basis in the clinical environment.

The keynote address fit quite well with the workshop that took place the previous evening. Maryellen Giger, Ph.D., and Robert Nishikawa, Ph.D., from the University of Chicago, conducted the workshop entitled "Using the Results of Human Perception Studies in the Development of Computer-aided Diagnosis." The workshop was also well attended and the discussion that resulted was quite lively and often controversial! Two very interesting points that brought up a lot of discussion were 1) differences between discrete and continuous rating scales for reporting diagnostic decisions, and 2) the utility of having the computer report on information that the human observer cannot perceive (e.g., higher-order texture measurements). Although discussion on both topics and from both sides of the arguments was intense at times, there was no clear resolution of the issues. As always, future research will hopefully lend support to one side or the other.

The conference itself presented a wide range of research topics. As in previous years, the issue of what statistical procedures are useful and appropriate was important, especially in the context of ROC analysis and its variants. The modeling visual signal detection sessions contained numerous interesting papers, covering the range from simulated, to quasi-simulated, to real medical images, and a variety of visual modeling parameters. Visual search was again a hot topic, with a number of eye-position studies being reported on from the U.S. and abroad. This year there were also quite a few technology assessment papers that looked at perception and performance issues in a wide variety of clinical tasks. It was interesting to hear talks on retinal screening, teledermatology, and other image-based areas outside of radiology that must deal with the same basic perceptual issues that we have dealt with in radiology for years.

This proceedings contains the papers that resulted from the conference presentations. They reflect the wide range of topics that the study of perception and performance touches on in the context of medical imaging. Many of the research topics themselves are quite narrow and specific, but the references provide the reader with means to delve further into the background of the topic, if they so choose.

Elizabeth A. Krupinski

Keynote Address

The Past and Future of Radiologic Error

Paul J. Friedman

Department of Radiology, University of California San Diego

Although radiographs are extremely important in clinical medicine, their interpretation is susceptible to significant error: mistakes in detection and interpretation result in a false negative rate of 30-40%. This figure has not changed with nearly two generations of research.

What are some of the contributing factors? First, consider the complexity of the radiologic images with all the variable human anatomy and potential pathology. The radiograph is a two-dimensional projection of a three-dimensional structure, so that there are many superimposed structures to be sorted out. This superimposition is eliminated with cross-sectional imaging techniques, such as computed tomography (CT) and magnetic resonance imaging (MRI), but at great cost. Further, their interpretation is complicated by the large number of images which must be mentally assembled to cover the entire subject.

The term "conspicuity" was coined to represent the potential of a radiographic finding to be detected, as influenced by its size, contrast, and background complexity. These are complex functions of not only the pathology but also the radiological technique. Suffice it to say that there is great variability in the conspicuity of the abnormalities to be detected in clinical practice.

Another major topic to consider is the physiological limitations of the human eye; specifically, the limited extent of foveal coverage with reduced contrast detection and detail resolution by the rest of the retina. The way a radiograph is examined is a technique learned by practice, and differs among practitoners. This search pattern, described by researchers who track eye movement, consists of fixations and rapid movements, so that the fovea covers only a minority of the film surface. Scanning by eye does not provide the systematic coverage of a television raster. Large shadows in the lungs can be readily detected by peripheral vision, but any lesion of low conspicuity must be looked at directly, with foveal vision, in order to be detected. How this is achieved is based on clinical understanding of where obscure findings should be sought.

Studies of the cases missed in clinical radiology (mainly studies of lung cancer detection) reveal two main troublesome regions in the chest: the periphery, where small lesions lurk; and the hilar region, whose deformity by tumor is poorly recognized, or which hide lesions behind them. I have noted the upper medial portions of the lungs are a difficult region in which to distinguish overlapping bone and vessel shadows from possible tumors. Regions hidden by the heart, because of relative underexposure, have less contrast available, and so peripheral vision isn't good enough. These considerations should be reflected in a well-tailored personal search pattern.

It has long been recognized that the clinical history affects search patterns, a form of bias. This will affect the likelihood of detection of a finding. On the other hand, the clinical information implies the prior probabilities that facilitate interpretation of a finding. Those who have advocated interpreting radiographs while ignorant of the clinical history capture only half the picture, however. The other half follows a directed search for radiographic findings, based on the differential diagnosis (clinically) of the patient's history and other findings. I advocate interpreting all films both with and without the history, sometimes requiring some mental gymnastics by the radiologist.

Part of the SPIE Conference on Image Perception and Performance
San Diego, California ● February 1999
SPIE Vol. 3663 ● 0277-786X/99/$10.00

One of the problems in proper utilization of the clinical history is that the clinical information provided on a radiology request is usually missing or wrong. This is a consequence of individuals other than the knowledgeable physician filling out the request forms, as well as certain misuse of computerized databases. For example, the patient's admitting diagnosis may appear as the clinical diagnosis for days after the clinicians have dismissed it since it is readily and mechanically available. An unintended consequence of tighter standards for reimbursing radiologic examinations is that the justification must meet certain standards. For example, a study to "rule out" something is not reimbursable. The individuals who enter the justification into the radiology computer know what kind of history is acceptable, and dutifully put in something appropriate, but not necessarily true, and rarely the true reason that would guide the radiologist's interpretation, as discussed above.

Other socioeconomic trends have undesirable effects from the point of view of reducing radiologic error. Managed care's financial incentives are nearly all negative from this perspective. Managed care discourages specialization by physicians, discourages patients from seeing specialists, and also discourages patients from seeing physicians altogether. This reduces the clinical skill needed to use imaging intelligently. Among radiologists, there is similar pressure to practice general rather than specialized radiology, reducing expertise within the discipline as well.

To what extent does the threat of malpractice action help reduce error in radiology? That would be difficult to quantify. Certainly, a minimal level of care is encouraged, but the diligence with which a radiologist studies an individual case is not likely to be affected. On the other hand my impression of the knowledge of malpractice lawyers (?and juries) is that they may mistake error for incompetence (or malpractice) without justification. The well-documented facts of radiological error are not well recognized by either the public or physicians in general, and not acknowledged by lawyers in this field.

Of course, most radiologic findings are nonspecific. They do not correspond to specific diseases or, in many cases, even to well-defined gross pathology. Many diagnoses are indirect or inductive by nature. Sometimes a number of minor findings add up to a likely diagnosis. Radiologic diagnosis is usually pattern recognition.

THE ROLE OF TECHNOLOGY

Technological advances can be both a help and a hindrance in the effort to reduce error. An example of an historic development, automatic film processing, provided uniform development and reduced patients' radiation exposure, resulting in better quality and consistency. This would have a beneficial effect on error. Phototiming of exposure has been very useful to encourage uniform and good film quality. Unfortunately, the subject is often positioned poorly with respect to the phototimer cells, so that exposure is still incorrect.

High kilovoltage radiographic technique results in better penetration and wider latitude, so that exposure is not so critical. These tremendous advantages outweigh a greater insensitivity to the detection of calcium. Scatter-absorbing grids improve contrast and detail, at the cost of using more radiation. The better the clean-up of scatter, the more useful radiation is removed from the x-ray beam, requiring some increase in patient exposure to achieve adequate film-blackening.

Beam-equalizing methods help achieve more uniform film density, solving the problem of looking at the lungs and the mediastinum with one exposure. This can be done with a simple beam-shaping Pb-lucite filter or (better) with a complex scanning system that adjusts beam intensity depending on how much radiation gets through a particular region. The filter, providing an extra dose of radiation to the dense mediastinum, is very useful, unless the patient is not centered perfectly, in which case one of the lungs will be quite overexposed. A relatively inexpensive way to equalize radiation density has been to use high and low sensitivity intensifying screens and matching film emulsions. There is a risk of failing to recognize underexposure, however, because film density looks adequate with the more sensitive (faster) screen-film pair, andthe lack of any detail from the slower screen-film pair may be inapparent. Underexposure, of course, promotes missing smaller lesions in the lung periphery.

The ultimate in technology may be the application of computers to radiology. Computed tomography was the first major application. By removing superimposed shadows and enabling a true cross-section to be seen, CT has revolutionized imaging. The sensitivity of CT images for many findings is much greater than plain radiography in the chest; in the abdomen, CT can be legitimately said to be infinitely better for many findings (which were simply not distinguishable on plain films).

Computed radiography and direct digital radiography sacrifice a little in image quality as the cost of automation but their potential to streamline the imaging process is substantial. With the addition of an electronic medical imaging system for readout, they also increase productivity, which may not decrease error by itself, but makes it possible to study images more carefully.

Having digital images makes computer manipulation possible. For example, computerized edge enhancement is good in CT of the lungs, less useful in radiographic chest imaging. On the other hand, noise suppression or smoothing of images has limited application of which I am aware. Removal of calcium, using dual exposures (getting rid of the ribs on a chest film!) can be extremely useful in allowing detection of underlying lesions; selecting for calcium can separate bone defects from overlying air shadows. False color has been used in nuclear medicine and proposed for general radiology, but color translation of the gray scale is not useful in radiography because it doesn't sort out image overlap. Computer identification of suspect findings may eliminate some false negative readings, at the risk of increasing false positives from the radiologist. The human eye and brain are not about to be superseded, fortunately, at least in chest radiology.

It is appropriate here to mention some research results that create some doubt about the advantages of having a computer (or a partially-trained assistant) point out suspicious regions on the film, allowing the radiologist to make the final decision. In a complicated but well-controlled experiment, comparing films previously selected for false positive findings with the same films containing artificially introduced nodules, pointing out a possible lesion resulted in a less accurate assessment than if the radiologist interpreted the film from scratch, with no indication of the region of interest. A similar result had been found, although challenged, some years before. No simple mechanism can explain this result, and it remains to be seen how new technology will be affected.

PACS (picture archiving & communication systems) are the latest advance. Combining digital images (usually obtained digitally, de novo) with fast networks, cheap digital archives, sophisticated prefetching, and large, bright workstations with user-friendly software, will be nirvana. PACS provide new convenience and efficiency, but incorporate a risky dependence on cutting edge technology. We have annoying crashes of computers of all kinds now; when they support patient images, such crashes could be disastrous.

With regard to error, PACS make it easier to retrieve old images and compare them (it answers many questions and eliminates some errors, when the diagnosis becomes obvious with comparison films or images). PACS provides easier access to current images for clinicians, but potentially less contact with radiologists, which is bad for their joint function. However, radiologist notations on the films will be available to the clinicians remotely as soon as they are drawn on the images.

Methods of reading, reporting, and communicating findings will change: most radiologists use stack or cine viewing of CT/MR images when using a workstation in contrast to spreading out the images as on a viewbox. The temptation to make a great many more images when the expense of filming them is eliminated, has already been noted in some centers! Reformatting, reconstructions, MIPs (maximum or minimum intensity projections) are all useful for complex CT anatomy/pathology, although time-consuming. (It's another case of technology making it possible to do new things, but at a considerable cost in time.)

Machine voice recognition of dictation will speed reporting and make it possible to have the report available by the time the clinician sees the films. Of course, it will also pressure the radiologist to treat all films as "STAT" readings, which will lower the opportunity to reflect on the images longer; however, immediate availability of past plain film and CT images should more than compensate for this problem. A change in the way radiology is practised is at hand.

Finally, I am enthusiastic about the potential of portable messaging devices and wireless technology to improve communication between radiologist and clinician. I am thinking about not only the transfer of radiologic interpretations back to a responsible referring physician, but also the opportunity to query the clinician about more clinical historic details. Perhaps accurate clinical information will become available! On the whole, the changes to be wrought by the adoption of new technology should only improve care and reduce error, and can be embraced with enthusiasm.

SELECTED REFERENCES

Casarett D, Helms C. Systems errors versus physicians' errors: finding the balance in medical education. Academic Medicine 1999; 74: 19-22.

Clark R, Anderson MB, Johnson BH, Moore DE, Herbert FD. Clinical value of radiologists' interpretations of perioperative radiographs of orthopedic patients. Orthopedics 1996; 19:1003-1007.

Davies HD, Wang EE, Manson D; Babyn P, Shuckett B. Reliability of the chest radiograph in the diagnosis of lower respiratory infections in young children. Pediatric Infectious Disease Journal 1996; 15:600-604.

DeCorato DR, Kagetsu NJ, Ablow RC. Off-hours interpretation of radiologic images of patients admitted to the emergency department: efficacy of teleradiology. AJR 1995; 165:1293-1296.

Doubilet P, Herman PG. Interpretation of radiographs: effect of clinical history. AJR 1981; 137: 1055-1058.

Forrest JV, Friedman PJ. Radiologic errors in patients with lung cancer. West J Med 1981; 134:485-490.

Garland LH. Studies on the accuracy of diagnostic procedures. AJR 1959; 82:25-38.

Groth-Peterson E, Lovgreen A, Thillemann J. On the reliability of the reading of photofluorograms and the value of dual reading. Acta Tuberc Scandinav 1952; 26:13-37.

Gurney JW. Missed lung cancer at CT: imaging findings in nine patients. Radiology 1996; 199:117-122.

Hessel SJ, Herman PG, Swensson RG. Improving performance by multiple interpretations of chest radiographs: Effectiveness and cost. Radiology 1978; 127:589-594.

Kundel HL, Wright DJ. The influence of prior knowledge on visual search strategies during the viewing of chest radiographs. Radiology 1969; 93:315-320.

Kundel HL, LaFollette PS. Visual search patterns and experience with radiological images. Radiology 1972; 103: 523-528.

Kundel HL, Nodine CF. A visual concept shapes image perception. Radiology 1983; 146: 363-368.

Loughran CF. Reporting of fracture radiographs by radiographers: the impact of a training programme. British Journal of Radiology 1994; 67:945-950.

Rigler LG, O'Loughlin BJ, Tucker RC. The duration of carcinoma of the lung. Dis Chest 1953; 23:50-71.

Ross PD, Huang C, Karpf D, Lydick E, Coel M, Hirsch L, Wasnich RD. Blinded reading of radiographs increases the frequency of errors in vertebral fracture detection. Journal of Bone and Mineral Research 1996; 11:1793-1800.

Smith MJ. Error and Variation in Diagnostic Radiology . 1967; Springfield, Illinois, Charles C. Thomas.

Swensson RG, Theodore GH. Search and nonsearch protocols for radiographic consultation. Radiology 1990; 177:851-856.

Thomas EL. Search Behavior. Radiol Clin North Am 1969; 7:403-417.

Veeze P. Rationale and Methods of Early Detection in Lung Cancer. 1968; Netherlands, Van Gorcum and Co.

Yerushalmy J. The statistical assessment of the variability in observer perception and description of roentgenographic pulmonary shadows. Radiol Clin North Am 1969; 7:381-392.

SESSION 1

Display Parameters and Performance I

Observer performance assessment of JPEG-compressed high-resolution chest images

Walter F. Good, Glenn Maitz, Jill King, Rose Gennari, David Gur

University of Pittsburgh, Pittsburgh, PA 15261

ABSTRACT

The JPEG compression algorithm was tested on a set of 529 chest radiographs that had been digitized at a spatial resolution of 100 μm and contrast sensitivity of 12 bits. Images were compressed using five fixed "psychovisual" quantization tables which produced average compression ratios in the range 15:1 to 61:1, and were then printed onto film. Six experienced radiologists read all cases from the laser printed film, in each of the five compressed modes as well as in the non-compressed mode. For comparison purposes, observers also read the same cases with reduced pixel resolutions of 200 μm and 400 μm. The specific task involved detecting masses, pneumothoraces, interstitial disease, alveolar infiltrates, and rib fractures. Over the range of compression ratios tested, for images digitized at 100 μm, we were unable to demonstrate any statistically significant decrease ($p>0.05$) in observer performance as measured by ROC techniques. However, the observers' subjective assessments of image quality did decrease significantly as image resolution was reduced and suggested a decreasing, but non-significant, trend as the compression ratio was increased. The seeming discrepancy between our failure to detect a reduction in observer performance, and other published studies, is likely due to: 1) the higher resolution at which we digitized our images; 2) the higher signal-to-noise ratio of our digitized films versus typical CR images; and 3) our particular choice of an optimized quantization scheme.

Keywords: Image compression, image processing, observer performance, chest imaging

1. INTRODUCTION

One of the major challenges that must be faced in our effort to adopt digital methods in radiology is how to deal with the vast amount of digital image data expected to be generated in future radiology departments. It is widely believed that some form of lossy data compression will be essential for handling this image data, though this introduces concerns about the impact of compression on the performance of radiologists. Since the problems of dealing with digital image data are universal, the Joint Photographic Experts Group (JPEG) was formed by the International Organization for Standardization (ISO) to address image compression issues, and it has adopted a widely used standard for general purpose image compression[1]. Although this standard does not specifically address radiological images, there will be significant benefits to radiology if the standard algorithm proves to be adequate for use on these images.

The JPEG algorithm, as applied in this study, is a block quantization version of the Cosine transform in which images are divided into 8×8 blocks and the Cosine transform is applied to each block individually, to produce an array of frequency coefficients. These derived frequency coefficients are then quantized by dividing by values from an 8×8 array of quantization factors and rounding the quotients to integral values. These quotients are aligned in a "zigzag" order and encoded by either Huffman coding or by adaptive arithmetic coding. In this process, the quantization factors that are applied to the frequency coefficients determine the compression ratio as well as the kinds of information lost or artifacts introduced.

One complication in applying JPEG standard compression to radiographic images arises because the default quantization values, which are provided in the standard, are not adequate for most purposes and hence, the standard encourages user specified quantization tables. But since the resulting image quality is determined by the quantization strategy employed, the design of these tables must be optimized for each particular kind of compression task.

Part of the SPIE Conference on Image Perception and Performance
San Diego, California • February 1999
SPIE Vol. 3663 • 0277-786X/99/$10.00

The primary goal being pursued in the study reported here was to determine the sensitivity of readers' performance to changes in the degree of compression for a suitably optimized version of the JPEG algorithm, and more specifically, to attempt to determine performance versus compression ratio curves for a variety of detection tasks.

2. METHODS

This study was designed as a historical prospective, multi-observer, multi-abnormality, reader performance (ROC) study, in which observer performance was measured over a range of compression ratios for the standard JPEG algorithm, as optimized in a previous project[2].

2.1. Case selection

A total of 529 high-quality chest images were selected and rated for quality by 2 radiologists experienced in chest interpretation. The set of 529 included 181 images positive for nodule, 119 positive for pneumothorax, 149 positive for interstitial disease, 77 with alveolar infiltrates and 76 with rib fractures; 124 were negative for all of the 5 abnormalities. The images were chosen so as to include, to the greatest extent, both difficult negative images and difficult positives in each category. Abnormal findings were verified independently by means of surgery, laboratory tests, other imaging modality reports, or in the case of interstitial disease, by agreement of certified B readers for pneumoconiosis. Negatives were verified through negative exams at least a year following the original negative finding. In selecting cases, we followed procedures which have been used successfully in our prior studies[3,4].

2.2. Film digitization

These 529 chest films (14 X 17 inch Kodak G films exposed with Lanex screens) were digitized at a spatial resolution of 100 μm with contrast sensitivity of 12 bits, to produce a 3504 X 4205 X 12 bit matrix, using a high-resolution film digitizer (Lumisys, Sunnyvale, CA). The modulation transfer function (MTF) of the digitizer at the Nyquist frequency of 5 lp/mm is 0.41 and 0.39 in the horizontal and vertical directions, respectively, with useful optical densities spanning the range 0.3 to 3.0.

2.3. Image compression

The digitized images were compressed as per our JPEG software to 5 increasing levels of compression as determined by psychovisual quantization tables. Quantization tables were calculated from methods described in Nill[6] and Ngan et al.[7] using visual system data from Kelly[8]. For the purpose of this calculation, we assumed that images would be displayed on laser-printed film and viewed initially from a distance equal to the diagonal of the film (56 cm). Our intent was that spatial frequencies were to be represented with equal "visual fidelity" at this viewing distance[6]. For this study, Huffman encoding was used to encode the quantized coefficients and all compression ratios were based on this. Huffman tables were derived from the statistics of individual quantized images rather than from ensemble statistics. Target compression ratios of 15:1, 21:1, 30:1, 42:1 and 60:1, were chosen, which ranged from below where previous studies by others[9-12] had failed to show any effect to well above the level where these studies had shown significant deterioration in image quality.

2.4. Image printing

The whole set of images (with and without compression) were laser printed . In addition, using a filtered pixel averaging algorithm[5], the non-compressed images were also printed at medium resolution of 200 μm per pixel and low resolution of 400 μm per pixel.

All images were printed at full size using a Kodak Ektascan laser printer (Kodak, Rochester, NY), from the digital source data onto Kodak's Ektascan EHN film; the printer's capabilities to store calibration tables and to perform scaling via an interpolation program allowed us to insure that the contrast response or the original film was maintained. We were able to demonstrate that the variations produced by the film processor were within acceptable limits.

2.5. Performance of study

Seven board certified radiologists, each with a minimum of 3 years experience interpreting chest films, blind to the study's aims, and who did not participate in the film selection and approval process, reviewed all 529 images in each of the 8 display modes described above. Generally, 40 cases in one mode were presented to a reader in a given session. To prevent learning effects, any of the 529 images would be seen a second time (regardless of mode changes) only after a span of 4 weeks. To facilitate the time delays, the images for a given session were selected by a specifically designed program that would choose randomly only from the pool of images available at the time for that reader, changing to a new mode for each session. Each film envelope and film were clearly marked with a unique number based on both mode and image number, and were pulled and stacked in the random order given by a list generated by the program. A linked program would display on a color monitor the scoring form, with the unique identifying number clearly marked with the same number appearing on the envelopes and film.

The reader was asked to specifically rate the likelihood of the presence of each of the five abnormalities on a 0 to 100 scale, with 0 indicating the absolute certainty of negative for the abnormality in question and 100 if absolutely certain the abnormality was present in the image. Each reader entered the answers into his/her database by using a mouse to click on their response to questions about image quality and comfort level (5 possible answers for each: from "excellent" to "unacceptable"; or from "very comfortable" to "extremely uncomfortable"); and to move a horizontal slider to choose from 0 to 100 in response to the questions about the presence of each of the 5 abnormalities. Secondary questions were also presented in response to an interstitial disease and/or nodule rating if it was greater than 30. When all the questions were answered, the rater clicked on a box at the bottom marked done that would bring up a new form with the number corresponding to the next film on the stack.

2.6. Data Analysis

Using our own programs each reader's data was prepared as input into the CLABROC program that includes among the calculations it performs: the area under the ROC curve (A_Z) for each of two sets of correlated data, the standard deviations of the areas, and the p-value indicating the statistical significance of the difference between the data sets. The area under the ROC curve was calculated for each abnormality, each reader, and for each compression mode and resolution mode, all paired with the non-compressed , high-resolution mode, yielding a total of 280 area calculations ($7 \times 5 \times 8$). As was noted, one reader was unable to complete the study and for this reader we performed analysis on the subsets of paired data for each mode that was complete. The study data was in all instances analyzed with and without this reader's results.

Although we performed paired t-tests on all 7 readers' results for each mode paired with the non-compressed mode to get a preliminary result and to emphasize certain aspects of the study results, current methods of analyzing multi-reader, multi-modality ROC studies take into account the variability of both the cases and the readers[13-15]. The method of Berbaum, et al.[15], employs a jackknifing technique to produce values that can be evaluated by analysis of variance (ANOVA); thereby including in the data analysis the variance due both to multiple cases and to multiple readers; a second method by Obuchowski employs estimates of case variance from the correlations between cases (correlations are calculated by the CLABROC program), to take into account case variation[13,14]. Both of these methods of analysis, as well as a trends test were used to evaluate the effect on observer performance of both the compression modes and the resolution modes.

Values of 0 through 4 were assigned to the image quality and comfort ratings, the low rating of 0 indicating "excellent image quality" and 4 representing "unacceptable image quality"; analogously, 0 is assigned to "very comfortable", with 4 assigned to "very uncomfortable". The estimate of the reading time for each image is taken directly from the database. This data was analyzed simply by taking the averages of these ordinal ratings and taking the average of the reading times. Time estimate of each image reading was recorded by the computer as the time in seconds between scoring form displays. Times exceeding 300 seconds (5 minutes) were excluded in an effort to discard excess times due to external factors such as telephone calls/discussions etc.

3. RESULTS

The results of the study are summarized in Table 1 in the form of the A_Z values averaged over the 6 readers who completed the entire study. By inspection it would appear that there are no obvious trends across the compression modes for any of the

5 abnormalities, while there is a suggestion of increased performance at the highest resolution for all but interstitial disease. However, there was no statistical significance among any of the modes ($p > 0.05$) by either of the two comprehensive methods described above for either the compression modes or the resolution modes. In Table 2, it can be seen that none of the 25 paired t-tests (5 modes $\times$ 5 abnormalities) on the CLABROC ROC areas, pairing the readers' non-compressed mode CLABROC output A_Z with those of each of the compressed modes' A_Z's , were statistically significant (all two-tailed p values > 0.05). Trend tests also yielded negative results.

From Table 3 it is clear that decreases in resolution were easily detected as reflected by readers' lower average rating for both the image quality and comfort level assessments. On the other hand, the compression levels are not distinguished even in this more subjective assessment. Interestingly however, the perceived decline in image quality and comfort level as resolution decreases is not mirrored by the average reading time, which is remarkably consistent across all modes at a reading rate of 50(+/- 20) seconds per image.

4. DISCUSSION

Although our subjective impression of our image set was that, even at the highest level of compression, image quality remained quite good, and this was confirmed by the subjective ratings of the observers in the study, the lack of a significant effect on observer performance at the higher compression ratios was rather unexpected. Previous studies by other groups have consistently reported decreases in performance for chest images compressed at ratios well below the upper ratio of 61:1 used in our study -- in some cases at ratios as low as 7:1.

Typical of these studies are those reported by Ishigaki[9], and MacMahon[10], Aberle[11] and Cox[12]. A review of the results of all of these studies clearly indicates a reduction trend with increasing compression ratios. In both the Ishigaki study and the Cox study, the reduction is notable (although not statistically significant for the Ishigaki study) even at low compression ratios. There are some important differences in technique between these previous studies and the study reported here. In general, these studies have used: 1) images having lower spatial resolution; 2) CR images characterized by a lower signal-to-noise ratio than our digitized films; and 3) 10 bit as opposed to our 12 bit contrast resolution. These factors, in addition to our particular choice of an optimized quantization scheme, can explain the seeming discrepancy between our failure to detect a reduction in observer performance at even the 61:1 compression ratio, and these other published studies which have detected differences at much lower compression ratios.

By digitizing our images at a resolution of 100 µm as opposed to the 200 µm resolutions common in other studies, we may essentially be increasing the redundancy in the data, and thus increasing compressibility. If a chest image does not contain appreciable high-frequency information then the additional data acquired when digitizing at the higher resolution will be largely redundant. In this case, an appropriately designed compression algorithm could remove this additional data without adversely reducing observer performance. This improvement in compressibility cannot generally be fully realized in practice because the process of digitization introduces pixel noise, which can increase the high frequency content of the digitized image, and is difficult to compress. In our particular case, there is also evidence that the higher resolution versions of our images contain significant information not present in lower resolution versions, so that not all of the additional information can be redundant. Specifically, the subjective image quality data reported above suggests that there is a discernable difference in image quality between the 100 µm and 200 µm images.

The Ishigaki and Cox studies both used CR images. The average signal-to-noise ratio of CR images is generally lower than for digitized films, though in both cases, this signal-to-noise ratio is locally density dependent. Noise, because of its random nature, increases the high-frequency content of images which can make the CR images more difficult to compress than digitized films. The fact that MacMahon and Aberle used digitized films instead of CR images may explain why their studies, like ours, seems to show less of a detrimental effect from compression. The sensitivity of the two-alternative forced choice protocol employed in the Cox study, combined with their use of very subtle synthetic "abnormalities", may account for their ability to demonstrate a significant result at compression ratios as low as 7:1. However, it is difficult to predict how their results relate to more realistic diagnostic tasks.

Our study deviated somewhat from common practice in that, when psychophysical quantization tables are traditionally used in studies of this sort, it is customary to force readers to view the images under the specific conditions that were assumed in the design of the quantization schemes. This maximizes the apparent benefit of psychophysical quantization but the results have little relevance to an unrestricted reading environment. In this study we expected that our readers would initially view images at approximately the distance designed into the psychovisual quantization tables, but then to modify their viewing distance, as needed, for particular films. We believe that if there is some feature in the image that merits a closer study, it is important that the feature be visible at the initial viewing distance, but once readers have detected a feature they should be free to examine it from what they consider to be an optimal distance.

The results discussed here suggest that, at the present time, there is substantial evidence that would support using the JPEG algorithm at a compression ratio up to about 20:1 for 200 μm digitized film images or somewhat higher for 100 μm digitized films. For CR images, the corresponding ratios will likely have to be reduced somewhat. Nevertheless, the relationship between observer performance, compression ratio and image resolution, as it relates to the JPEG algorithm, and specifically the question of the maximum compression ratio that should be used in a particular situation, need further study.

ACKNOWLEDGEMENTS

The authors thank Robert Slifko and Howard Rockette for assisting in the design and performance of this study. This work is sponsored in part by grants CA60259, CA66594 and CA67947 from the National Cancer Institute and LM06236 from the National Library of Medicine, National Institutes of Health.

REFERENCES

1   Joint Photographic Experts Group (JPEG). JPEG Technical Specification, Revision 5 (Document No. JPEG8R5 or JTC1/SC2/WG8 N933). ISO Central Secretariat, 1990
2   JM Holbert, M Staiger, TS Chang, JD Towers, CA Britton: Selection of processing algorithms for digital image compression -- a rank order study. Academic Radiology 1995; 2:273-6
3   FL Thaete, CR Fuhrman, JH Oliver, CA Britton, WL Campbell, JH Feist, WH Straub, PL Davis, MB Plunkett: Digital radiography and conventional imaging of the chest. AJR 1994; 162:575-581
4   BS Slasky, MS Rosenthal, CR Fuhrman, D Sashin, FL Thaete, JH Feist, MA Costa-Greco, KM Harris, HD Curtin, JH Sumkin:. Primary diagnosis of chest images in a PACS environment. Proc SPIE 1990; 1234:120-125
5   CC Shaw, J Herron, D Gur: Pixel averaging versus digitization using larger apertures -- a comparison of the spatial resolution properties. Proc SPIE 1992; 1651:128-133
6   NB Nill: A visual model weighted cosine transform for image compression and quality assessment. IEEE Trans Commun 1985;COM-33:551-7
7   KN Ngan, KS Leong, S Harcharan: Cosine transform coding incorporating human visual system model. Proc SPIE 1986; 707:165-171
8   DH Kelley: Visual contrast sensitivity. Opt Acta 1977; 24:107-129
9   T Ishigaki, S Sakuma, M Ikeda, Y Itoh, M Suzuki, S Iwai: Clinical evaluation of irreversible image compression: Analysis of chest imaging with computed radiography. Radiology 1990; 175:739-743
10 H MacMahon, K Doi, S Sanada, SM Montner, ML Giger, CE Metz, N Nakamori, FF Yin, XW Xu, H Yonekawa, H Takeuchi: Data compression: Effect on diagnostic accuracy in digital chest radiography. Radiology 1991; 178:175-179
11 DR Aberle, F Gleeson, JW Sayre, K Brown, et al: The effect of irreversible compression on diagnostic accuracy in thoracic imaging. Invest Radiol 1993; 28(5)398-403
12 GG Cox, LT Cook, MF Insana, MA McFadden, TJ Hall, LA Harrison, DA Eckard, NL Martin: The effects of lossy compression on the detection of subtle pulmonary nodules. Med Phys 1996; 23:127-132
13 N Obuchowski: Hypothesis testing in multireader ROC studies. American Statistical Association meeting, Atlanta, GA, August, 1991
14 NA Obuchowski: Estimators of variance components in multireader ROC studies. Presented at the Annual Meeting of the Biometric Society Joint meetings with the Institute of Mathematical Statistics and the American Statistical Association, Houston, TX, March 1991; pg 118
15 DD Dorfman, KS Berbaum, CE Metz: Receiver operating characteristic analysis -- generalization to the population of readers and patients with the jackknife method. Invest Radiol1992; 2(9)723-31

Abnormality		Subsampled		Non-compressed	Compressed				
		400 μm	200 μm	100 μm	15:1	21:1	34:1	40:1	61:1
Interstitial Dis.	Avg. A_z	0.73	0.73	0.73	0.73	0.72	0.76	0.74	0.75
(n=149)	st.d.	0.05	0.05	0.03	0.03	0.04	0.04	0.04	0.03
Nodule	Avg. A_z	0.83	0.83	0.84	0.84	0.84	0.83	0.84	0.82
(n=181)	st.d.	0.03	0.03	0.04	0.03	0.05	0.03	0.03	0.02
Pneumothorax	Avg. A_z	0.91	0.92	0.93	0.93	0.91	0.91	0.92	0.91
(n=119)	st.d.	0.07	0.06	0.05	0.05	0.06	0.06	0.06	0.06
Rib Fractures	Avg. A_z	0.84	0.82	0.85	0.83	0.85	0.85	0.84	0.85
(n=77)	st.d.	0.07	0.06	0.05	0.07	0.07	0.05	0.03	0.06
Alveolar Infiltrates	Avg. A_z	0.86	0.87	0.87	0.87	0.86	0.85	0.88	0.87
(n=76)	st.d.	0.05	0.04	0.04	0.04	0.05	0.05	0.03	0.05

Table 1: Average observer performance, A_z, and standard deviations for six readers who completed ROC study. For the task of detecting each specific abnormality, performance changes between modes were inconsistent and not significant.

Abnormality	Compression ratios				
	15:1	21:1	34:1	40:1	61:1
Interstitial Disease	0.70	0.42	0.08	0.45	0.15
Nodule	0.29	0.88	0.73	0.30	0.32
Pneumothorax	0.61	0.07	0.24	0.16	0.19
Rib Fractures	0.59	0.48	0.20	0.41	0.86
Alveolar Infiltrates	0.14	0.76	0.76	0.33	0.69

Table 2: Two-tailed p-values for paired t-tests comparing non-compressed with compressed modes.

		Subsampled		Non-compressed	Compressed				
		400 μm	200 μm	100 μm	15:1	21:1	34:1	40:1	61:1
Image Quality	Avg.	2.42	2.26	2.15	2.16	2.16	2.14	2.18	2.20
	st.d.	0.22	0.22	0.31	0.27	0.26	0.25	0.31	0.30
Comfort Level	Avg.	2.14	2.01	1.86	1.88	1.87	1.87	1.91	1.89
	st.d.	0.52	0.47	0.41	0.40	0.40	0.40	0.38	0.44
Reading Time (sec)	Avg.	50	51	52	50	51	52	52	52
	st.d.	21	20	21	20	18	21	21	19

Table 3: Average time required to read images, and subjective assessments of image quality. The time required to read images is largely independent of the image mode. On the other hand, both the observers opinions on image quality and on degree of comfort in using the images for the specified diagnostic tasks, appear to change in the expected direction. Image quality and comfort levels were measured on a scale of 0 (Excellent, Very comfortable) to 4 (Unacceptable, Very uncomfortable).

ACCEPTABLE COMPRESSION RATIOS FOR CR IMAGES FOR PACS ARCHIVES

Bijoy M. Misra[a], Philip F. Judy , Francine L. Jacobson,
William B. Hanlon and Scott D. Davis

Brigham and Women's Hospital, Harvard Medical School
55 Francis Street, Boston, MA 02215

[a]Faculty of Arts and Sciences, Harvard University, Cambridge, MA 02138.
(email:bmisra@bwh.harvard.edu)

ABSTRACT

We make a preliminary study with a ROC experiment to determine the acceptable levels of image compression that may be utilized for PACS archives. CR images of 1760x2140 pixel size and 10 bit depth are studied. The experiment uses wavelet algorithm for image compression and printed films for image viewing. The "internal standard" experiment results in an acceptable value of compression ratio of 6 for imperceptible difference $(d_a'=1)$ between the compressed and the uncompressed image. Such ratio would lead a storage reduction factor of 9.6 for these images. The information capacity of the CR images may be extrapolated to be 40 bits per millimeter of viewing area.

1. INTRODUCTION

The cost efficiency of softcopy reading and the utility of teleradiology have lately focussed attention to the issues of electronic storage, transport and retrieval of radiology images (1,2). The problems of image storage and transport are effectively facilitated by resorting to image compression techniques (3), while the retrieval is accomplished through image reconstruction, the latter being compromised by the amount of loss of information through the process of compression (4,5,6).

Besides the residual scatter and noise in the images, the CR image may contain information, the brightness values of which are perceptually redundant. One can subject the image to compression to remove any unnecessary brightness values and to be able to recreate the clinical information from a reduced number of pixel values. While the reconstructed image can be perceptually equivalent to the original image, it is not physically equivalent and is stated to have gone through "lossy compression" (7,8). The physical loss of image information is a function of the amount of compression and the algorithm used. Different modalities in radiology may respond to different degrees of compression depending on the modes of capturing image and the clinical value of information in the image(9).

We will examine the question of image compression for chest CR images in this paper with special focus towards the PACS(Picture Archival and Communication System) archives. From the ACR/NEMA point of view(10), a PACS archive is a repository of compressed images that form an image library and any particular image is recalled from the repository for reference and comparison at a later time. The offline media library is designed to be a repository of images until the legal period for image referral is exhausted. When the request for an image is received, the library is to deliver a compressed version of the image, which can then be reconstructed by the requesting client, by using appropriate reconstruction software. Our goal is to determine the maximum stretch of the compression ratio at which the reconstructed image would be perceptually indifferent from the original image. Following ACR/NEMA definitions (10), the compression ratio is defined as the ratio of the file size of the original image to that of the compressed image.

A good summary of the state of research in image compression has been compiled as a SCAR report (11). Principally, two distinct types of compression techniques are applied: DCT (12,13,14)and wavelets (15,16,17). All the earlier research in compression has been done using digitized films with a view towards application in teleradiology. The digitization is accomplished at a resolution ranging from 150 microns to 50 microns, the resulting digitized to a desired compression ratio and then reconstructed. The reconstructed image may be viewed on a CRT monitor or can be printed on a laser printer. Depending on the fineness of resolution (image size) and viewing methods, the acceptable compression ratio without discernible information degradation has been reported in the range of 4 to 40 (12-17).

In this paper, we approach the problem in two distinctly different ways. First, in the spirit of a PACS archive, we consider the actual CR images and not the digitized film, thus reducing the possibility of artifacts in the uncompressed image. Secondly, we develop ROC procedure for an experiment through which we may examine the perceptual and diagnostic degradation in the reconstructed image using the printed film as the standard. By queuing the reconstructed image to print in identical manner to the uncompressed image, we simulate the scenario of representation of the archival image in the original format.

The results in this paper will be of interest to PACS planners and radiologists, who would be interested in the long term storage of digital information for reference and teaching. The paradigm of accomplishing a primary reading of the soft copy image on a CRT monitor and viewing a reconstructed image on a similar workstation with the appropriate tools of leveling, windowing and magnification will be taken up in a future paper.

2. MATERIALS AND METHODS

2.1 Images

The materials for our study consisted of printed films of CR chest images collected and processed at the Ambulatory Division of Brigham and Women's Hospital. The following tasks constitute the collection:

  (i) selection of patient cases
  (ii) transporting the images to research workstation
  (iii) compression
  (iv) reconstructing the images, relabelling and retransporting
  (v) printing the images in triplicates.

We describe each of the steps and the methods below.

2.1.1 Selection of patient cases

2.1.1.1 Imaging Device

Images were obtained from the Fuji FCR 9501 (Model CR-IR 325) storage phosphor device. The high resolution screen elements are captured by a ST-V screen and processed through the standard Fuji processing algorithms. The final image is captured at 10 bits in 1760x2140 resolution at 5 pixels/mm sampling rate(18). The image is then processed on a GE ACRQA workstation for unsharp masking and other enhancements for radiological interpretation(19). A DICOM label for the image is created separately at the ACRQA workstation. The label file and the pixel file constitute the image for a case.

2.1.1.2 Cases

A trained radiologist (FLJ) studied all images captured on June 17, 1997 and selected fourteen images based on over all features and variety of diagnosis. Out of these fourteen cases, seven images were finally selected with a view to a spectrum of sensitivity parameters (sensitivity, $S = 200/exposure(mR)$). The sensitivity values for the seven cases ranged from 183 to 318. This included two male cases and five female cases. A list of extracts from the reports is reproduced in Table 1.

Table 1

Image no.	M/F	Specificity	Diagnosis
1	F	283	Normal
2	M	236	Normal
3	M	210	Blunting of Left Posterior Sulcus
4	F	215	Normal
5	F	318	Low lung volume, Cardiomegaly
6	F	183	Normal
7	F	215	Moderate Lung Volume, Normal

2.1.2 Transporting the images to research workstation

At the GE ACRQA workstation, the image is stored as a pair of files: a DICOM header file and a 1760x2140 pixel file. Each pixel occupying 2 bytes of memory, the size of the pixel file is 7,732,800 bytes. The DICOM tags are added in the filenames to identify each set of files. The medical ID number and the time of capture of the image are distinguishable in the filename and are used to select particular patient cases in the image library. The selected images are then transported to the compression workstation through normal FTP protocol. With a fully operational PACS system, these steps may be reducedby a simple "DICOM send" from the dispatching workstation to the receiving workstation.

2.1.3 Compression

Image compression was accomplished by "AccuPress for Radiology" wavelet compression software distributed by Aware, Inc. (Bedford, Ma). The details of the method and several studies with the application of the software have been published (20, 21, 22). The algorithm operates in three stages. In the first stage, two dimensional wavelet transforms are created by using Daubechies filters up to 15 taps in length. The transforms are created using an adaptive Mallat tree. The second step involves quantization, which has the effect of zeroing out perceptually uninteresting sub-bands and reducing precision in others. In the final stage, run length and Huffman coding techniques are applied to further reduce the size of the quantized data. The compression ratios are targeted towards the actual pixel values in the image, a compression of 10:1 to the 10 bit image would yield 1 bit per pixel compressed file. Compression ratios of 6, 10, 15, 20 and 25 were utilized in the study resulting in effective compression of the file size in the ratios of 9.6, 16, 24, 32 and 40. With seven cases, we have thirty-five compressed images obtained through the procedure. The minimum compression accomplishable by AccuPress software is limited at 6. The average cpu time for compression on a Sparcstation 2 is about 3 minutes.

2.1.4 Reconstructing the images, relabelling and retransporting

The compressed images are reconstructed back using "AccuPress decompress" algorithm. The average cpu time for decompression is about a minute. The DICOM file headers were modified to remove the patient names and to add compression tags to the header. The modified header file and the reconstructed pixel file were transported back to the ACRQA workstation to be queued for print. By modifying the patient name in the file header, it is easy to keep track of the printed film from the laser printer. We may also note in passing that the reduced decompression time makes the image delivery from the archive an efficient process.

2.1.5 Printing images in triplicates

2.1.5.1 Print device

The printing device that is used in the experiment is a Kodak 390lp model laser printer operating at 79 microns pitch. The printer is similar in its characteristics to the more popular Kodak 2180 laser printer. The 10 bit image from ACRA workstation is mapped to a 12 bit scale using a proprietary Kodak look-up table. the 1760x2140 image is then extrapolated to a 4096x5120 pixel print file using a cubic extrapolation algorithm.

2.1.5.2 Triplicate prints

All original images and the reconstructed images were printed in triplicates to create the database for the ROC experiment. All printing was completed in two consecutive evening sessions. The appropriate case numbers and the compression ratios were printed in lieu of the patient ID field for recognition. 126 images comprising of triplicates of seven original images and thirty five reconstructed images form the database for the experiment.

2.2　ROC Experiment

2.2.1 Internal Standard

The experiment was done by randomizing all images and viewing them in sequence with an ordinal scoring for perception and diagnosis. The full set of 126 images was broken into subsets of eighteen images each and each subset was viewed by an observer in one sitting. The task for the observer was to formulate an "internal standard" on the basis of the image quality to draw up a psychophysical ordinal scale. A four point perception rating scale and a three point diagnosis rating scale was used.

2.2.1.1　Perception ratings

The four perception ratings were:

1. Uncompressed original
2. Just perceptible that lossy compression occurred
3. Noticeable that lossy compression occurred
4. Obvious that lossy compression occurred

2.2.1.2　Diagnosis ratings

The three diagnosis ratings were:

1. Completely adequate diagnostic information retained in the compressed image
2. Most diagnostic information retained in the compressed image
3. Compressed image is unacceptable for diagnostic purposes

2.2.1.3　Observations

Three radiologists and four physicists participated in the experiment. All observers were given short training sessions and were allowed to view a sample set of images before scoring. The observers were allowed to vary distance from the pictures and utilize a magnifying lens if desired. All images were viewed under controlled lighting conditions in the Perception Laboratory of Brigham and Women's Hospital. An observer could complete all observations in one sitting the total time varying between one and half to two hours. All observers were called back for a second reading after a lapse of about two weeks.

2.2.2　Analysis

All data were analyzed by the BWH MROC code (23). The code is an extension of the original ROC code of Dorfman and Alf (24), generalized for a distribution of stimuli. The scoring data for each observer were first tabulated through an Excel spreadsheet and the elements of the contingency matrix were read over to the MROC program. The data were then analyzed for frequency and arranged in a normal distribution. The maximum likelihood estimates for the normal deviates are then determined to result in an ROC curve for each stimulus for each observer. Depending on the area under the ROC curve, each curve is given an index of discrimination and these indices of discrimination for each observer are plotted against the stimuli.

3. RESULTS

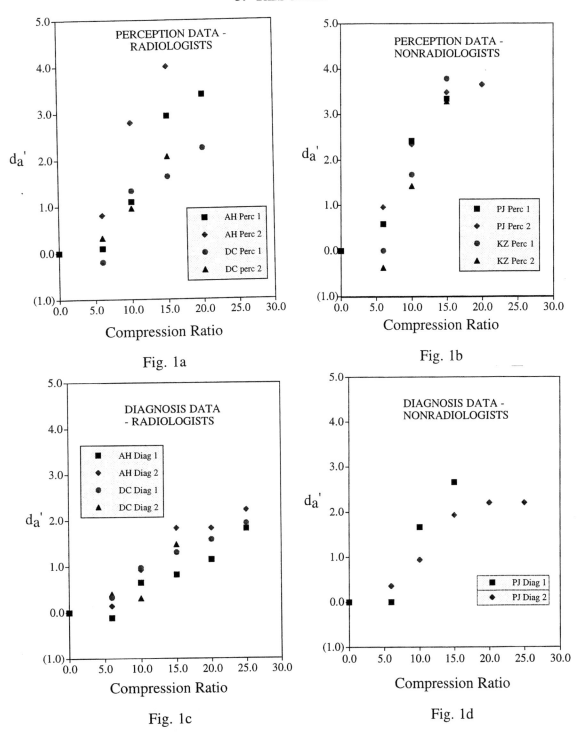

Fig. 1a

Fig. 1b

Fig. 1c

Fig. 1d

Fig.1 The results of perception and diagnosis ROC experiments for radiologists and nonradiologists. (a) perception data for radiologists, (b) perception data for noradiologists,(c) diagnosis data for the radiologists and (d) diagnosis data for the nonradiologists

3.1 Perception and Diagnosis

The perception and diagnosis results for the radiologists and the nonradiologists are separately presented in fig 1a, fig 1b, fig 1c, fig 1d. We observe that the trend for the d_a' values in perception data tend to be higher than those in the diagnosis data. The degradation in diagnosis most likely saturates at a compression ratio of 15. Higher d_a' values provide better facility for the observer to distinguish the uncompressed images from the compressed images. We observe in the perception data that the d_a' value can reach values of 4 for a compression ratio of 15. We observe in the diagnosis data that the d_a' values may cluster around 2. Several observers' data, being perfect scores, could not be fit through the ROC procedures.

3.2 Perception plus Diagnosis

MROC calculations of the d_a' parameters for a stimulus assumes the uniform ordinal scoring scale and hence we can create a new distribution by summing the perception and diagnosis scores for each observer for each stimulus. This new variable p+d captures the information from both the perception rating and also from the diagnosis rating. MROC analysis of p+d values are plotted in figure 2. The average of the d_a' values for an individual stimulus and the best linear fit of the data is shown in the figure.

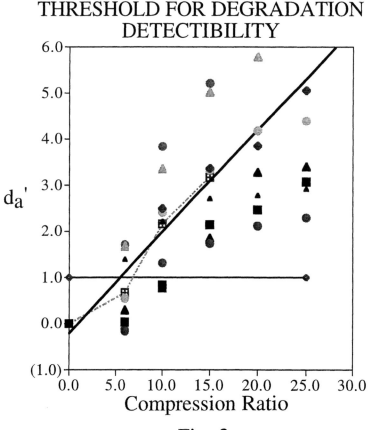

Fig. 2

3.3 Criterion for imperceptible difference

The horizontal line in figure 2 is a line of constant magnitude for $d_a' = 1$. The criterion serves as a boundary between areas of indistinguishability and those of distinguishability in a ROC framework(25). Observations below $d_a' = 1$ would have imperceptible difference.

While for some observers, an image compressed at a compression ratio 10 might appear indistinguishable, the average compression ratio for $d_a' = 1$ criterion is approximately 6. (We have to remind ourselves that the minimum compression ratio achieved by the Aware AccuRad software is also 6.)

4. DISCUSSION

Various recent works have approached the problem of data compression of radiologic images (12-17). The digitized films have been known to allow a high compression ratio since the data size itself is very large. It is also observed that the image artifacts are not strong impediments for radiologists to read images for adequate diagnosis (14, 17).

4.1 Information capacity for a CR image

With high resolution digitizing, the digitized film allows a larger redundancy for compression. One would surmise that there exists a critical threshold of information capacity for an image depending on its spatial resolution. For a 200μ pixel 10bit CR image, such a threshold is arrived at 1.6bits per pixel. A proportionality is likely to exist between the acceptable bit capacity threshold and the pixel size in the image. Assuming such proportionality, one can hypothesize that the threshold of information capacity per millimeter of film viewing area would have a limit of 40 bits. We may verify this hypothesis by working on different modalities that have different image capture methods.

4.2 Image storage consideration

An acceptable image compression ratio of 6 for 10 bit image results in a value of 9.6 in terms of the storage ratio for the 1760x2140 pixel images. With the low resolution and low bit depth, this may serve as the lower limit of the compression ratio for the Fuji CR images.

4.3 Reference standard experiment

The results of an earlier experiment where all images of a particular patient were viewed by observers in comparison to the original image of the patient side by side were presented earlier at the 7th Far West Image Perception Conference. The acceptable compression ratio under such criterion reduces to 4, close to the lossless compression ratio reported in literature (26).

4.3 Future work

Compression ratios chosen for the experiment are based on earlier work(unpublished) to transport CR images on to CRT monitors. No image artifacts are noticed on 8bit greyscale monitors even when the compression ratio was very high (around

50). We noticed serious image degradation when we printed the images and then verified the degradation on the screen by utilizing magnification on high resolution monitors. A tighter set of compression ratios would be required to prevent the perception saturation as is noticed on these images. Such a study is under progress.

ACKNOWLEDGEMENTS

We are thankful to Dr. Arthur Burgess for many helpful discussions. Our thanks are due to Dr. Keith W. Dreyer, Dr. Ramin Khorasani and Dr. Stephen Seltzer for their encouragement and support. BM wishes to thank Partners' Healthcare in Boston for providing consulting support while working on this project.

REFERENCES

1. N. H. Strickland, "Some Cost-Effective Considerations For PACS: A Radiological Perspective", The British Journal of Radiology, 69, pp 1089-1098, 1996.

2 E. Siegel and R. Shannon, "The Rationale for Image Compression", in *Understanding Compression,* SCAR, pp 11-15, 1997.

3. E. Siegel, "Economic and Clinical Impact of Filmless Operation in a Multifacility Environment", Journal of Digital Imaging, 11, pp 42-47, 1998.

4. E.C.Reiter, "Cost Consideration for Image Compression", in *Understanding Compression,* SCAR, pp 25-28, 1997.

5. M.A.Goldberg, "Recommendations for the Use of Image Compression", in *Understanding Compression,* SCAR, pp 29-36, 1997.

6. M.A.Goldberg, M.Pivavarov, W.W.Mayo-Smith, M.P.Bhalla, J.G.Blickman, R.T.Bramson, G.W.L.bolard, H.J.Llewellyn and E. Halpern, "Application of Wavelet Compression to Digitized Radiographs", American Journal of Radiology, 163, pp 463-468, 1994.

7. T. Ishigaki, S.Sakunia, M.Ikada, Y.Itoh, M.Suzuki and S.Iwai, "Clinical evaluation of Irreversible Image Compression: Analysis of Chest Imaging with Computed Radiography", Radiology, 175, pp 739-743, 1990.

8. H.McMohan, K.Doi, S.Sanada, S.M.Montner, M.L.Giger, C.R.Metz, N.Nakamori, F.Yin, X. Xu, H.Yonekawa and H.Takeuchi, "Data Compression - Effect in Diagnostic Accuracy in Digital Chest Radiography", Radiology, 178, pp 175-179, 1991.

9. R.M.Allman and D.Goodenough, "Compression and Image Quality", in *Understanding Compression*, SCAR, 1997.

10. NEMA, "Data Compression Standard", ACR/NEMA PS2-1989, Washington DC, 1989.

11. P. G. Drew, Ed., "Understanding Compression", SCAR, Merrifield, VA, 1997.

12. S.Lo and H.K.Huang, Compression of Radiological Images with 512, 1024 and 2048 Matrices", Radiology, 161, pp 519-525, 1986.

13. D.R.Aberle, F.Gleeson, J.W.Sayre, K.Brown, P.Batra, D.A.Young, B.K.Stewart, B.K.T.Ho and H.K.Huang, "The Effect of Irreversible Image Compression in Diagnostic Accuracy in Thoracic Imaging", Investigative Radiology, 28, pp 398-403, 1993.

14. G.G.Cox, L.T.Cook, M.F.Insana, M.A.McFadden, T.J.Hall, L.A.Harrison, D.A.Eckard and N.L.Martin, "The Effects of Lossy Compression on the Detection of Subtle Pulmonary Nodules", Medical physics, 23, pp 127-132, 1996.

15. P.W.Jones, S.Daily, R.S.Gaborski and M. Rabbani, "Comparative Study of Weavelet and DCT Decompositions with Equivalent Quantization and Encoding Strategies for Medical Images", SPIE 2431, pp 571-581, 1995.

16. M.P.Eckert, "Lossy Compression Using Wavelets, Block DCT, and Lapped Orthogonal Transforms Optimized with a Perceptual model", SPIE 3031, pp 339-350, 1997.

17. V.Savcenko, B.J.Erickson, P.M.Pallison, K.P.Persons, A.Manduca, T.E.Hartman, G.F.Harms and L.R.Brown, "Detection of Subtle Abnormalities on Chest Radiographs after Irreversible Compression", Radiology, 206, pp 609-616, 1998.

18. J. A. Siebert (Chair), "Acceptance Testing and Quality Control of Computed Radiography Imaging Systems", Report of Tak Group #10, AAPM, 1997.

19. GE Medical systems, "Advantage CR QA Quality Assurance Workstation Operation Manual", 1996.

20. J.Huffman and A.Cohen, "Wavelet Technology for Radiology Image Processing, V: Lossy Compression of Plain Films", Aware Inc., 1993.

21. Aware Inc., "Wavelet Image Compression Software User's Guide", 14 pp, 1994.

22. E. Reiter, "Wavelet Compression of Medical Imaging", Telemedicine Journal, 2, pp 131-137, 1996.

23. M.F.Kijewiski, R.G.swenson and P.F.Judy, "Analysis of Rating Data from Multiple-Alternative Tasks", Journal of Mathematical Psychology, 33, pp 428-451, 1989.

24. D.D.Dorfman and E. Alf, "Maximum-Likelihood Estimation of Parameters of Signal-Detection Theory and Determination of Confidence intervals - Rating-Method Data", Journal of Mathematical Psychology, 6, pp 487-496, 1969.

25. P.F.Judy, R.G.Swenson, R.D.Nawfel, K.H. Chan and S.E. Seltzer, "Contrast Detail Curves for Liver CT", Medical Physics, 19, pp 1167-1174, 1992.

26 J.Kivijarvi, T.Ojala, T.Kaukoranta, A.Kuba, L.Nyul and O.Nevalainen, "A Comparison of Lossless Compression Methods for Medical Images", Computerized Medical Imaging and Graphics, 22, pp 323-339, 1998.

The Effect of De-Noising on the Consistency of Manually Defined Borders

Xuli Zong[*a], Edward A. Geiser[b], Donald A. Conetta[c]

[a]GE Corporate Research and Development, Schenectady, NY 12301

[b]Department of Medicine, University of Florida, Gainesville, FL 32610

[c]Division of Cardiology, Univ. of Florida HSC Jacksonville, Jacksonville, FL 32209

ABSTRACT

This paper presents experimental results and analysis for a study of the effect of de-noising on the consistency and reliability of manually-defined borders of echocardiograms. De-Noising and image enhancement have been performed on a test data set of 60 sequences from an echocardiographic database exhibiting diverse image quality. Both endocardial and epicardial borders of end diastolic and end systolic frames were manually identified for original and enhanced images based on image perception and wall motion information. Statistical analysis was performed on the identified borders. The experimental results show that de-noising and image enhancement help to improve the consistency of the manually-defined borders for the data set.

Keywords: Speckle reduction, de-noising, contrast enhancement, image enhancement, image perception, border detection, manual border identification, performance measurement, ultrasound images, echocardiograms

1. INTRODUCTION

Manual border identification with myocardial wall motion analysis in echocardiographic images remains a reliable tool for clinic research. Because of considerable difference in image quality of echocardiograms, automated or semi-automated border detection algorithms succeed on some images and fail to produce satisfactory results on other images. Noise and artifacts often cause signal and image degradations in various medical imaging modalities. Image formation using coherent waves, as are used in ultrasound images, results in a granular pattern known as speckle. The granular pattern is correlated with the surface roughness (structures) of an object (tissues) being imaged and is also related to imaging characteristics. Goodman[1] presented an analysis of speckle properties under coherent irradiance. Abbott and Thurstone[2] pointed out the primary differences between laser and ultrasound speckle in terms of coherent interference and speckle production. For speckle reduction, earlier techniques include temporal averaging,[1,2] median filtering,[3] and homomorphic Wiener filtering.[4] Similar to temporal averaging, the speckle reduction technique[5] used frequency and/or angle diversity to generate multiple uncorrelated synthetic-aperture radar images which were summed incoherently to reduce speckle. Hokland and Taxt[6] reported a technique which decomposed a coherent image into three components, one of which, subresolvable quasi-periodic scatter, causes speckle noise. The component was eliminated by a harmonic analysis algorithm. Moulin et al.[7] presented an algorithm based on the maximum-likelihood principle and a wavelet regularization procedure for the logarithm of a radar image to reduce speckle. Guo et al.[8] reported a wavelet-based method for speckle reduction. In this study, we have applied a previously developed de-noising method[9,10] on original noisy images for speckle reduction and contrast enhancement along boundaries of importance to cardiologists, such as endocardial and epicardial boundaries.

Myocardial border detection, wall thickness, and wall motion analysis provide important information regarding heart size and function for clinical diagnosis.[11–15] Several approaches for border detection of the left ventricle (LV) have shown partial success in either identifying the endocardial boundary,[16,17] the center point of the LV and partial boundary points,[18,19] or epicardial boundary detection.[20] A method for automatic identification of papillary muscles has also been reported.[21] An improved active contour model (balloons) using energy minimizing principles has also been developed for ventricle detection in magnetic resonance and ultrasound images.[22] In this method, an initial curve which does not have to be close to the extracted feature needs to be specified. Chalana et al.[23] reported another extension of active contour models for cardiac boundary detection. In these (and most other) approaches,

---

*Correspondence: Email: zong@crd.ge.com; Telephone: 518 387 6115; Fax: 518 387 6923

Part of the SPIE Conference on Image Perception and Performance
San Diego, California • February 1999
SPIE Vol. 3663 • 0277-786X/99/$10.00

human knowledge of the approximate shape of endocardial and epicardial boundaries and/or a computer generated center point of the LV have been used successfully to initiate boundary detection. Thus, modeling and analysis of the LV shape[24-26] have played important roles in some boundary detection methods. Most of these methods measure their performance against expert, manually-defined borders, sometime referred to as a "gold standard"[23] or "ground truth".

Our study on clinical images was conducted to investigate the effect of de-noising on the consistency and reliability of expert manually-defined borders of the left ventricle in two-dimensional short-axis echocardiographic images. Experimental results indicate the algorithm is promising. Borders defined by experts exhibit less variation after de-noising. It seems that in echocardiograms, where real borders are seldom clearly visible and frequently incomplete, expert borders usually indicate image positions where real borders are likely to exist. When two expert borders agree with each other, the range of real borders is more likely limited around the two expert borders. This study of clinical images shows that de-noising with feature enhancement improves the consistency of manually-defined borders by expert observers.

The rest of the paper is organized as follows. In Section 2, we present methods employed in the study. Each step of the whole procedure is explained. Experimental results and analysis are presented in Section 3. We calculate statistical results for several quantitative measurements and show the visual effect of de-noising with feature enhancement and manually-defined borders by two expert observers. Section 4 concludes this paper based on our experimental analysis.

2. METHODOLOGY

The study was organized and conducted in six major steps. First, the test images were selected from a large database of echocardiographic images with diverse quality, including 60 total image sequences of two-dimensional short-axis echocardiograms of the LV of 30 patients. Two sequences per patient, and 16 frames per sequence, were chosen. Half of the test images were rated as good quality in terms of border information visible to a cardiologist while the rest were considered as poor quality. In the second step, the end diastolic and end systolic frames were identified for each sequence. In Step 3, we have applied a de-noising method previously developed[9,10] on all noisy echocardiographic images for speckle reduction and contrast enhancement along boundaries of importance to cardiologists, such as endocardial and epicardial boundaries. The 120 sequences of images, 60 original sequences plus 60 de-noised sequences, were randomized in Step 4 into a single list of images identified by a random identification (ID) number while keeping the two sequences of each patient in the same order as they appear in the original image list. The reason that we kept the two sequences of each patient one after another was that expert observers have this information in the clinical setting and learn from the first sequence of each patient. The expert observers drawing the borders were informed only that the two sequences belonged to the same patient. In Step 5, expert observers were only required to identify the left ventricular endocardial (Endo) and epicardial (Epi) borders of the end diastolic (ED) and end systolic (ES) frames in each sequence based on their expertise and border motion when viewing the video loop of each sequence. Statistical analysis of the manually-defined borders for the original and de-noised images was performed in the last step.

The selection of the test data set was carried out by a sonographer who knew the echocardiographic image database well. This sonographer also performed the identification of the ED and ES frames. The algorithm for speckle reduction and contrast enhancement of echocardiographic images was a wavelet-based approach.[10] Within a framework of multiscale wavelet analysis, wavelet shrinkage techniques were applied to eliminate noise while preserving the sharpness of salient features. In addition, nonlinear processing of feature energy was carried out to enhance contrast within local structures and along object boundaries. In the method, we adopt regularized soft thresholding (wavelet shrinkage) to remove noise energy within the finer scales and nonlinear processing of feature energy to enhance contrast. Hard thresholding is incorporated for preserving features while removing small noise perturbations within the middle levels of analysis. The algorithm was shown to be capable of not only reducing speckle, but also enhancing features of diagnostic importance, such as myocardial walls in 2-D echocardiograms obtained from the parasternal short-axis view.

The de-noising operation was accomplished through a batch processing with a single set of de-noising and enhancement parameters used to process all the test echocardiographic images in this study. It is suggested based on this study that a single value set of parameters should be enough for de-noising and enhancing a class of images with a similar noise pattern for noise reduction and selected features for enhancement.

Table 1. Quantitative measurements of manually-defined borders between two expert observers

		All Test Images		Good Images		Poor Images	
		Ori	Enh	Ori	Enh	Ori	Enh
MDistDiff	Endo (in mm)	2.105 0.084	1.817 0.274	1.597 0.120	1.532 0.197	2.612 0.142	2.101 0.365
	Epi (in mm)	1.785 0.150	1.674 0.172	1.398 0.107	1.589 0.138	2.171 0.218	1.760 0.216
MAreaDiff	Endo (in cm^2)	2.373 1.901	1.889 1.605	1.660 1.614	1.454 1.161	3.087 1.916	2.324 1.868
	Epi (in cm^2)	2.568 2.406	2.080 1.847	1.582 1.341	1.954 1.709	3.553 2.822	2.206 1.994

Table 2. Percentage improvement computed from Table 1

		All Test Images	Good Images	Poor Images
MDistDiff	Endo	13.68%	4.07%	19.56%
	Epi	6.22%	-13.66%	18.93%
MAreaDiff	Endo	20.40%	12.41%	24.72%
	Epi	19.00%	-23.51%	37.91%

Steps of the study

The major steps of this study are summarized as follows:

1. Select test images, 60 sequences of 2-D short-axis echocardiographic images of the 30 patients. Choose 2 sequences from each patient echo with 16 frames per sequence. Fifteen patient studies, 30 sequences, were judged to be good quality while the remaining 15 patient studies (30 sequences) were rated to be of poor quality.

2. Identify ED and ES frames for each systolic sequence.

3. Process the test images using the de-noising algorithm.

4. Randomize the original and de-noised image sequences, while keeping the two original or de-noised sequences of each patient together.

5. Present the randomized image sequences to two expert observers to manually define Endo and Epi borders at ED and ES.

6. Compare the borders defined by the two observers, by performing a statistical analysis to determine the impact of the de-noising algorithm on the consistency and reliability.

3. EXPERIMENTAL RESULT ANALYSIS AND DISCUSSION

If the manually-defined borders by expert observers differ in a substantial amount in terms of inter-observer distances, then the real borders are more likely to have a large difference from one or both of the expert borders. On the other hand, if two borders manually defined by two expert observers are very close to each other, then the real border should be close to one or both of them. In the second case, the two expert borders can be considered to be more reliable compared to the first case. Expert borders in this context are referred to as the reliable identification of real borders when more border information is present or as a close guess of real borders when not enough border information is visible. When the image quality is poor and there is a considerable amount of border information drop out, the guess error will more likely be increased. If low contrast along borders and/or border information in an image is corrupted by noise, such as speckle, de-noising and feature enhancement techniques may play a role in improving the quality of images to make manually-defined borders by expert observers more consistent and reliable.

The set of test images included in our study of clinical images was selected from an echocardiographic database exhibiting a wide range of image quality. Sixty, 16-frame sequences of 2-D short-axis echocardiographic images were selected. For more details about how these echocardiographic image sequences were acquired, we refer the reader to.[18] Quantitative measurements were calculated in terms of the mean of absolute border differences (MDistDiff) in

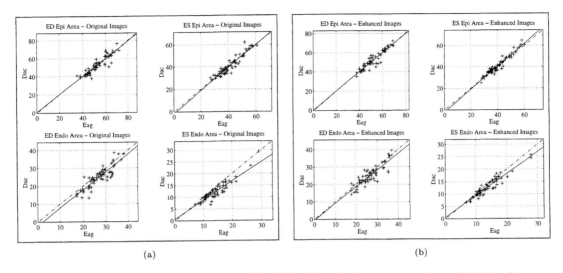

(a)   (b)

Figure 1. Area correlation between manually-defined borders by two expert cardiologist observers.

mm and the mean of border area differences (MAreaDiff) in cm^2. The border difference was measured by its close approximation in 64 radial directional differences from an estimated center[18] of the left ventricle. The consistency of manually-defined expert borders on poor quality images were improved after de-noising. The statistical means and standard deviations of quantitative measurements of two sets of expert manually-defined borders are shown in Table 1. The statistical computation results listed under the column "Ori" are the quantitative measurements between two sets of expert borders on the original images while the results under the column "Enh" are based on the de-noised and enhanced images.

Overall percentage improvement computed from Table 1 is shown in Table 2. In general, the quantitative measurements of border distance differences agree with the area differences. Border distance differences and area differences show improved agreement between two expert observers on all and poor images after de-noising. A slight improvement for Endo border agreement on good quality images after de-noising is also observed while Epi border agreement on de-noised images becomes slightly worse than on the original images.

Figure 1 shows the area correlation between two sets of manually-defined borders by expert observers. The four diagrams in Figure 1(a) present the correlation of ED Epi border areas, ES Epi border areas, ED Endo border areas, and ES Endo border areas on the original noisy images. The four diagrams in Figure 1(b) show similar results for the de-noised images with features restored or enhanced. The solid lines in the figure are the linear regression lines, while the dash and dotted lines are (lines of identity) ideal regression lines. From the diagrams, it is clear that the points which represent the two expert border areas on the de-noised image are, in general, close to the ideal regression line. Additional improvement can be seen on the Endo area correlation for the de-noised images. Noisy border information (low signal-to-noise ratio (SNR)) affects border interpolation by human observers for the manually-defined borders. After de-noising, Endo border information in terms of SNR is improved, so the expert border areas tend to agree with each other, especially ES Endo areas.

Figure 2 shows the fractional area change (FAC) between manually-defined borders by two expert cardiologist observers. Figure 2(a) shows FAC on original images while Figure 2(b) presents FAC on enhanced images. Based on the definition of FAC,

$$FAC = \frac{Area_{ED\_Endo} - Area_{ES\_Endo}}{Area_{ED\_Endo}},$$

there are a few factors affecting FAC. First, the difference $Area_{ED\_Endo} - Area_{ES\_Endo}$ is affected by the changes of both $Area_{ED\_Endo}$ and $Area_{ES\_Endo}$. The zooming (scale or normalizing) factor ($\frac{1}{Area_{ED\_Endo}}$) also plays an important role. Here smaller MDistDiff and MAreaDiff do not directly translate to a more correlated FACs. In fact, the FACs based on the two expert borders on enhanced images is slightly less correlated compared to the FACs computed for original images in this study.

Figure 3 shows the distributions of mean border differences on the original images; (a) the distribution of Epi ED border differences, (b) the distribution of Epi ES border differences, (c) the distribution of Endo ED border

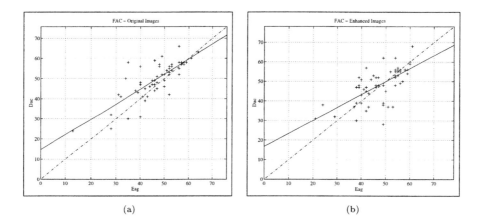

Figure 2. Fractional area change (FAC) between manually-defined borders by two expert cardiologist observers. (a) FAC on original images. (b) FAC on enhanced images.

Table 3. Quantitative measurements of the mean of area differences for the manually-defined borders of each observer between two cycles

		All Test Images		Good Images		Poor Images	
		Ori	Enh	Ori	Enh	Ori	Enh
Dac –	Endo (in cm^2)	1.8637	1.9350	1.4413	1.9440	2.2860	1.9260
	Epi (in cm^2)	3.5245	3.0677	3.4860	2.9560	3.5630	3.1793
Eag –	Endo (in cm^2)	2.2025	1.9140	1.6047	1.7620	2.8003	2.0660
	Epi (in cm^2)	3.1973	3.0702	2.6513	2.3907	3.7433	3.7497

differences, and (d) the distribution of Endo ES border differences. Figures 4(a)-(d) show the distributions of mean border differences on the enhanced images, similar to Figures 3(a)-(d). The solid lines in Figures 3 and 4 are the linear fitting lines in a least-squares sense. With the same scale for both Figures 3 and 4, Figure 4 shows that border distance differences for enhanced images have smaller means and standard deviations than the corresponding differences for the original noisy images as shown in Figure 3. The linear regression lines for the borders of de-noised and enhanced images are more close to the center line (the border difference mean).

Table 3 shows the quantitative measurements of the intra-observer mean of border area differences (MAreaDiff in cm^2). "Eag" and "Dac" are the IDs for two expert observers. These measurements are calculated on the borders for all test images, good quality images, and poor images separately between the two cycles of each patient.

Quantitative measurements of intra-observer border differences are shown in Tables 4 and 5. These measurements show the impact of de-noising the images on how each observer defines the borders. Table 4 shows the quantitative measurements of intra-observer border differences on good original versus enhanced images. Similarly, Table 5 refers to the measured impact on the borders of all poor quality images. Tables 4 and 5 should be interpreted as relative magnitudes. In other words, if the mean intra-observer difference is large, the de-noising had a greater impact on changing the border position than if the intra-observer difference is small.

Figure 5 shows an example of de-noising and image enhancement. Figure 6 shows the same images as Figures 5 with two expert manually-defined borders overlaid. Significant overall improvement on the agreement of two expert borders is visible from the overlaid borders of the enhanced images compared to the original images, as shown visually in Figure 6 and quantitatively in Table 6. The Endo borders have more improvement than the Epi borders based on quantitative measurements and visual appearance.

4. CONCLUSIONS

In this paper, we have presented experimental results which show that de-noising and image enhancement help to improve the consistency of manually-defined borders of clinical echocardiographic images by expert observers. A test

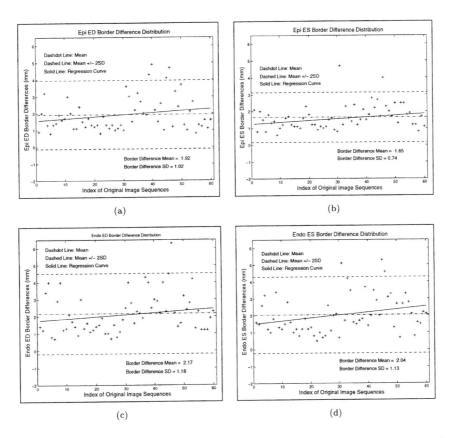

Figure 3. Border difference variation on the original images. (a) Distribution of Epi ED border differences. (b) Distribution of Epi ES border differences. (c) Distribution of Endo ED border differences. (d) Distribution of Endo ES border differences. The solid lines are the linear fitting lines in a least-squares sense.

Table 4. Quantitative measurements of intra-observer border differences on good original versus enhanced images

	Epi-ED	Epi-ES	Endo-ED	Endo-ES
Dac – MDistDiff (in mm)	1.4371	1.4006	1.3348	1.2527
MAreaDiff (in cm^2)	1.7420	1.6687	1.2237	0.8343
Eag – MDistDiff (in mm)	1.4463	1.1099	1.2298	1.0212
MAreaDiff (in cm^2)	2.0113	1.4107	1.1790	0.7510

Table 5. Quantitative measurements of intra-observer border differences on poor original versus enhanced images

	Epi-ED	Epi-ES	Endo-ED	Endo-ES
Dac – MDistDiff (in mm)	1.9702	1.8170	1.8959	1.4138
MAreaDiff (in cm^2)	2.7447	2.9130	2.1357	1.0310
Eag – MDistDiff (in mm)	1.5161	1.4492	1.4726	1.2686
MAreaDiff (in cm^2)	2.3037	2.1893	1.5473	1.0883

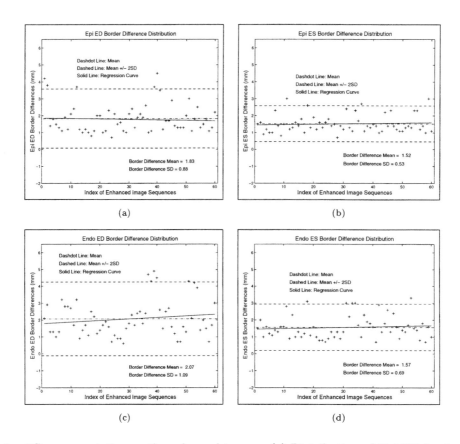

Figure 4. Border difference variation on the enhanced images. (a) Distribution of Epi ED border differences. (b) Distribution of Epi ES border differences. (c) Distribution of Endo ED border differences. (d) Distribution of Endo ES border differences. The solid lines are the linear fitting lines.

Table 6. Quantitative measurements of inter-observer mean border differences in *mm* on original versus enhanced images, as shown in Figure 6

	Epi-ED	Epi-ES	Endo-ED	Endo-ES
Ori	4.7	4.0	6.3	4.6
Enh	1.4	2.3	1.2	1.3

data set from a large database has been randomized and presented to cardiologists to identify the endocardial and epicardial borders at ED and ES. Half of the test data had good quality while the other half had poor quality.

Statistical analysis shows improvement in terms of the mean of absolute border differences and mean border area differences of de-noised images compared to their original images. The greatest impact is on the expert borders drawn on images with poor image quality.

REFERENCES

1. J. W. Goodman, "Some fundamental properties of speckle," *J. Opt. Soc. Am.* **66**(11), pp. 1145–1150, 1976.
2. J. G. Abbott and F. L. Thurstone, "Acoustic speckle: theory and experimental analysis," *Ultrasonic Imaging* **1**, pp. 303–324, 1979.
3. R. N. Czerwinski, D. L. Jones, and W. D. O'Brien, Jr. "Ultrasound speckle reduction by directional median filtering," in *Proceedings of ICIP*, vol. I, pp. 358–361, (Washington, D.C.), 1995.
4. A. K. Jain, *Fundamentals of Digital Image Processing*, Prentice-Hall, Inc., Englewood Cliffs, New Jersey, 1989.
5. L. J. Porcello, N. G. Massey, R. B. Innes, and J. M. Marks, "Speckle reduction in synthetic-aperture radars," *J. Opt. Soc. Am.* **66**(11), pp. 1305–1311, 1976.

6. J. H. Hokland and T. Taxt, "Ultrasound speckle reduction using harmonic oscillator models," *IEEE Transactions on Ultrasonics, Ferroelectrics, and Frequency Control* **41**, pp. 215–224, Mar. 1994.

7. P. Moulin, "A wavelet regularization method for diffuse radar-target imaging and speckle-noise reduction," *J. of Mathematical Imaging and Vision* **3**(1), pp. 123–134, 1993.

8. H. Guo, J. E. Odegard, M. Lang, R. A. Gopinath, I. W. Selesnick, and C. S. Burrus, "Wavelet based speckle reduction with application to SAR based ATD/R," in *Proceedings of ICIP*, vol. I, pp. 75–79, (Austin, TX), 1994.

9. X. Zong, E. A. Geiser, A. F. Laine, and D. C. Wilson, "Homomorphic wavelet shrinkage and feature emphasis for speckle reduction and enhancement of echocardiographic images," in *Medical Imaging: Image Processing*, Proceedings of SPIE, vol. 2710, pp. 658–667, (Newport Beach, CA), 1996.

10. X. Zong, A. F. Laine, and E. A. Geiser, "Speckle reduction and contrast enhancement of echocardiograms via multiscale nonlinear processing," *IEEE Transactions on Medical Imaging* **17**(4), pp. 532–540, 1998.

11. J. W. Klingler, Jr., C. L. Vaughan, T. D. Fraker, and L. T. Andrews, "Segmentation of echocardiographic images using mathematical morphology," *IEEE Transactions on Biomedical Engineering* **35**, pp. 925–934, Nov. 1988.

12. E. A. Geiser, D. C. Wilson, J. M. Billett, and G. L. Gibby, "Automated segmentation of the left ventricular region of search from short axis 2-dimensional echocardiograms," *Circulation Supplement III* **82**(4), p. III68, 1990.

13. D. C. Wilson, E. A. Geiser, J. M. Billett, and D. A. Conetta, "Computer identification of left ventricular endocardium from 2-dimensional short axis echocardiograms," *Journal of American College of Cardiology* **17**(2), p. 264A, 1991.

14. E. A. Geiser, "Edge detection and wall motion analysis," in *Echocardiography: An International Review*, J. Chambers and M. J. Monaghan, eds., pp. 71–82, Oxford University Press, Oxford, 1993.

15. J. M. B. Dias and J. M. N. Leitão, "Wall position and thickness estimation from sequences of echocardiographic images," *IEEE Transactions on Medical Imaging* **15**, pp. 25–38, Feb. 1996.

16. N. Friedland and D. Adam, "Automatic ventricular cavity boundary detection from sequential ultrasound images using simulated annealing," *IEEE Transactions on Medical Imaging* **8**, pp. 344–353, Dec. 1989.

17. P. R. Detmer, G. Bashein, and R. W. Martin, "Matched filter identification of left-ventricular endocardial borders in transesophageal echocardiograms," *IEEE Transactions on Medical Imaging* **9**(4), pp. 396–403, 1990.

18. D. C. Wilson and E. A. Geiser, "Automatic center point determination in two-dimensional short-axis echocardiographic images," *Pattern Recognition* **25**, pp. 893–900, Sept. 1992.

19. D. C. Wilson, E. A. Geiser, and J.-H. Li, "Feature extraction in two-dimensional short-axis echocardiographic images," *J. of Mathematical Imaging and Vision* (3), pp. 285–298, 1993.

20. J. Feng, W. Lin, and C. Chen, "Epicardial boundary detection using fuzzy reasoning," *IEEE Transactions on Medical Imaging* **10**, pp. 187–199, June 1991.

21. T. Karras, D. C. Wilson, E. A. Geiser, and D. A. Conetta, "Automatic identification of papillary muscles in left-ventricular short-axis echocardiographic images," *IEEE Transactions on Biomedical Engineering* **43**, pp. 460–470, May 1996.

22. L. D. Cohen, "On active contour models and balloons," *CVGIP: Image Understanding* **53**, pp. 211–218, Mar. 1991.

23. V. Chalana, D. T. Linker, D. R. Haynor, and Y. Kim, "A multiple active contour model for cardiac boundary detection on echocardiographic sequences," *IEEE Transactions on Medical Imaging* **15**(3), pp. 290–298, 1996.

24. J. Duncan, R. Owen, P. Anandan, L. Staib, T. McCauley, A. Salazar, and F. Lee, "Shape-based tracking of left ventricular wall motion," in *IEEE Computers in Cardiology*, pp. 41–44, 1990.

25. C. Chen, T. Huang, and M. Arrott, "Modeling, analysis, and visualization of left ventrical shape and motion by hierarchical decomposition," *IEEE Trans. Pattern Anal. Mach. Intell.* **16**, pp. 342–356, Apr. 1994.

26. A. Laine and X. Zong, "Border identification of echocardiograms via multiscale edge detection and shape modeling," in *Proceedings of ICIP*, vol. III, pp. 287–290, (Lausanne, Switzerland), 1996.

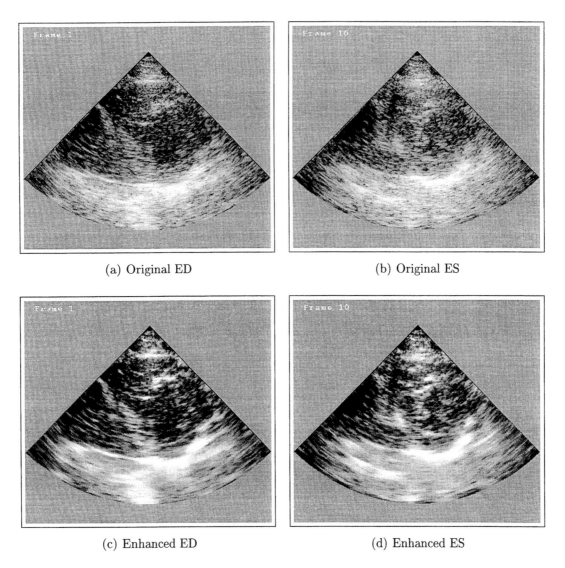

(a) Original ED

(b) Original ES

(c) Enhanced ED

(d) Enhanced ES

Figure 5. De-noising and image enhancement: (a) An original ED frame; (b) An original ES frame; (c) The enhanced ED frame; (c) The enhanced ES frame.

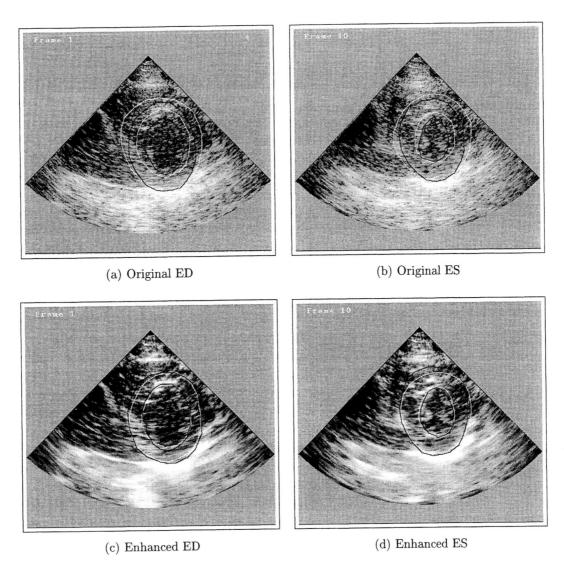

(a) Original ED

(b) Original ES

(c) Enhanced ED

(d) Enhanced ES

Figure 6. Image and border display: (a) An original ED frame with manually-defined borders overlaid; (b) An original ES frame with manually-defined borders overlaid; (c) The enhanced ED frame with manually-defined borders overlaid; (c) The enhanced ES frame with manually-defined borders overlaid. Black and white borders were drawn by the two observers.

Clinical Validation Studies on Clinical Workstation Prototypes

Bert Verdonck, Karel C. Strasters, Frans A. Gerritsen

Philips Medical Systems Nederland B.V., EasyVision Advanced Development,
P.O.Box 10.000, NL-5680 DA Best, The Netherlands,
tel +31 40 27 62 456, {Bert.Verdonck, Karel.Strasters, Frans.Gerritsen}@best.ms.philips.com

ABSTRACT

This paper reports on our experience with setting up and analyzing clinical validation studies for new or improved medical image processing algorithms. This is illustrated with two specific examples: (1) clinical validation of a motion correction algorithm to improve the image quality of digital subtraction angiography (DSA) imaging and (2) clinical validation of an overview image reconstruction algorithm for translated X-ray image sequences (bolus chase reconstruction, spine imaging, colon image map or leg bone imaging).

1. OVERVIEW OF CLINICAL VALIDATION METHODOLOGY

The first step in our method is to clearly define the target of the study: What is the gold standard (if any)? Which alternative algorithms are to be investigated? What are the degrees of freedom (algorithm parameters)? Which clinical applications are to be involved? Which thesis do we advance? Which claim do we try to support? Which image properties should be evaluated?

This opens a tedious hunt for relevant clinical patient image data with considerable attention for capturing a large variety in clinical protocols, image acquisition parameters, anatomical variation, etc. This quickly leads to a need for 50 to 200 patient cases. While some standard case-archives primarily contain "nice and well-behaved" show-case images, we are clearly also interested in gathering "error-prone" images and images of day-to-day clinical quality.

We build dedicated comparison tools with basic viewing functionality (to allow interactive modification of zoom, contrast, brightness, edge enhancement), based on our commercially available workstation (EasyVision, Philips Medical Systems). We ask the observer to score the image quality (esthetics) and the clinical relevance (clinical value). Depending on the application, additional questions might also be asked: amount of image noise, presence of artefacts, ... Comparative scoring is done on a 5-grade scale (much worse, worse, similar, better, best). Observers can indicate some regions of interest and add textual comments on their judgement. We typically work with at least 10 observers: clinical experts who are used to work with the kind of images under investigation.

The results are subjected to statistical analysis. Since it is difficult to come to a statistically significant conclusion for each individual case based on observations from 10 experts only, series of similar cases are combined in order to increase the statistical population. The primary task is then to challenge the null hypotheses that the new or improved algorithm does not lead to an improvement (e.g. by using a two sided t-test corrected for non-continuity of the scores). Further analysis of the score distributions and statistics of the answers on the additional questions complete the study.

2. CASE 1: MOTION CORRECTION FOR DSA

Our validation framework has been successfully applied to compare four automatic motion correction algorithms and the conventional manual pixel shifting of digital subtraction angiography images.

2.1. Algorithm

The algorithm details have been described extensively in a series of other papers by Buzug et al. [1-5]. Here we will only summarize the algorithm in short. The aim is to correct the mask image for motion that has occurred between the acquisition of the mask and the contrast images. This can considerably improve the quality of the subtracted image. Figure 1 shows an example of the renal vascular tree, from left to right: mask, contrast and subtracted image (on a region of interest).

The conventional way to improve DSA image quality is to interactively shift one of both images while observing the improvement or degradation of the subtracted image. However, this can be a tedious task and in this way one can only correct for translational movements.

The new procedure estimates the displacement automatically and more accurately by using a two-step procedure. First a series of square templates (one is superimposed on the image on the left of figure 1) is translated and compared by using

34

Part of the SPIE Conference on Image Perception and Performance
San Diego, California ● February 1999
SPIE Vol. 3663 ● 0277-786X/99/$10.00

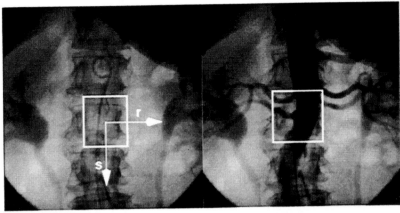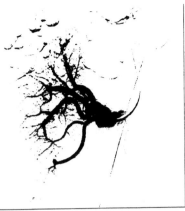

Figure 1: Mask image with a template that can be translated along the r and s axes.

Contrast image with the automatically and optimally translated template.

Region of interest of the subtracted image.

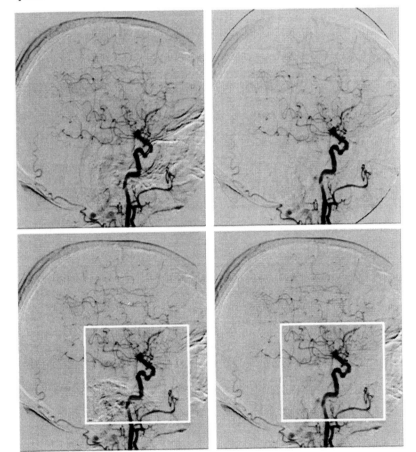

Figure 2: Subtracted cerebral lateral X-ray angiogram. Results of image subtraction after motion correction with 4 variants of the automatic algorithms:

a. Auto shift on entire image
b. Auto warp on entire image
c. Auto shift on a rectangular ROI
d. Auto warp on a rectangular ROI

result of a.	result of b.
result of c.	result of d.

some similarity measure. The translation that maximizes the similarity measure is selected. Then a global affine transformation is fit to the set of template displacements. The transformation can be detailed as follows:

$$\begin{cases} x_{\text{Contrast}} = a_{00} + a_{01} x_{\text{Mask}} + a_{02} y_{\text{Mask}} \\ y_{\text{Contrast}} = a_{10} + a_{11} x_{\text{Mask}} + a_{12} y_{\text{Mask}} \end{cases}$$

where $(x_{Contrast}, y_{Contrast})$ and (x_{Mask}, y_{Mask}) are corresponding coordinates in both images and a_{ij} are the estimated parameters of the affine transformation. This transformation will be used to deform or "warp" the mask image in order to let it fit better to the contrast image.

2.2. Validation aims and tools

Thorough *technical validation* of the algorithm already occurred before clinical validation started. This included experiments with simulated motions, evaluation of different similarity measures, warping transformations and several algorithm parameters (template size, number of templates, etc.). The results are reported in the papers by Buzug et al. [1-5].

Four variants of the algorithm remained after the technical validation phase (illustrated in figure 2 on a cerebral angiogram):

1. Auto-shift (translation only) on the entire image.
2. Auto-warp (affine transform) on the entire image.
3. Auto-shift on a user selected rectangular region of interest (ROI).
4. Auto-warp on a user selected rectangular region of interest.

It was then decided to start *clinical validation* in order to answer the following questions:

- Under which circumstances and in how many cases does the algorithm fail?
- What is the amount of quality improvement compared to manual shifting (the current clinical practice)?
- Which of the four algorithm variants is the most effective (one single or are several variants complementary)?

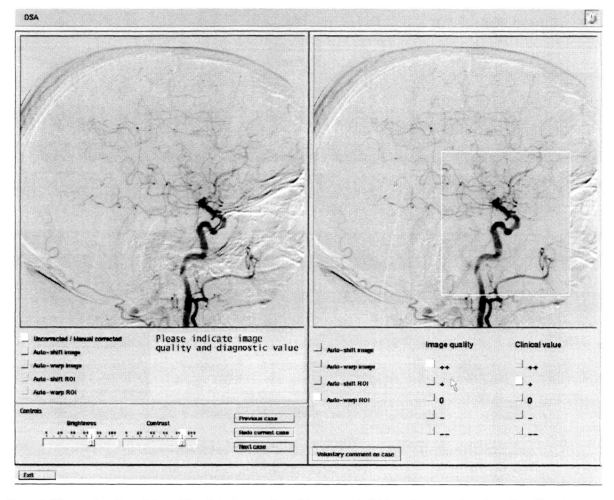

Figure 3: The user interface of the tool for clinical comparison of the automatic DSA motion correction alternatives. The viewports at the top of the screen show the manually shifted subtraction or one of the four automatically corrected results. The clinical expert is asked to enter the comparison scores with the controls in the lower right.

Clinical data was gathered and categorized into four clinical application areas (cerebral, thorax, abdomen, peripheral) and two Philips acquisition modality segments (high end, cardio/vascular Integris systems and mid range, universal R/F systems). The cases were selected in order to assure an almost equal distribution among these categories.

An on-screen validation tool was built on a clinical prototype environment, based on the EasyVision platform, and therefore had a similar look-and-feel as the commercially available workstation. This shortened the learning curve of the clinical experts. The evaluation tool implemented the following functionality (see also figure 3):

1. Observer identification: by entering initials.
2. Patient case selector: automated data retrieval in a random order.
3. Selection by the observer of a rectangular ROI for two out of four algorithms.
4. Two large viewports showing freely selectable images out of the following: the manual shifted subtraction and one of the four automatically shifted or warped subtractions. Each combination of image pairs could therefore be displayed and compared directly.
5. Image enhancement: contrast & brightness.
6. On-screen multiple-choice questionnaire.
7. Text box for free textual comments.
8. Saving of results: ROI position, scores and textual comments.

The observers were asked to compare and score the image quality as well as the clinical value of each of the 4 automatically corrected subtractions. The scores were selected from a 5-grade, linear scale: from much worse (-- or -2), worse (- or -1), no difference (0), better (+ or +1), to much better (++ or +2).

A clear distinction was made between the pure *image quality* or "esthetic appearance" and its *clinical value:* the interest or importance of this quality improvement, i.e. does this quality improvement also improves the clinical (diagnostic) value of the image.

Five specialists from four different clinical sites and five Philips application specialists each observed and scored 62 cases. There were 16 cerebral (10 + 6, i.e. Integris + universal R/F), 12 thoracal (5 + 7), 16 abdominal (7 + 9) and 18 peripheral (8 + 10) cases.

2.3. Statistical analysis

First some basic statistics were calculated over all cases and observers, per application area and per acquisition system:

- Absolute scores of the 4 automatic algorithms compared to manual shift: minimum, maximum and mean scores.
- Score differences among the 4 algorithm variants: minimum, maximum and mean signed differences.

The statistical significance was determined for the rejection of the null hypothesis that "there is no difference between the automated method and the manually shifted reference image", or that "there is no difference between variant x and variant y of the automated methods".

The significance was determined in the following ways: first by using a hypothesis that the distribution was normally (Gaussian) distributed around 0 (no difference) and, second, with a stronger hypothesis that the distribution was uniform (each score is equally likely). The latter turns into multi-nomial distributions of 5th order (5 scores) or 9th order (all possible combinations of score differences). For the normal distribution a standard t-test (corrected for discrete scores, reference [7] p. 146) was used. The significance levels that were obtained using the uniform distribution showed that similar conclusions could be drawn using the normal distribution if the acceptance levels were sufficiently low: $p < 0.001$.

Table 1 shows some results of calculation of the statistical significance using normal distributions over the following groups: all cases, Integris cases only, universal R/F cases only and all cases per application area. The statistics are shown for the scores of the four algorithms with respect to the manually shifted subtraction and, in the last column, for the score difference between the auto-warp algorithm on a ROI and on the entire image. The values of significant results ($p < 0,001$) are highlighted in bold face.

This table learns that:

- On the average, the automatic shift on the entire image had small, but statistically significant, lower quality than the manually shifted subtraction.
- The automatic shift on a ROI was sometimes better, sometimes worse than the manually shifted subtraction. These very small differences were not statistically significant (p values between 0,001 and 0,5).
- The auto-warp on the entire image and on a ROI resulted in higher image quality. These improvements were statistically significant for most groups. The differences between both auto-warp variants were not statistically significant.
- All of the above conclusions could not be drawn for the thorax images. They were somewhat less convincing for the abdominal images.

		Table 1: image quality comparisons				
		auto-shift image versus manual	auto-warp image versus manual	auto-shift ROI versus manual	auto-warp ROI versus manual	auto-warp: ROI versus image
Integris	average	**-0,213**	**0,699**	0,182	**0,626**	-0,073
	prob H0	**2,72E-04**	**1,73E-32**	1,10E-03	**4,66E-26**	0,16
Universal R/F	average	**-0,818**	**0,312**	0,003	**0,460**	0,148
	prob H0	**3,83E-36**	**2,97E-08**	1,00	**2,13E-15**	0,006
Cerebral	average	**-0,775**	**0,801**	0,245	**0,768**	-0,033
	prob H0	**1,52E-17**	**6,55E-18**	4,15E-03	**4,93E-19**	0,70
Thorax	average	-0,339	0,165	-0,157	0,087	-0,078
	prob H0	2,35E-03	0,042	0,095	0,316	0,437
Abdomen	average	**-0,361**	0,116	-0,055	**0,281**	0,164
	prob H0	**8,92E-07**	0,143	0,462	**3,31E-04**	0,029
Peripheral	average	**-0,552**	**0,812**	0,255	**0,885**	0,073
	prob H0	**2,46E-10**	**8,59E-32**	1,55E-03	**1,62E-30**	0,316
All	average	**-0,519**	**0,503**	0,092	**0,542**	0,038
	prob H0	**3,33E-31**	**1,13E-34**	0,02	**3,10E-39**	0,32

The analysis of the clinical value scores lead to similar statistically significant results, although with somewhat smaller quality differences [5].

Finally, the success rate of each automatic algorithm has been calculated (table 2). The success rate, or "no worse rate", is the portion of cases with similar-or-better image quality averaged over a group of cases and over all observers. The font size of the numbers in this table increases for more convincing results.

	Table 2: Success rates (no-worse rates) for image quality			
	auto-shift image	auto-shift ROI	auto-warp image	auto-warp ROI
Integris	67%	**80%**	**90%**	**91%**
Universal R/F	41%	74%	79%	**86%**
Thorax	50%	68%	77%	**81%**
Abdominal	67%	**80%**	75%	**85%**
Peripheral	56%	79%	**95%**	**96%**
Cerebral	43%	78%	**86%**	**91%**
All	54%	77%	**84%**	**89%**

This second table learns that:

- The success rates are higher for Integris than for Universal R/F systems.
- The automatic algorithms are most successful in the peripheral and cerebral areas.
- The auto-warp algorithms clearly outperform the auto-shift algorithms.
- Working on regions of interest is more successful than working on the entire image.

2.4. Major results

The major conclusions of this study may be briefly summarized as follows:

- Automatic warping improves DSA image quality and clinical value with respect to manual and automatic shifting.
- The improvements are most pronounced for cerebral and peripheral applications.
- The results for Integris systems are slightly better than for Universal R/F systems (the reason is unclear).
- The observers found no significant difference between auto-warp on the whole image or on a ROI: none of the measured differences is statistically significant. The success rate is however somewhat higher for the auto-warp on a ROI.

These conclusions answer the questions for which the study was set up. Moreover, the study created a high degree of confidence in the algorithm's effectiveness. After this study, the auto-warp algorithm on the entire image became commercially available as part of the vascular processing package of the EasyVision workstation (Philips Medical Systems).

The study resulted in a huge amount of observation data that has not been analyzed to the full extent: e.g. inter-observer differences in scoring and ROI selection, outlier analysis, etc. Eventhough the study has been performed thoroughly and the results have been presented clearly and convincingly it is remarkable to note that some customers and marketing people still do not accept the results and only have faith in their own judgement. Finally it should be noted that this kind of study is somewhat expensive, due to the important time efforts for data collection, scoring and analysis.

3. CASE 2: IMPROVED X-RAY TRANSLATION RECONSTRUCTION

The same validation framework is currently used for the validation of an improved algorithm for translation image reconstruction in different clinical applications: bolus chase reconstruction, spine and leg bone reconstruction, colon map.

3.1. Algorithm

The translation reconstruction algorithm creates one long overview image out of a vertically translated series of X-ray projection images. This principle is illustrated in figure 4 for the spine application: the series of small image intensifier X-ray images (on the left) is combined into one long overview image (on the right) which shows the entire spinal column [6]. The algorithm matches each pair of consecutive images and merges or pastes overlapping stripes of each image pair into the overview image.

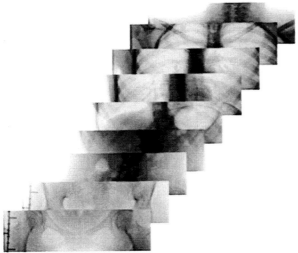 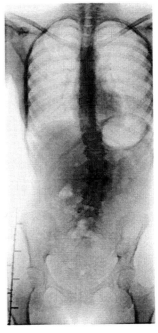

Figure 4: Translation reconstruction of a series of X-ray image intensifier images of the human spine. The series of original images is shown on the left. The resulting overview image is shown on the right. Similar overviews can be reconstructed to visualize other anatomy which does not fit into a single image intensifier picture: peripheral vascularity, peripheral bones and the colon.

However, the overview images sometimes suffer from a parallax problem. Unsharp and doubled edges may occur on object parts that are at different depths with respect to the image intensifier. The problem degrades when the step between images increases and the objects are thicker or further apart with respect to the X-ray source-to-detector axis.

The algorithm improvements that are subject to clinical evaluation try to reduce these parallax effects while at the same time increasing the reliability of the reconstruction process. This is possible by subdividing the image into smaller regions that are optimally focussed at the depth of their anatomical content. Figure 5 shows a small part of a bolus chase reconstruction of the contrast filled blood vessels in the lower limbs. Figure 6 shows the result of the new and improved algorithm. Remark how the ruler and blood vessel edges become sharper and the doubled contours disappear.

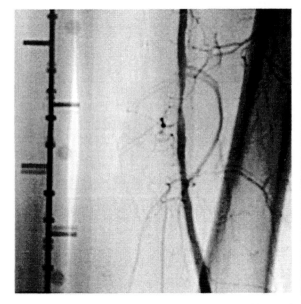

Figure 5: Part of a bolus chase overview image with blood vessels in the lower limbs and a ruler. Remark the doubling of ruler tick marks and blood vessels.

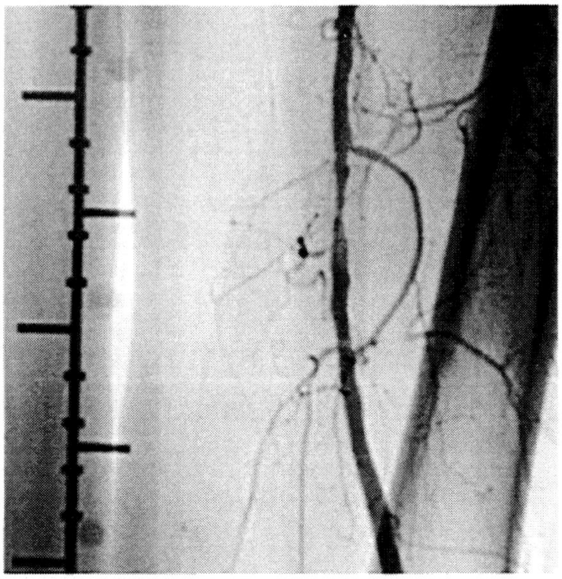

Figure 6: Result of reconstruction of the same part as shown in figure 5, but using the new algorithm.

3.2. Validation aims

We now want to evaluate the performance of the new reconstruction algorithm compared to the old one. No other algorithm variants exist and all algorithmic parameters have been fixed after technical validation. The concrete aims of the study can be summarized as follows:

- Evaluate the quality of the new reconstruction results as a function of the diagnostic purpose: does the overview image exhibit sufficient quality in order to satisfy the reasons for which it was made? These quality criteria can therefore be different for each of the clinical application areas.
- Compare the quality of the results of both algorithms.
- Check for the presence and importance of reconstruction artefacts.
- Check for the presence of artefacts that can be confused with pathology, since such artefacts must of course be avoided.

3.3. Validation method and tools

We initially considered to set up a film-based quality assessment. Film is still the regular format for most of the referring physicians. It allows easier comparison with conventional radiography. Finally, light boxes are available everywhere so that no special equipment or software is needed.

However, we decided to implement a screen based approach as we did with the DSA validation study described before. This allows variable and (extremely) large zooming into selected details and flexible contrast / brightness adjustments. The observers can indicate ROIs interactively to highlight the locations with problems. An integrated and on-line questionnaire automates the assessment of the scoring results.

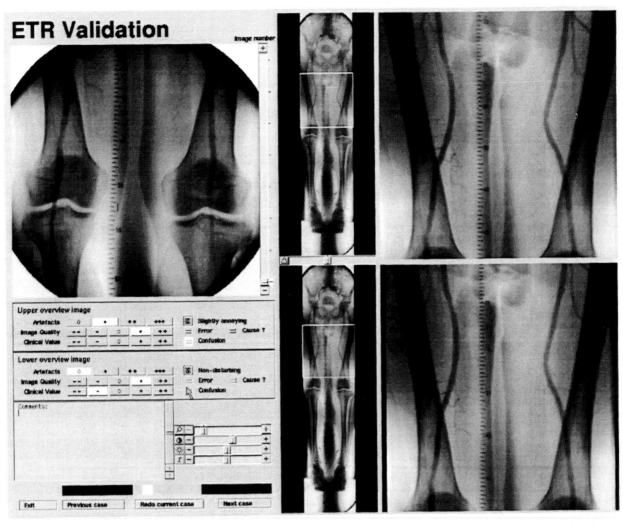

Figure 7: Screen capture of a user interface for direct clinical comparison of two different reconstruction results: two overview images in the center of the screen for navigation, corresponding zoomed images on the right, corresponding original image on the upper left, scoring buttons, text comments and image visualization settings on the lower left.

An initial prototype for direct comparison of both reconstructions is shown in the screenshot in figure 7. The reconstructions are shown in the viewports on the upper and lower right parts of the screen. A zoombox on the overview image allows to selectively zoom in. The entire overview image remains on screen for navigation purposes (in the center of the screen). The viewports on the right of these overviews show the zoomed parts. The center of zoom and the zoom factor are identical for the upper and lower case. The viewport on the top left of the screen contains the original image that corresponds with the position of the zoombox. The original image serves as ground truth in case of confusion or doubt. The lower left of the screen allows to capture the quality scores, artefact indicators and leaves room for free textual comments.

This way of working is partly blinded since there is no indication of which algorithm reconstructed which overview image. The overview images are shown in the upper or lower viewport in a random order. However, the kind of artefacts often allows to guess which algorithm created which overview image, especially when you know that both reconstructions are on screen simultaneously. Moreover, we already decided to score each overview independently and to calculate the score differences afterwards. This eliminates the need to have both overview images on the screen simultaneously.

So we came to a second prototype, for completely blinded comparisons, as shown in figure 8. Only one overview image is shown at a time. All cases and reconstruction types are presented in a random order. A larger part of the screen is now free to show larger parts of the image. The original images and scoring buttons are hidden in some pop-up panels. This example illustrates how the observer can indicate problem areas with rectangular boxes and annotate the type of problem.

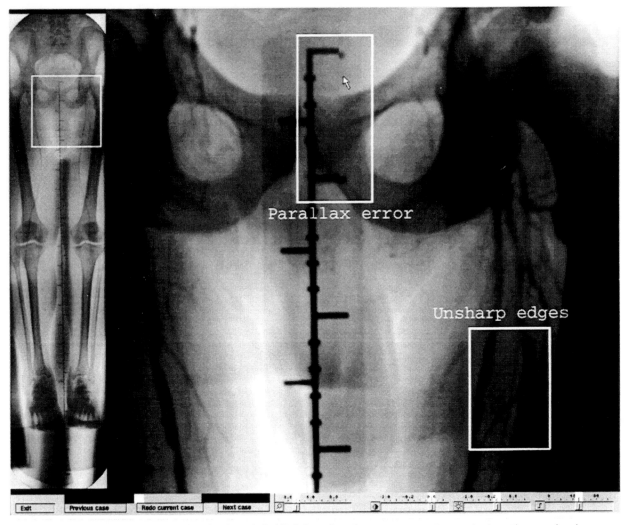

Figure 8: Screen capture of a user interface for the entirely blinded scoring of some reconstruction result: the entire overview image is shown on the left for navigation, the largest viewport shows the zoomed part of the overview image, image visualization controls are in the bottom tool bar. The original image and scoring buttons are displayed in pop-up panels.

3.4. Evaluation parameters

The overall evaluation of the reconstruction result depends on the following parameters:

- Image quality: the overall quality, independent from the clinical purpose (very bad, bad, modest, good, very good).
- Clinical value: the success of the overview image to fulfill the clinical need for which it was made (5 grades from complete failure to extremely useful).
- The amount (none, single, some, many, omnipresent) and importance (none, negligible, small, heavy, unacceptable) of artefacts.

A more detailed and localized analysis of the problems within the overview images can be obtained from the standardized indications: regions of interest (rectangles) that highlight problems such as reconstruction artefacts, artefacts leading to confusion, obscure artefacts, etc.

3.5. Observations: observers and cases

The observers have been selected among specialists per clinical application (the referring physicians: vascular, orthopedic or other surgeons) and among generalists (radiologists and Philips' clinical scientists or application specialists).

Clinical cases have been collected per application category: bolus chase (1 and 2 legs), spine (frontal and lateral), leg bones (1 and 2 legs) and colon. The selection of cases per category has been made in order to include as much cases as possible with variable pathology from as much as possible different clinical sites. The latter is needed to ensure that all practical acquisition protocols are represented into the validation image database.

We are currently appointing 5 observers to compare 30 clinical cases per application category.

4. CONCLUSIONS

The paper reports on the clinical validation efforts that are indispensable on the way to translate a research idea into a commercial product. We commented on clinical data gathering, setting up dedicated comparison user interfaces and statistical analysis of the results.

The first example case on automatic motion correction for DSA has been completed successfully. The second example case on an improved translation reconstruction algorithm has been designed and implemented and the scoring will start shortly. We hope to be able to present the results of this second study at a later occasion.

Some of the important lessons that we have learned up to now can be summarized as follows:

- Clearly define the aims of the study before starting the observations since this can reduce the complexity of the validation task significantly (comparison tool setup, observer time, statistical data analysis).

- Plan a sufficient amount of time to collect and select data in order to make the variability of the clinical cases as rich as possible.

- Clearly clarify the clinical meaning of the comparison parameters that need to be scored: e.g. the difference between image quality and clinical value.

- Select the desired statistics beforehand in order to estimate the needed amount of observations (cases and observers).

It is clear that the efforts for these studies depend on a cost / benefit compromise. The study must be set up as a function of the validation aims. The analysis and processing of a large number of cases can be a secondary goal. External players stimulate us more and more to do high quality validations: the clinical customer, product marketing, FDA, CE, ISO-procedures, etc. Finally, a carefully designed and trustworthy validation study that confirms the success of a new algorithm helps us to earn credibility and clinical acceptance.

Validation studies are essential to the objective evaluation of new or improved image processing methods for both product decision makers and clinical customers. Our validation framework based on clinical workstation prototypes has proven to provide such indispensable information.

ACKNOWLEDGEMENTS

We are grateful to the people who worked on the algorithms, who provided clinical data and who participated in the validation scoring sessions: T. M. Buzug and J. Weese from Philips Research Hamburg; S. Devillers and S. Makram-Ebeid from Philips Research Paris; A. van Eeuwijk, S. Lobregt, R. Nijlunsing and several application specialists from Philips Medical Systems Nederland; all clinical sites, radiologists and surgeons. Images for this publication were provided by Dr. L. J. Schultze Kool, University Hospital Leiden (The Netherlands) and Dr. P. Lefere, Het Stedelijk Ziekenhuis Roeselare (Belgium).

REFERENCES

1. T. M. Buzug and J. Weese, "Improving DSA images with an automatic algorithm based on template matching and an entropy measure", *Proceedings of CAR'96*, eds. H. U. Lemke et al., p. 145, Elsevier, Amsterdam, 1996.

2. T. M. Buzug, J. Weese, C. Fassnacht and C. Lorenz, "Using an entropy similarity measure to enhance the quality of DSA images with an algorithm based on template matching", *VNC'96, Lecture Notes in Computer Science* 1131, p. 235, Springer, Berlin, 1996.

3. T. M. Buzug, J. Weese, C. Fassnacht and C. Lorenz, "Image registration: convex functions for histogram-based similarity measures", *CVRMed/MRCAS'97, Lecture Notes in Computer Science* 1205, p. 203, Springer, Berlin, 1997.

4. T. M. Buzug and J. Weese, "Image registration for DSA quality enhancement", *Computerized Medical Imaging and Graphics* 22, pp. 103-113, 1998.

5. T. M. Buzug, K. C. Strasters, J. Weese and B. Verdonck, "A new registration approach for digital subtraction angiography: methodology and clinical evaluation study", *submitted to IEEE Trans. Med. Imaging*, 1998.

6. A. H. W. van Eeuwijk, S. Lobregt and F. A. Gerritsen, "A novel method for digital X-ray imaging of the complete spine", *CVRMed/MRCAS'97, Lecture Notes in Computer Science* 1205, pp. 521-530, Springer, Berlin, 1997.

7. G. W. Snedecor and W. G. Cochran, *Statistical methods*, 8th edition, Iowa state university press, 1989.

Effects of radiation dose and display contrast on low contrast phantom image visibility.

Charles C Chamberlain, Walter Huda, Andrij R Wojtowycz

Department of Radiology
SUNY Health Science Center at Syracuse
750 East Adams Street, Syracuse, NY 13210

ABSTRACT

Computed radiography (CR) radiographs were generated of a low contrast phantom with 5 mm diameter disks. The radiation exposure incident on the imaging plate was varied from ~0.1 mR to ~10 mR, with the phantom images printed to film using a range of display contrast settings. Changing the radiation exposure by two orders of magnitude had only a modest effect on disk detection performance (~20%), and much less than predicted by signal detection theory for the perception of noise limited objects. For images generated at ~1 and ~10 mR, increasing the display contrast markedly improved the disk detection performance (~50%). There was approximate agreement between the experimental data and the corresponding theoretical predictions for the detection of contrast limited objects. For the contrast detail phantom employed in this study, disk detection was primarily contrast limited, with image noise being relatively unimportant. Lesion detection with an anthropomorphic phantom containing a structured background would be unlikely to change this conclusion, since noise is expected to be *most* important for low contrast objects viewed against a uniform background. Contrast enhancement, as opposed to increasing radiation exposure, is therefore the method of choice for improving the detection of 5 mm diameter sized low contrast lesions in CR images.

Key words: Image perception, quantum mottle, image noise, image contrast, radiation dose, contrast enhancement, computed radiography, digital radiography

1. INTRODUCTION

Computed Radiography (CR) makes use of photostimulable phosphor technology to produce a digital radiograph[1]. CR systems are linear over four orders of magnitude of radiation exposure and therefore permit the incident radiation intensity to be selected by the operator[1,2]. The resulting digital images also permit image enhancement to be performed, including the modification of display contrast by the use of a variable window and level selection.

Computed Radiography radiographs were generated of a low contrast phantom with 5 mm diameter disks. The radiation incident on the imaging plate was varied over two orders of magnitude, with the phantom images displayed using a range of window settings. A systematic study was made of the relative importance of radiation dose and display contrast enhancement for the detection of low contrast disks in a uniform background. The results obtained will help to establish the appropriate amount of radiation to be used in the acquisition of digital radiographic images, as well as the relative importance of image display for CR radiography.

Part of the SPIE Conference on Image Perception and Performance
San Diego, California ● February 1999
SPIE Vol. 3663 ● 0277-786X/99/$10.00

2. THEORY

For a disk of uniform thickness t, the image contrast C is given by the term (μ x t) where μ is the linear attenuation coefficient. If the level of quantum mottle is σ_q, the contrast to noise ratio (CNR) is given by

$$CNR = (\mu \text{ x } t)/(\sigma_q^2 + \sigma_e^2 + \ldots\ldots)^{1/2} \qquad (1)$$

where σ_e is the electronic noise, and the remaining terms in the denominator relate to (any) additional noise sources, including σ_i, the internal noise level of the observer[3]. For an image where σ_q is dominant source of image mottle, the image noise is proportional to $X^{(-0.5)}$, where X is the radiation exposure.

The contrast to noise ratio at the threshold of detection, CNR_t, is the value which will (just) result in the detection of disks of diameter t. When quantum mottle is the dominant noise, then the value of CNR_t is given by

$$CNR_t = (\mu \text{ x } t)/ \sigma_q \qquad (2)$$

and the detection performance will increase with increasing radiation exposure[4]. Under these conditions, the detection threshold value (t) will be proportional to $X^{-0.5}$. It is important to note that for a quantum noise limited image, changing the display contrast (γ) will *not* affect the detection threshold value, because adjusting the value of γ *equally* affects the magnitude of displayed image signal (contrast) and image noise.

A contrast limited image is one where the dominant source of noise is the internal noise (σ_i). For contrast limited objects, the value of the CNR_t is given by

$$CNR_t = \gamma \text{ x } (\mu \text{ x } t)/ \sigma_i \qquad (3)$$

and where the value of image contrast may be adjusted by changing the image display contrast γ[5]. For images where σ_i is the dominant source of noise, performance should improve with a narrowing of the window width, but be independent of radiation exposure. For a contrast limited image, a doubling of the image display contrast would reduce the (detection threshold) disk thickness by a factor of two.

3. METHOD

3.1. Image acquisition

A low contrast phantom was constructed with 5 mm diameter disks. The phantom consisted of an array of 20 columns of 5 mm diameter holes, with 10 rows of holes in each column. There were two components to the phantom: (i) an acrylic wedge (Z = 6.51; ρ = 1.19 g cm^{-3}) with a thickness of 1.5 mm at one end and 0.5 mm at the other end and (ii) a rectangular block of a constant thickness made of polycarbonate (Z = 6.33; ρ = 1.20 g cm^{-3}). In this way, the thickness of each column consisting of 10 rows was varied from one edge of the phantom to the other. The thickness of the polycarbonate could be varied for any given experiment to ensure that the composite phantom would always include holes on both sides of the visual "detection threshold" thickness (mg cm^{-2}). Figure 1 shows a schematic diagram of the low contrast phantom.

Phantom images were obtained with the contrast detail phantom placed on top of a slab of scattering material (acrylic) located on top of a CR plate. A small air gap was made between the scattering acrylic slab and the CR plate to permit the measurement of the exposure level incident on the detector. Phantom images were obtained with *no* grid, to reduce disk visibility because of the presence of scatter. Exposures were made with a Philips generator, 4 mm added Cu filtration, 140 kVp and an SID of 126 cm. Figure 2 shows a schematic drawing of the experimental set up to generate the phantom images. Table 1 summarizes the experimental information pertaining to the measured radiation exposure level incident on the photostimulable phosphor receptor.

Table 1. Summary of measured radiation exposures.

mAs value	Nominal exposure (mR)	Measured exposure (mR)	Exposure precision (%)
0.5 mAs	0.1 mR	0.144 mR	7.4%
3.2 mAs	1.0 mR	1.16 mR	3.9%
32 mAs	10 mR	12.1 mR	1.7%

3.2 Image processing

Exposed cassettes were processed in a FUJI 9000 CR system. The experiment utilized 24 x 30 cm imaging plates, which were all processed in a single session to minimize the experimental uncertainties. All CR plates were processed using the Test Pattern option, with no edge enhancement, and a linear "look up" table (i.e., $GT = A$)[2]. The GS processing parameter was empirically adjusted to generate a nominal constant film density of ~ 1.5. The GA parameter, which defines the level of contrast in the resultant image[2], was set at four different values of contrast enhancement (i.e., GA = 1; GA = 2; GA = 3; GA = 4). Film contrast was measured directly by including a 17 mm thick slab of polycarbonate adjacent to the low contrast phantom. Figure 3 shows an image of the phantom generated at a high contrast to permit the visualization of all 200 disks in the phantom, as well as the adjacent 17 mm thick slab of polycarbonate.

3.3 Image assessment

Images were read in a darkened room, with the radiographic images masked to all stray light. Two experienced readers were used, and the films were all reviewed in a single session. The visibility of each hole in the phantom image was scored on a five point scale: 0 corresponded to "not visible"; 3 was "average visibility"; and 5 was "excellent visibility". The threshold thickness, t mg cm^{-2}, was determined by interpolation for any column where the total score for the column was 50% (i.e., a score of 25 where 50 was the maximum possible). The readers made a conscious effort to maintain the same criterion when assessing disk visibility for all the images in this experimental study.

4. RESULTS

4.1. CR film density and contrast

Table 2 summarizes the mean film densities obtained for the CR images generated at radiation exposures ranging from ~0.1 mR to ~10 mR, and processed using GA values ranging from GA=1 to GA=4. As expected, the film density of the phantom images was constant, except at the lowest exposure and GA settings where the signal intensities were insufficient to generate the required film density value of ~1.5. For any given value of GA and radiation exposure, the film density was constant to within ~2% of the mean density. For the 8 sets of experiments summarized in Table 2, the overall mean (± standard deviation) film density was 1.51 ± 0.06, which corresponds to an overall 4% variation in image film density.

Table 2. Mean film density summary.

Nominal exposure	GA = 1	GA = 2	GA = 4
~0.1 mR	*	1.42 ± 0.02	1.54 ± 0.02
~1 mR	1.52 ± 0.03	1.51 ± 0.04	1.43 ± 0.05
~10 mR	1.59 ± 0.03	1.57 ± 0.02	1.52 ± 0.03

*Maximum film density was only 1.17 ± 0.02 (data excluded from further analysis)

Figure 4 shows the relationship between image contrast and the GA parameter. The solid lines are least squares data fit which have been constrained to go through the origin. As expected for this linear characteristic curve, there is a linear relationship between GA and image contrast. The relatively large error bars are a direct consequence of the low image contrast for the 17 mm thick slab of polycarbonate, which ranged from ~0.03 at GA=1, to ~0.12 at GA=4. The data shown in Figure 4 show that increasing the GA parameter from GA=1 to GA=4 resulted in an increase in display contrast of a factor of approximately four.

4.2. Detection performance

Figure 5 shows how the measured detection threshold thickness (t mg cm^{-2}) varied with radiation exposure and which are plotted as solid lines. Data is presented for two values of the GA parameter (GA=2 and GA=4). Increasing the radiation exposure by two orders of magnitude reduced the average disk thickness, at the visual detection threshold, by about 20%. Also depicted on these figures are the corresponding theoretical predictions (dashed lines) of signal detection theory on the assumption that quantum noise is the dominant source of noise, and that signal detection is noise limited[6,7].

Figure 6 shows how the measured detection threshold thickness (t mg cm^{-2}) varied with the GA parameter used to process the acquired phantom images (solid lines). At both radiation exposure levels investigated (i.e. ~1 mR and ~10 mR), there was a significant improvement in imaging performance with increasing GA value (i.e., image contrast). Increasing the GA parameter from GA=1 to GA=4 resulted in an average reduction in disk thickness, at the visual detection threshold, of about 50%. Also depicted in these figures are the corresponding theoretical predictions for a contrast limited imaging system (dashed lines), where the observer is the dominant source of noise.

5. DISCUSSION

The results depicted in Table 2 show that for this digital CR system, the film density is *independent* of the radiation exposure used to generate the phantom image. Image density was generally constant, at a value of ~1.5, even though the incident radiation exposure varied by a factor of a hundred. Display contrast was adjustable by manipulating the GA parameter, and in these experiments the display contrast varied by a factor of approximately four. This ability to modify the image density and contrast is a common feature of all digital imaging modalities, and a major advantage in comparison to conventional screen-film radiography.

The data presented in Figure 5 depict that changing the level of radiation exposure has very little effect on imaging performance. Changing the radiation exposure by two orders of magnitude improved disk detection performance by a relatively modest amount. These results suggest that image noise is of little importance for the detection of 5 mm diameter disks in a uniform background. It is of interest to note that relatively modest changes in the radiation exposures in chest radiology can have a significant impact in the perceived level of image mottle in pediatric chest x-rays[8]. However, it is important to differentiate between a perceived level of mottle, and any corresponding differences in observer detection performance.

Increasing the display contrast by a factor of four significantly improved the detection of low contrast disks, and the disk thickness at the threshold of visibility was reduced by about a factor of two. The trends shown for the experimental data and theory in Figure 6 are generally very similar, and indicate that detection performance is significantly affected by the display contrast used to view the images. Comparison of the data in Figures 5 and 6 also shows that changes in display contrast are much more important to detection performance than any modifications to the radiation exposure. These combined results therefore suggest that for this specific visual task, signal detection is essentially contrast limited, and that noise is not a significant factor[5]. If this finding is generally true, improved lesion detection will occur as a result of image processing algorithms which attempt to improve local image contrast[9].

For current photostimulable phosphor technology operated in the clinical exposure region (i.e., ~1 mR), contrast effects are much more important than noise effects for the visibility of 5 mm diameter disks in a uniform background. In clinical radiology, lesion conspicuity is most likely limited by the complexity of the background structure in radiographs, such as the rib cage in chest x-rays[10,11]. Use of an anthropomorphic phantom with a more clinically realistic background, however, would be unlikely to change this conclusion given that (random) noise is expected to be *most* important for low contrast objects viewed against a uniform background[4,7]. As a result, it is contrast enhancement, as opposed to increasing radiation exposure, which is the method of choice for improving low contrast circular disks in CR images.

Two recent studies which compared screen-film with digital radiology using simple low contrast phantoms, have both shown that digital radiography was significantly superior to screen-film[12,13]. Digital detectors de-couple image capture from image display, and permit an *independent* optimization of each component of the imaging chain. Improved imaging performance could be achieved by changing the technique factors of image acquisition (i.e., kVp and mAs) or by changing the way images are displayed (i.e. window and level settings of the display image). The results obtained in this study suggest that for 5 mm diameter disks, it is image display that is of much greater importance, and that modifying image acquisition techniques is of less importance.

Digital radiology is currently replacing screen-film radiography in routine clinical practice and practical choices will need to be made regarding the best way to acquire and display digital images. Greater attention will therefore need to be given to image acquisition and image display factors, and how performance in digital radiography can be optimized. In the future, however, it will be necessary to conduct experimental investigations using anthropomorphic phantoms, together with more clinically relevant lesions, than the simple low contrast phantom used in this study[14].

6. CONCLUSIONS

1. The use of a digital (CR) radiographic imaging system permitted the image density to be maintained at a constant value ($\pm$ 4%) when the radiation exposure was varied by two orders of magnitude.

2. The CR system permitted image contrast to be varied by a factor of four by modification of the display contrast parameter (γ).

3. Changing the radiation exposure by a factor of 100 had a small effect (~20%) on detection performance (disk thickness at the detection threshold).

4. Changing the display contrast by a factor of four had a relatively large effect (~50%) on detection performance (disk thickness at the detection threshold).

5. Low contrast lesions (5 mm diameter) in a uniform background are primarily contrast limited, and not noise limited.

6. Improving the detection of 5 mm low contrast disks in digital radiographs will likely require improved image processing, as opposed to any modification of radiographic technique factors.

ACKNOWLEDGEMENTS

The authors would like to thank Frank Kline for expertly manufacturing the low contrast phantom used in this study. We also wish to acknowledge useful discussion on medical imaging with Drs Zhenxue Jing and Robert F Wagner.

REFERENCES

1. Kato H "*Photostimulable phosphor radiography design considerations*" American Association of Physicists in Medicine Medical Physics Monograph 20 (1991 Summer School Proceedings) American Institute of Physics 1994 731-777.

2. Siebert JA "*Photostimulable Phosphor System Acceptance Testing*" American Association of Physicists in Medicine Medical Physics Monograph 20 (1991 Summer School Proceedings) American Institute of Physics 1994 771-800.

3. Ohara K, Chan H-P, Doi K, Giger ML and Fujita H "Investigation of basic imaging properties in digital radiography: 8. Detection of simulated low contrast objects in digital subtraction angiographic images" *Med Phys* 13 (1986) 304-311.

4. Rose A "*Vision: Human and electronic*" Plenum Press (NY-London) 1974.

5. Vyborny CJ and Schmidt RA "Technical image quality and the visibility of mammographic detail" RSNA Categorical Course in Physics, 103-111 (1994).

6. Green DM and Swets JA "Signal detection theory and psychophysics" Robert E Krieger Publishing Company (Huntingdon, NY) 1974.

7. Hendee WR and Wells PNT "*The Perception of Visual Information*" Springer-Verlag (New York) 1992.

8. Huda W, Slone RM, Belden CJ, Williams JL, Cumming WA and Palmer CK "Mottle on computed radiographs of the chest in pediatric patients" *Radiology* **199**, 249-252 (1996).

9. Laine AF, Schuler S, Fan J and Huda W "Mammographic feature enhancement by multiscale analysis". *IEEE Transactions on Medical Imaging* **13**, 725-740 (1994).

10. Kundel HL and Revesz G "Lesion conspicuity, structured noise, and film reader error" *AJR* **126**, 1233-1238 (1976).

11. Kundel HL, Nodine CF, Thickman D, Carmody D, and Toto L "Nodule detection with and without a chest image" *Invest Radiol* **20**, 94-99 (1985).

12. Qu G, Huda W, Laine AF, Steinbach BG, and Honeyman JC "Can digital mammography improve low-contrast lesion detection?" *Digital Mammography 96*, K. Doi, M.L. Giger, R.M. Nishikawa, and R.A. Schmidt (editors) 451-454 (1996).

13. Liu H, Fajardo LL, Barrett JR, and Baxter RA "Contrast-detail detectability analysis: comparison of a digital spot mammography system and an analog screen-film mammography system" *Acad Radiol* **4**, 197-203 (1997).

14. Huda W, Jing Z, Qu G, Steinbach BG and Honeyman JC "How do radiographic technique factors affect detection performance in digital mammography?" *Radiology* 209 (1998) 160

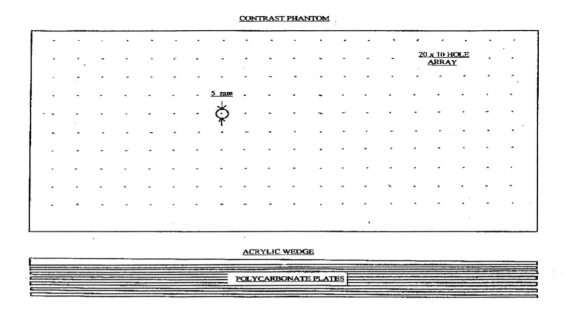

Figure 1. Schematic diagram showing the design characteristics of the low contrast phantom.

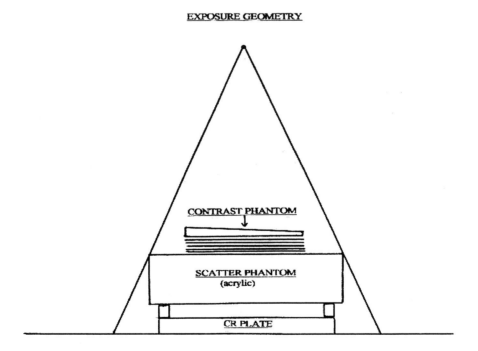

Figure 2. Schematic diagram of the experimental arrangement used to radiograph the low contrast phantom.

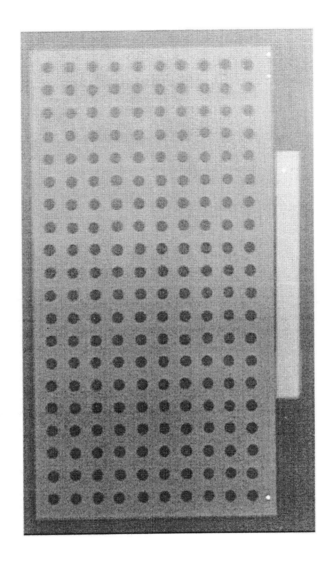

Figure 3. Radiograph of the low contrast phantom showing all 20 holes, and the 17 mm thick slab of polycarbonate adjacent to the phantom.

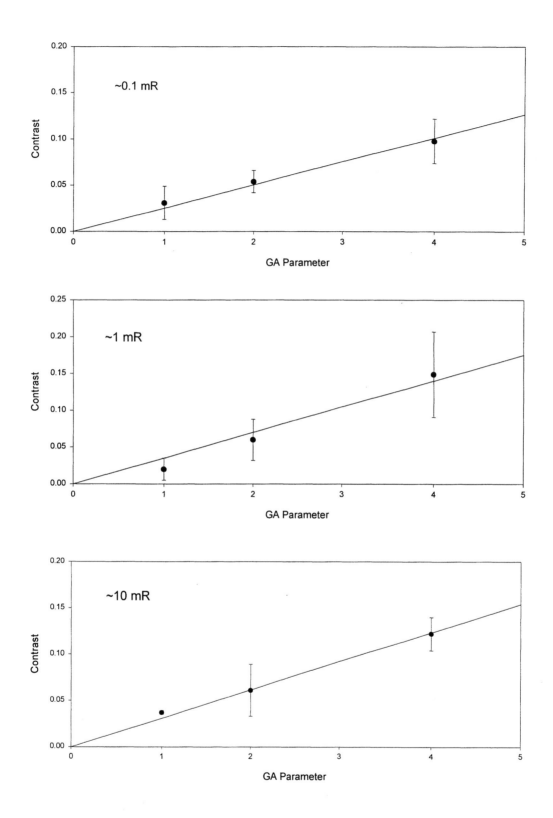

Figure 4. Measured film contrast versus the selected computed radiography GA (contrast) parameter.

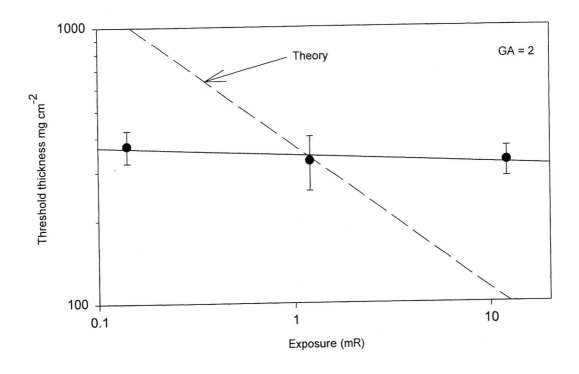

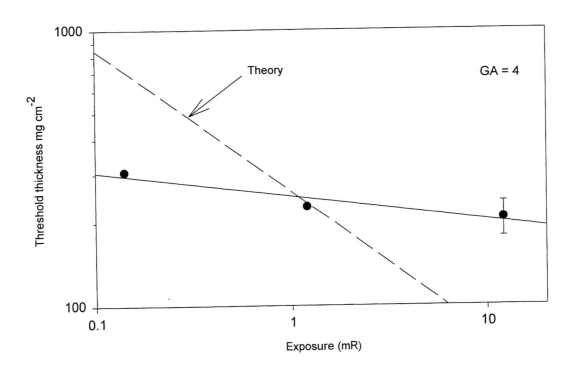

Figure 5. Hole thickness at the threshold of visibility (mg/cm2) versus detector exposure (mR)

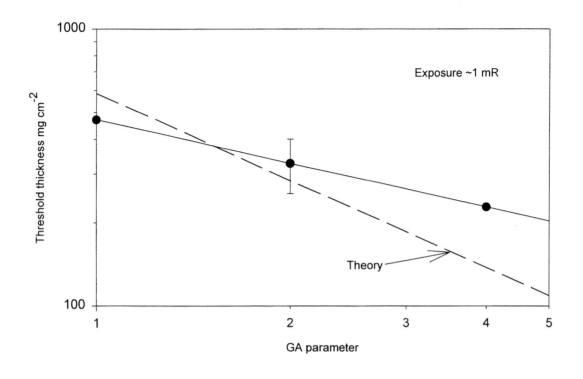

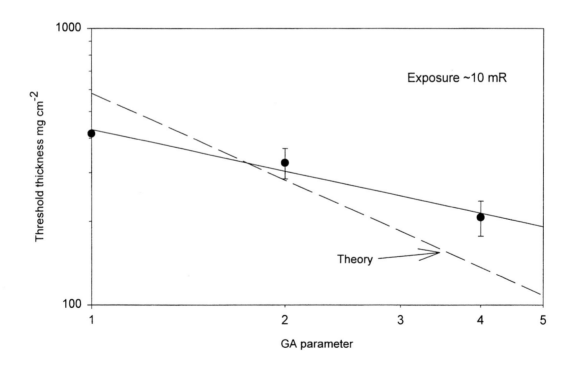

Figure 6. Hole thickness at the threshold of visibility (mg/cm^2) versus GA (contrast) parameter

SESSION 2

Display Parameters and Performance II

Radiologists' ability of using computer-aided diagnosis (CAD) to improve breast biopsy recommendations

Yulei Jiang[*] and Robert M. Nishikawa

Kurt Rossmann Laboratories for Radiologic Image Research,
Department of Radiology, The University of Chicago, Chicago, IL 60637

ABSTRACT

An important issue in developing computer-aided diagnosis (CAD) methods is to demonstrate the ability of a computer aid to improve diagnostic accuracy when used by radiologists. A related issue to that is to understand how radiologists' decision-making is influenced by the computer aid. We conducted an observer performance study designed to address these issues for a computerized classification scheme for malignant and benign clustered microcalcifications in mammograms. Results of the study showed that radiologists' diagnostic performance improved significantly when they used the computer aid. The results also showed that radiologists were able to incorporate the computer aid—a quantitative analysis of the mammogram—effectively in their decision-making.

Keywords: Computer-aided diagnosis (CAD), medical decision-making, Observer performance study, diagnosis, breast cancer, mammography, digital mammography, clustered microcalcifications, classification, artificial neural networks (ANNs).

1. INTRODUCTION

Computer-aided diagnosis (CAD) has the potential of improving diagnostic accuracy. However, before CAD can be applied to clinical practice and before the potential benefits of CAD can be realized, laboratory observer performance studies[1-4] and clinical trials[5] must be done to show that CAD can indeed improve diagnostic accuracy. It is also important to investigate, in these observer studies and clinical trials, how a computer aid influences radiologists' decision-making. Since it is unlikely that a computer aid would help a radiologist's decision-making in every patient, it is important to identify the cases that a computer aid would likely influence a radiologist's diagnostic opinion and to understand whether that influence would result in a correct diagnosis.

Computer aids can take several different forms[1, 6-12]. The ability of a computer aid to influence radiologists' decision-making will likely depend on the forms of the computer aid. In this paper, we study one particular form of a computer aid: quantitative advice. Specifically, we have developed a computer scheme to classify clustered microcalcifications in mammograms as malignant or benign. The output of this computer scheme is a likelihood-of-malignancy estimate (LME). The LME advises a radiologist, quantitatively, on the likelihood that a microcalcification cluster represents a malignancy.

We conducted an observer performance study to compare radiologists' diagnostic accuracy with and without our computer aid (i.e., the LME). The task was to differentiate malignant from benign clustered microcalcifications and to make appropriate clinical-management recommendations. Results of the study clearly showed that radiologists were significantly more accurate, both in terms of diagnostic confidence and in terms of biopsy recommendations, when they used our computer aid. The details of the observer study and the main conclusion from it have been described elsewhere[4]. The purpose of this paper is to analyze, from the data of the observer study, the effects of LME on influencing radiologists' decision of clinical-management recommendations.

---

[*] Correspondence: e-mail: y-jiang@uchicago.edu; phone: (773) 834-3467; fax: (773) 702-0371.

Part of the SPIE Conference on Image Perception and Performance
San Diego, California • February 1999
SPIE Vol. 3663 • 0277-786X/99/$10.00

56

2. OBSERVER PERFORMANCE STUDY

The objective of the observer performance study was to measure, comparatively, the diagnostic performance of radiologists in differentiating between malignant and benign clustered microcalcifications with and without our computer aid. Therefore, a set of mammograms was read by a group of radiologists *twice*: once without aid and once with aid. The observers consisted of ten radiologists with experience in mammography. Five of the observers were attending radiologists who read mammograms as part of their clinical practice. The other five observers were radiology residents from our institution who had completed as least one rotation in mammography. None of the observers read the study cases before the experiment. The mammograms consisted of 104 cases of consecutive biopsies for suspicious clustered microcalcifications. Forty-six cases contained cancer and 58 contained benign lesions. In all cases, a microcalcification cluster was the only significant lesion. Mammograms of each case consisted of both standard and magnification views.

The computer aid in the study was the LME—the computer-estimated likelihood of malignancy. A schematic diagram of our technique that produced the LME is shown in Fig. 1. The LME was computed by an artificial neural network (ANN) based on an analysis of eight image features extracted from mammograms. The image features describe, quantitatively, the appearance of both the cluster and of the individual microcalcifications. They correlate qualitatively with radiologists' perceptual experience in the interpretation of microcalcifications and, as such, provide a basis for the computation of the LME. A more detailed description of the technique and the features can be found elsewhere[11]. Note that only standard-view mammograms were analyzed by our technique to compute the LME, even though the observers also read the magnification mammograms. Also note that the LME was obtained from the output of the ANN through a transformation so that it represented a probability[4].

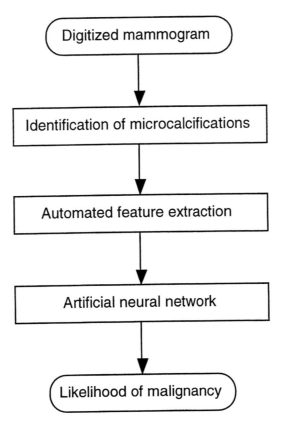

Figure 1. Schematic diagram of our computer technique for the classification of malignant and benign clustered microcalcifications.

Since the objective of the study was to measure the effect of the computer aid on the observers' performance, it was imperative that the observers use the computer aid. For this reason, we instructed the observers to consider the LME when it was provided. To assist them in using this unfamiliar tool, they were informed that the performance of our technique (i.e., the LME) could be better than the performance of radiologists, based on results from a previous study[11]. They were also told that if a threshold of 0.3 was applied to the LME, such that higher values of LME was associated with decision to biopsy, then a performance of 90% sensitivity and 47% positive predictive value (PPV) can be derived. Up to 25 training cases was read by the observers with feed back of histologic diagnosis before the actual experiment.

Two types of data were collected from the observers: their confidence that a microcalcification cluster was malignant and their choice of clinical recommendation for the microcalcifications. There were four choices of clinical recommendations: (a) surgical biopsy, (b) alternative tissue sampling, (c) short-term follow-up, and (d) routine follow-up. However, in the analysis of this paper, the four choices were grouped into two sub-categories: biopsy (choices a and b) and follow-up (choices c and d). The recommendations of biopsy versus follow-up are the clinically critical decision and, thus, underlie our analysis. The finer selection of four recommendation choices was used in the experiment to avoid ambiguities.

3. DATA ANALYSIS

The observers' diagnostic accuracy was measured by their ROC curves computed from their confidence data. A combined ROC curve was obtained by pooling all observers' individual ROC curves (by averaging the binormal model's a and b parameters) for the no-aid and for the with-aid performance. Sensitivity and specificity of biopsy decisions were calculated based on their choices of recommendations. Sensitivity was defined as the fraction of cancer cases recommended for biopsy, and specificity was defined as the fraction of benign cases recommended for follow-up.

The data of biopsy decisions were also used to analyze how LME influenced the observers' decision-making. In this analysis, we computed the probability of event x as a result of the LME, where x represented, e.g., upgrading the clinical decision to biopsy or downgrading the clinical decision to follow-up or making no change to the decision. The probability was computed using the following formula.

$$ \mathbf{P}\ \{x \,|\, \text{LME}\}\ =\ \frac{\mathbf{M}\ \{x \,|\, \text{LME}\}}{\mathbf{N}\ \{\text{cases} \,|\, \text{LME}\}\ \times\ \mathbf{K}\ \{\text{readers}\}}\ \times\ 100\%, $$

where $\mathbf{P}$ is the probability, $\mathbf{M}$ is the number of observations for event x, $\mathbf{N}$ is the number of cases, and $\mathbf{K}$ is the number of observers. In this paper, we report the results obtained from all observers ($\mathbf{K} = 10$), because separate analyses of the attending ($\mathbf{K} = 5$) and resident ($\mathbf{K} = 5$) radiologists yielded similar results.

4. RESULTS

1. Comparison of accuracy

Diagnostic accuracy of the observers with the computer aid was significantly better than their accuracy without the computer aid. The average area under the ROC curve (A_z) increased from 0.61 of no-aid to 0.75 of with aid (p < .0001). The average sensitivity increased from 73.5% to 87.4% and the average specificity increased from 31.6% to 41.9%. The corresponding (hypothetical) positive biopsy yield increased from 46% to 55%[4].

2. Overall biopsy rate

The probability to recommend biopsy was both 71% with and without the computer aid. Therefore, the gain in sensitivity was not a result of sending more patients to biopsy. Rather, the gain in sensitivity must have been achieved by sending more cancer cases to biopsy and sending fewer benign cases to biopsy.

3. Probability of changing versus *not* changing a recommendation

There was no difference between the overall probability of upgrading a decision to biopsy or downgrading a decision to follow-up (16% in both cases). However, the probability of making a change in either direction was smaller than the probability of not making a change (31% versus 69%). Therefore, the entire increase in diagnostic accuracy was obtained from approximately one third of cases.

4. Probability of changing a recommendation

The probability of changing a recommendation was strongly dependent on LME. The probability of upgrading a decision to biopsy was 27% when LME was greater than 0.60 but was only 4% when LME was less than 0.3. The probability of downgrading a decision to follow-up was the opposite: it was 3% for LME > 0.6 and was 39% for LME < 0.30. Please note that LME is itself a probability; it is not expressed as a percentage here for reason of clarity.

The probability of upgrading a recommendation to biopsy (LME > 0.6) was the same for actual cancer and for actual benign cases (26% and 28% respectively). This result could imply that the observers were willing to upgrade their decision to biopsy when the LME was high, regardless of their own suspicion. This result was consistent with the current focus in mammography practice to diagnose early-stage cancers. However, the probability of downgrading a recommendation to follow-up (LME < 0.3) was lower for actual cancer cases than for actual benign cases (22% and 42% respectively). This result could imply that the observers were less willing to downgrade their decision to follow-up if their own suspicion was high, even when the LME was low. This result was consistent with the willingness of radiologists to recommend biopsy in clinical practice with even a moderate level of suspicion.

5. SUMMARY AND CONCLUSIONS

Our results clearly showed that our computer aid—the estimate of likelihood of malignancy (LME)—can significantly improve radiologists' diagnostic accuracy and can improve radiologists' biopsy recommendations.

Our results also showed that radiologists are able to incorporate the LME—a quantitative aid—effectively into their decision making. Radiologists are more likely to upgrade their decision to biopsy with high LME (> 0.6) and they are more likely to downgrade their decision to follow-up with low LME (< 0.3). Their decisions to upgrade to biopsy are likely to be indiscriminate for actual cancer and for actual benign cases. However, their decisions to downgrade to follow-up are less likely to occur for actual cancer cases than for actual benign cases.

ACKNOWLEDGEMENTS

This work was done as part of the International Digital Mammography Development Group (IDMDG) and was funded in part by NCI/NIH through a grant CA 60187.

REFERENCES

1. D. J. Getty, R. M. Pickett, C. J. D'Orsi and J. A. Swets, "Enhanced interpretation of diagnostic images," *Invest Radiol* **23**, pp. 240-252, 1988.
2. H.-P. Chan, K. Doi, C. J. Vyborny, R. A. Schmidt, C. E. Metz, K. L. Lam, T. Ogura, Y. Wu and H. MacMahon, "Improvement in radiologists' detection of clustered microcalcifications on mammograms: the potential of computer-aided diagnosis," *Invest Radiol* **25**, pp. 1102-1110, 1990.
3. W. P. Kegelmeyer, J. M. Pruneda, P. D. Bourland, A. Hillis, M. W. Riggs and M. L. Nipper, "Computer-aided mammographic screening for spiculated lesions," *Radiology* **191**, pp. 331-337, 1994.
4. Y. Jiang, R. M. Nishikawa, R. A. Schmidt, C. E. Metz, M. L. Giger and K. Doi, "Improving breast cancer diagnosis with computer-aided diagnosis," *Acad Radiol* **6**, pp. 22-33, 1999.
5. R. M. Nishikawa, M. L. Giger, D. E. Wolverton, R. A. Schmidt, C. E. Comstock, J. Papaioannou, S. A. Collins and K. Doi, "Prospective testing of a clinical mammography workstation for CAD: analysis of the first 10,000 cases," in *Digital Mammography*, edited by N. Karssemeijer, M. Thijssen, J. Hendriks and L. van Erning (Kluwer Academic Publishers, Dordrecht, 1998), pp. 401-406.
6. H. A. Swett, P. R. Fisher, A. I. Cohn, P. L. Miller and P. G. Mutalik, "Expert system-controlled image display," *Radiology* **172**, pp. 487-493, 1989.

7.   J. Sklansky, E. Y. Tao, C. J. Ornes and A. C. Disher, "Visualizing a database in mammographic screening," (Abstract) *Radiology* **209 (P)**, pp. 392, 1998.

8.   J. A. Baker, P. J. Kornguth, J. Y. Lo, M. E. Williford and C. E. J. Floyd, "Breast cancer: prediction with artificial neural network based on BI_RADS standard lexicon," *Radiology* **196**, pp. 817-822, 1995.

9.   R. M. Nishikawa, M. L. Giger, K. Doi, C. J. Vyborny and R. A. Schmidt, "Computer-aided detection of clustered microcalcifications on digital mammograms," *Med Biol Eng Comput* **33**, pp. 174-178, 1995.

10. P. Taylor, J. Fox and A. Todd-Pokropek, "Evaluation of a decision aid for the classification of microcalcifications," in *Digital Mammography,* edited by N. Karssemeijer, M. Thijssen, J. Hendriks and L. van Erning (Kluwer Academic Publishers, Dordrecht, 1998), pp. 237-244.

11. Y. Jiang, R. M. Nishikawa, D. E. Wolverton, C. E. Metz, M. L. Giger, R. A. Schmidt, C. J. Vyborny and K. Doi, "Malignant and benign clustered microcalcifications: automated feature analysis and classification," *Radiology* **198**, pp. 671-678, 1996.

12. H. P. Chan, B. Sahiner, N. Petrick, M. A. Helvie, K. L. Lam, D. D. Adler and M. M. Goodsitt, "Computerized classification of malignant and benign microcalcifications on mammograms: texture analysis using an artificial neural network," *Phys Med Biol* **42**, pp. 549-567, 1997.

A Computer Algorithm for Automated Detection and Quantification of Microaneurysms and Hemorrhages (HMAs) in Color Retinal Images

Samuel C. Lee[*a], Yiming Wang[a], Elisa T. Lee[b]

[a]School of Electrical and Computer Engineering, Univ. of Oklahoma, Norman, OK 73019

[b]College of Public Health, Health Sciences Center, Univ. of Oklahoma/Oklahoma City

ABSTRACT

This paper presents a computer algorithm for automatic quantification of HMAs in a color retinal image. The algorithm begins with an image quality test. If the image is determined to be useful (normal), image processing and pattern recognition techniques are then applied. The image processing techniques employed are designed to achieve three purposes, image enhancement, noise removal, and most importantly, image normalization. It is followed by the detection of (1) optic disc and macula, (2) flame and blot hemorrhages, and (3) dot hemorrhages and microaneurysms. A special polar coordinate system centered at the macula is proposed. Such a coordinate system is particularly attractive in describing the location of a lesion relative to the center of the macula. In addition, it can be viewed as a "spider net" and thus can be used to catch hemorrhages of large size, e.g., flame and blot hemorrhages, the way a spider net to catch insects. The spider net, however, will not work for the detection of microaneurysms and dot hemorrhages, because their sizes are too small to be caught by the net. A method specially designed for the detection of microaneurysms and dot hemorrhages is presented. It uses a sequence of seven automatically globally-thresholded binary images, obtained from the pre-processed normalized image, and a set of matched filters using only binary coefficients for differentiating HMAs and blood vessels. At the end, a computer printout of list of all the HMAs detected and their sizes and locations is given. Over four hundred color fundus photographs including standard fundus photographs are used to test the system. It should be pointed out that the sensitivity of this system can be adjusted by the user. By comparing the computer detected and quantified HMAs with the manual counts, it is found that the results are quite satisfactory. Therefore, we conclude that with the sensitivity of the system adjusted to human experts, this system can provide an automatic, objective, and repeatable way to quantify HMAs accurately.

Keywords: Retinal Lesions, Automated Quantification, Count, Image Normalization, Global Threshold, Matched Filters

1. INTRODUTION

Recently, there have been a considerable interest in automated detection and quantification of microaneurysms in fluorescein angiograms[1-4]. This is because manual counting procedures[5] are laborious, time-consuming and subject to human error. Digitization of the fundus images enables the application of computer processing techniques to the images, first to discriminate automatically the microaneurysms from the other features and second to count the number of microaneurysms present. Computers are well suited to problems involving the extraction of quantitative information from such images because of their ability to process data in fast and efficient manner with a high degree of reproducibility[6-9]. Klein et al[10] studied the relationship of change in the number of retinal microaneurysms to the 10-year progression to significant retinopathy, proliferative retinopathy, and clinically significant macula edema. They concluded that microaneurysm counts using stereoscopic color fundus photographs are an early important measure of progress of retinopathy and may serve as a surrogate end point for severe change in some clinical trials. Hellsted[11] conducted an analysis of the formation and disappearance rates of individual microaneurysms in mild background retinopathy. Their

---

[*] Correspondence: Email: samlee@mailhost.ecn.ou.edu; Telephone: 405 325 4289; Fax: 405 325 7066

Part of the SPIE Conference on Image Perception and Performance
San Diego, California ● February 1999
SPIE Vol. 3663 ● 0277-786X/99/$10.00

study showed that background diabetic retinopathy is a dynamic process. In their study, a significant proportion of microaneurysms present disappeared within 2 years. This is compensated for by formation of new microaneurysms, the resultant net changes in microaneurysm counts being small. Microaneurysm formation and disappearance rates are new variables of diabetic retinopathy and may prove to be more sensitive indicators of progression patterns of background diabetic retinopathy than microaneurysm count changes.

The purpose of this paper is to present a fully automated digital image processing system, which provides an objective and repeatable way to detect and quantify microaneurysms and hemorrhages in digital color fundus photographs. The algorithm flowchart is shown in Figure 1.

2. IMAGE PROCESSING

The digital retinal images (Figure 2a) used in this study are obtained by scanning the standard 35mm color fundus photo slides taken at the 45° field of view by fundus camera with 512 x 512 pixels. Each pixel consists of 3 bytes of data, which give the R(red), G(green), and B(blue) values of the pixel, ranging from 0 - 255. The first step in the processing of such an image is to check its image quality. If it does not meet some minimum image quality criteria, for example, too dark, too bright, totally out of focus, etc., the system will not process it further. A detailed discussion on the automatic image quality measure of a color fundus photo was given in [12]. Hence it will nit be presented here.

After the image passes the quality test (i.e., it is determined to be a useful image for medical diagnosis), we then apply an image normalization and enhancement operation to the image. This operation also transforms the given color image into a red-free (green) image as shown in Figure 2c. The histograms of the image before and after the operation are shown in Figure 2b and 2d, respectively. The image quality index values Q of the images before and after the operation are found to be 0.54 and 0.91[12], with $Q = 0$ being the poorest and $Q = 1.0$ the best. It is seen that the quality of the given image has been improved considerably after this image processing. Now the image is ready for automated detection and quantification of HMAs.

3. AUTOMATED DETECTION OF OPTIC DISC, MACULA, BLOOD VESSELS, AND HMAs

Based on the local reflectance (intensities), color, shape, edge and spatial distribution information exhibited in the enhanced image, we have developed pattern recognition techniques to detect the two essential features, the optic disc and the macula, and the HMA lesions. The optic disc is located at the area where the average intensity is the highest in the image; whereas the macula is located at the area with low average intensity. Both of them are of round shape and hence could be detected using matched filters. The other important retinal feature is the blood vessels. For the automated detection of blood vessels in retinal images, see reference [13].

The macula provides human's primary vision, clinically, it is important to know the location of a lesion, related to the center of the macula. This information can provide physicians the severity of the effects of the lesion to the patient's vision. For this reason, a new image coordinate system is introduced. It uses the center of the macula as the origin of the system. Figure 2a shows a retinal image containing flame, blot, dot hemorrhages and microaneurysms. These lesions are grouped into two groups. Lesions of large size – blot or flame hemorrhages are in one and lesion of small size – dot hemorrhages and microaneurysms are in the other. Two pattern recognition algorithms are designed for detecting them. The first algorithm is based on the use of a "spider net" to catch large-size hemorrhages (blot and flame hemorrhages) very quickly. The net is originated at the center of the macula. The angular and radial resolutions of the net may vary. An example of such net is shown in Figure 3a, of which the angular resolution is 5°, and the radial resolution is 10 pixels. The polar coordinates of each "knot" (cross section) of the net is indicated by $k(\rho, \theta)$, where $\rho = 10, 20, 30, ..., 300$, and $\theta = 5°, 10°, 15°,..., 360°$. For a 3 x 3 neighboring cross sections of a knot $k(\rho, \theta)$, the coordinates are $k(\rho+10, \theta-5°)$, $k(\rho, \theta-5°)$, $k(\rho-10, \theta-5°)$, $k(\rho+10, \theta°)$, $k(\rho-10, \theta°)$, $k(\rho+10, \theta+5°)$, $k(\rho, \theta+5°)$, $k(\rho-10, \theta+5°)$. This net will be used later in our experiment. From Figures 4, 3b and 3c it is seen that the net patterns of the blot and flame hemorrhages are distinguishable from those of other retinal objects including vessels.

The spider net method will not work for the detection of the dot hemorrhages and microaneurysms because their sizes are too small to be caught by the net. A new scheme for detecting these lesions are needed. This method consists of three steps:

1) Automatic determination of global thresholds from the improved red-free (green) image for obtaining a sequence of binary images.
2) Image segmentation to separate image objects (blood vessels, HMAs, etc.) from the image background.
3) Detection of HMAs using binary matched filters.

The details of this procedure can be found in [14]. An example of detecting HMAs using this procedure is given in Figure 5.

4. EXPERIMENTS AND RESULTS

Over four hundred color fundus photographs including standard fundus photographs were used to assess the detectability and reliability of this computer algorithm. Two sample diagnostic reports are shown in Figure 6. Note that on the top of the report, the coordinates of the optic disc (X_o, Y_o) and the macula (X_m, Y_m) are indicated. It is followed by the list of all HMAs detected. For each HMA, both its location and size are indicated. These results were manually verified and found in good agreement with the manual counts.

5. CONCLUSION

A computer algorithm for automated detection of HMAs in color fundus photographs has been presented. Standard fundus photographs were used to test the accuracy of the algorithm. The sensitivity of this automated system is designed to be adjustable by the user, whereby the user's manual count can be closely matched by the machine count. The results were found to be satisfactory. This automated HMA counting technique provides an objective and repeatable way not only to quantify HMAs, but also to compute HMA count changes and other clinically significant quantities, such as microaneurysm formation and disappearance rates in clinical trials and epidemiology studies.

ACKNOWLEDGEMENT

The study is supported by a grant (Grant number U10EY09898) from the National Eye Institute. The authors wish to thank Dr. Ronald Kingsley and Dana Russell for their assistance.

REFERENCES

1. Spencer, T, Phillips RP, Sharp PF, and Forrester JV. Automated detection and quantification of microaneurysms in fluorescein angiograms. *Graef's Archive Clinical and Experimental Ophthalmology* (1992) 230: 36 - 41.
2. Hellstedt T, Vesti E, and Immonen I. Identification of individual microaneurysms: a comparison between fluorescein angiograms and red-free and color photographs. *Graef's Archive Clinical and Experimental Ophthalmology* (1996) 234, suppl 1: S13-7.
3. Spencer T, Olson JA, McHardy KC, Sharp PF, and Forrester JV. An image-processing strategy for the segmentation and quantification of microaneurysms in fluorescein angiograms of the ocular fundus. *Computer and Biomedical Research* (1996) 29(4): 284-302.
4. Cree MJ, Olson JA, McHardy KC, Sharp PF, and Forrester JV. A fully automated comparative microaneurysm digital detection system. *Eye* (1997) 11 (Pt 5): 622-8.
5. baudoin CE, Maneschi F, Quentel G, Soubrane G, Hayes T, Jones G, Coscas G, and Kohner EM. Quantitative evaluation of fluorescein angiograms: microaneurysm counts. *Diabetes* (1983) 32, suppl 2: 8-13.
6. Fribert TR, Rehkopf PG, Warnicki JW, and Eller AW. Use of directly acquired digital fundus and fluorescein images in the diagnosis of retinal disease. *Retina* (1987) 7:246-251.

7. GoldBaum MH, Chatterjee S, Chaudhuri S, and Katz N. Digital image processing for ophthalmology. In: Masters BR (ed) Noninvasive diagnostic techniques in ophthalmology. *Springer. New York Berlin Heidelberg* (1990) pp 548-568.

8. Peli E. Electro-optic fundus imaging. *Surv Ophthalmology* (1989) 34: 113-122.

9. Rehkopf PG and Warnicki JW. Ophthalmic image processing. In: Masters BR (ed) Noninvasive diagnostic techniques in ophthalmology. *Springer. New Yrok Berlin Heidelberg* (1990) pp 1-16.

10. Klein R , Meuer SM, Moss SE, and Klein BE. Retinal microaneurysms counts and 10-year progression of diabetic retinopathy. *Arch Ophthalmology* (1995) 113 (11): 1386-91.

11. Hellstedt T and Immonen I. Disappearance and formation rates of microaneurysms in early diabetic retinopathy. *British Journal of Ophthalmology* (1996) 80 (2): 135-9.

12. Lee SC, Wang Y, and Lee ET. Automatic retinal image quality assessment and enhancement. *Medical Imaging 1999*. San Diego, CA. (3661-170)

13. Wang Y and Lee SC. A fast method for automatic detection of blood vessels in retinal images. *31st Asilomar Conference on Signals, Systems, and Computers*. Pacific Grove, CA. (Nov. 1997) WA8b-4.

14. Lee SC and Wang Y. A general algorithm for recognizing small, vague, and imagery-alike objects in a nonuniformly illuminated medical diagnostic image. *32nd Asilomar Conference on Signals, Systems, and Computers*. Pacific Grove, CA. (Nov. 1998)

Algorithm Flowchart

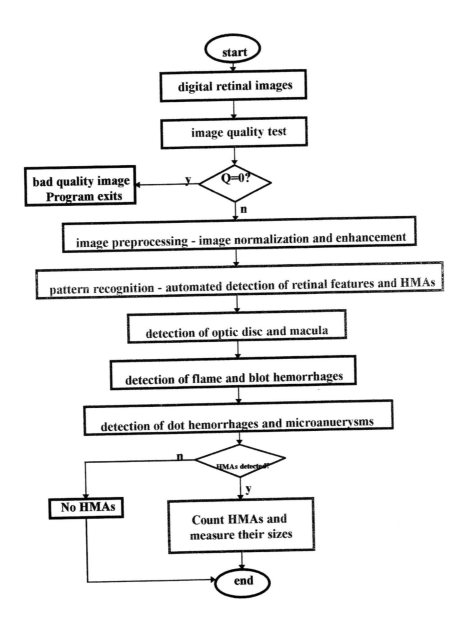

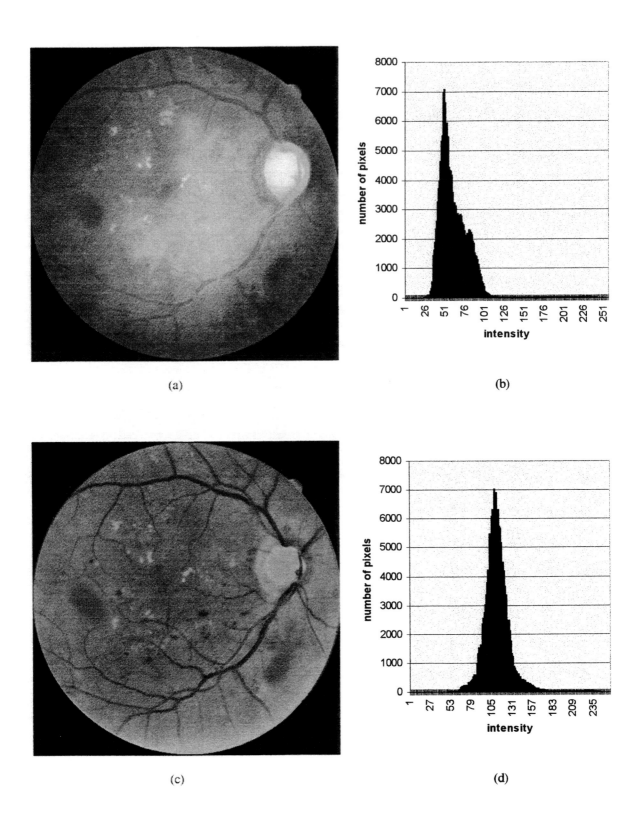

Figure 2. (a) Original image containing HMAs. (b) Intensity histogram of (a)
(c) Normalized image of (a). (d) Intensity of histogram of (c)

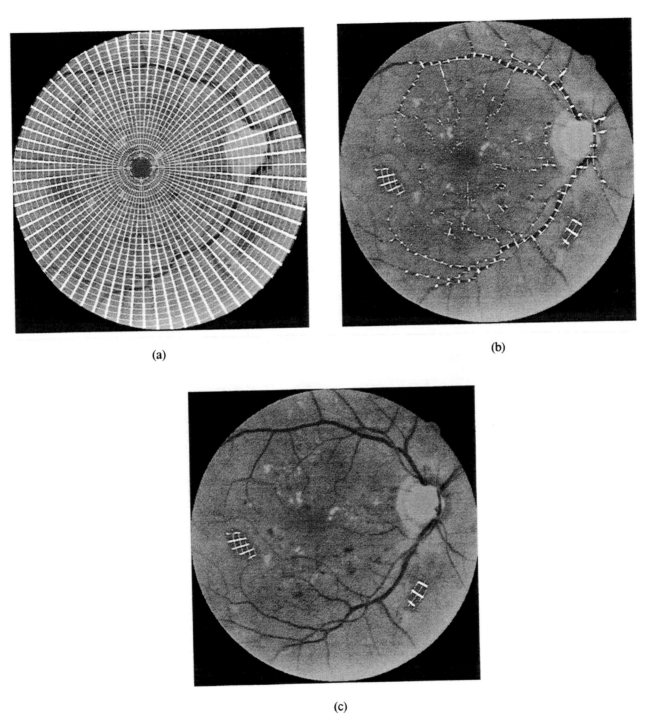

(a)

(b)

(c)

Figure 3. (a) Construction of the spider net.
(b) The net pattern of the flame hemorrhages superimposed by the spider net.
(c) Result of the flame hemorrhages detection.

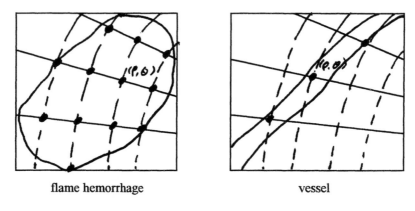

flame hemorrhage   vessel

Figure 4. Net pattern of the blot and flame hemorrhages.

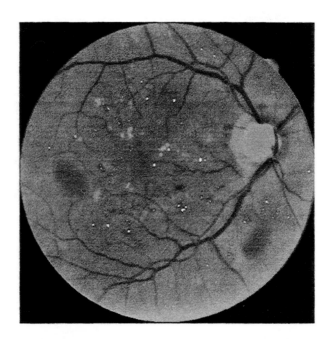

Figure 5. Result of HMA (dot hemorrhages and microaneurysms) detection.

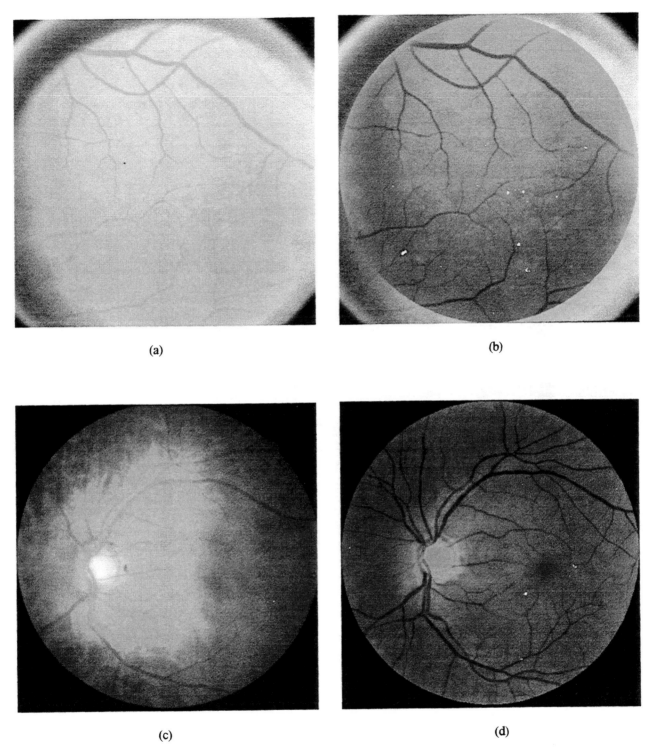

(a)

(b)

(c)

(d)

Figure 6.(a) Standard photo 1a. (b) Result of HMA detection of (a).
(c)Test sample image. (d) Result of HMA detection of (c).
(e)Printout diagnostic report of standard photo 1a in (a).
(f) Printout diagnostic report of test sample image in (c).
Note that the white spots in (b) and (d) indicate the detected HMAs.

The optic disk and the macula were not found in this image.

RESULT OF DIAGNOSIS FOR STANDARD PHOTO 1A:

The following HMAs were found:

Lesion	location	SIZE (pixels)
HMA:	(375 225)	1
HMA:	(105 251)	1
HMA:	(353 266)	1
HMA:	(304 277)	2
HMA:	(150 290)	6
HMA:	(305 293)	2
HMA:	(309 305)	5
HMA:	(323 310)	3
HMA:	(253 333)	3
HMA:	(190 406)	2
HMA:	(301 150)	4
HMA:	(215 241)	4
HMA:	(245 285)	2
HMA:	(82 287)	4
HMA:	(317 295)	5
HMA:	(293 296)	7
HMA:	(368 303)	3
HMA:	(294 314)	2
HMA:	(309 373)	4
HMA:	(278 379)	2
HMA:	(133 383)	51

The total number of HMAs is 21and the total area of HMAs is 114 pixels.

Figure 6 (e)

The coordinates of the optical disc(Xo,Yo) and macula(Xm,Ym) indicated by the normal screen coordinate system were found to be:

(Xo,Yo)=(158, 265)
(Xm,Ym)=(355, 283)

RESULT OF DIAGNOSIS FOR SAMPLE TEST IMAGE:

The following HMAs were found:

lesion	S-location*	M-location**	SIZE(PIXELS)
HMA:	(421 236)	(66 47)	1
HMA:	(481 256)	(126 27)	1
HMA:	(477 260)	(122 23)	1
HMA:	(471 321)	(116 -38)	1
HMA:	(337 385)	(-18 -102)	1
HMA:	(309 141)	(-46 142)	5
HMA:	(472 150)	(117 133)	3
HMA:	(14 243)	(-341 40)	3
HMA:	(397 277)	(42 6)	6
HMA:	(399 276)	(44 7)	2
HMA:	(401 279)	(46 4)	6
HMA:	(391 294)	(36 -11)	2
HMA:	(314 321)	(-41 -38)	12
HMA:	(75 408)	(-280 -125)	7
HMA:	(77 412)	(-278 -129)	2
HMA:	(188 423)	(-167 -140)	2
HMA:	(303 427)	(-52 -144)	2
HMA:	(362 464)	(7 -181)	2

* S-location -- location indicated by the normal screen coordinate system.
**M-location -- location indicated by the macula-centered coordinate system.

The total number of HMAs is 18 and the total area of HMA is 59 pixels

Figure 6. (f).

SESSION 3

ROC and Other Performance Methodologies

Using Incomplete and Imprecise Localization Data on Images to Improve Estimates of Detection Accuracy

Richard G. Swensson,* Glenn Maitz, Jill L. King, David Gur

Department of Radiology, The University of Pittsburgh, Pittsburgh, PA 15261

ABSTRACT

We tested new analytic procedures for combining an observer's image-ratings of lesion-likelihood with localization reports that are incomplete (unavailable on images rated as "normal") and/or imprecise (possibly scored as "correct" by chance), and for fitting a constrained ROC formulation to the rating data alone. Eight radiologist readers in a previous study had rated the likelihood of nodular lesions on each of 250 chest-film cases (39 with subtle nodules, 36 with "typical" nodules and 175 normal cases) that were presented in two display modes (original films or on video workstation). Ratings in the four positive categories (2 to 5) were accompanied by reports that grossly localized the suspected nodules into one of 7 film-regions (upper, middle or lower portions of left or right lung field, or retrocardiac), but there was no localization for the cases rated as "normal" (category 1). In each of 29 sets of data, we estimated the area below the ROC curve (A_z) and its standard error using three different fits: 1) the usual ROC formulation, 2) the constrained ROC formulation and 3) the new procedure that included incomplete and imprecise localization data (I&I). Estimates of A_z from the usual and constrained ROC fits were quite similar unless the standard ROC exhibited an upward "hook," but standard errors of A_z were always the same or smaller for the constrained ROC fit. The I&I fit that included localization data often estimated A_z to be either larger or smaller than the usual or constrained ROC fits that considered only the rating data, but its A_z had substantially smaller standard errors in 28 of the 29 sets of observer data.

Keywords: Localization, LROC, ROC analysis, Observer performance, Detection accuracy, Estimation error

1. INTRODUCTION

A recent analysis of performance[1] combines the ratings of images for lesion-likelihood with a reader's localization of the "most likely" lesion, presumed to be complete (given on every image) and precise (unambiguously correct or incorrect). This statistical procedure concurrently fits the Receiver Operating Characteristic (ROC) curve (detection rates for abnormal vs. normal images) and the "Localization Response" (LROC) curve whose ordinate measures the *fraction of detected abnormal images whose lesions were correctly localized*. The additional information from lesion localization substantially improves statistical estimates of detection accuracy, like area below the fitted ROC curve (A_z), decreasing the standard error of estimated A_z by roughly the same amount as a two to fourfold increase in the case sample sizes.[1,2] Hitherto, however, that statistical procedure has required an observer's precise localization of a possible lesion on every image, which has limited its utility in clinical imaging tasks. This paper reports and tests an extended fitting procedure that can be applied when the localization of abnormalities is incomplete (not performed for images regarded as "normal") or imprecise (might be scored as "correct" by chance), or both. The extended procedure can also be used to fit a constrained formulation of the ROC curve to the rating data alone (ignoring any localization reports).

1.1. The Extended Model for Detection and Localization

The statistical model assumes that an observer's latent rating variable (V) and first-choice localization report both depend on the *maximally-suspicious* finding on the image. On abnormal images, V is assumed to be $\text{Max}[X_n \text{ or } X_L]$, the likelihood of abnormality evaluated at the location of the most suspicious normal finding (X_n) or at the actual lesion location (X_L), whichever is the larger. In addition, the model assumes that X_n has the same probability distribution whether or not the image also contains an actual lesion ($V = X_n$ on a normal image). The extended model assumes that an observer's first-choice localization on an abnormal image is always "correct" if determined by the actual lesion (when $X_L > X_n$), but that it may also

---

*Correspondence: Email: rswensson@radserv.arad.upmc.edu; Telephone: 412 648-3148; Fax: 412 648-9127

74

Part of the SPIE Conference on Image Perception and Performance
San Diego, California • February 1999
SPIE Vol. 3663 • 0277-786X/99/$10.00

be scored as correct "by chance" (when $X_n > X_L$) with some specified *prior probability* q. Let TP(Z) and FP(Z) be the respective conditional probabilities of true-positive and false-positive decisions at detection threshold Z, and let CL(Z) be the joint probability of a true-positive decision at Z that is also scored as a correct localization The extended model's assumptions imply that:

$$FP(Z) \equiv 1 - \text{Prob}\{X_n \leq Z\} = 1 - G(Z),$$ (1a)

$$TP(Z) \equiv 1 - \text{Prob}\{X_n \leq Z\} \times \text{Prob}\{X_L \leq Z\} = 1 - G(Z) \times F([Z - \mu]/\sigma),$$ (1b)

and $$CL(Z) \equiv \text{Prob}\{X_L > Z \text{ and } X_n \leq Z\} + q \times \text{Prob}\{X_n > Z \text{ and } X_L \leq Z\}$$

$$= (1/\sigma)\int_Z^\infty f([X - \mu]/\sigma) \times G(X)dX + q\int_Z^\infty g(X) \times F([X - \mu]/\sigma)dX$$ (1c)

with $$CL(Z) = TP(Z) - (1 - q) \times \text{Prob}\{X_n > Z \text{ and } X_L \leq Z\}$$

$$= TP(Z) - (1 - q) \times \int_0^{FP(Z)} \left[\frac{1 - TP(X)}{1 - FP(X)}\right] dFP(X),$$ (1d)

where the probability density functions f(t) and g(t) are each standardized to have a mean of zero and standard deviation of 1.0, with respective cumulative distribution functions F(t) and G(t), and where μ and σ are the two free parameters that specify the mean and standard deviation for the distribution of X_L relative to that of X_n.

Equations 1a and 1b determine a constrained formulation for the ROC curve,[1] because (whatever the distribution forms) TP(Z) ≥ FP(Z) and the ROC curve can never exhibit an upward "hook." This constrained formulation defines the true-positive probability in terms of the (implicit) probability distribution for a maximum of the two explicit latent variables—i.e., Prob{Max[X_n and X_L] ≤ Z} = G(Z) x F([Z-μ]/σ). In contrast, the usual formulation of the ROC curve assumes some explicit, two-parameter form for the latent rating variable (X_a) on sampled images that contain actual abnormalities. That usual ROC curve is defined as:

$$FP(Z) \equiv 1 - \text{Prob}\{X_n \leq Z\} = 1 - G(Z)$$ (2a)

$$\text{and } TP(Z) \equiv 1 - \text{Prob}\{X_a \leq Z\} = 1 - H(BZ-A).$$ (2b)

where the rating variable X_a has mean A/B and standard deviation $(1/B)$, and where G(t) and H(t) are both standardized cumulative probability distributions. Maximum-likelihood procedures that fit this usual ROC formulation (Eqs. 2a and 2b) to rating data typically assume standard normal distributions for both G(t) and H(t).[3,4,5] Similarly, standard normal distributions for G(t) and F(t) are assumed by the present maximum-likelihood procedure that fits the constrained formulation of the ROC curve (Eqs. 1a and 1b). Once this constrained ROC has been specified by the (assumed or estimated) values of μ and σ, however, then Eqs. 1c and 1d are also completely determined.

Equations 1a and 1c define the LROC curve. The rightmost term in Eq. 1c vanishes when $q = 0$, which then represents the case of precise localization for CL(Z), as assumed by the original detection and localization model.[1] Except for the multiplier (1-q), Eq. 1d is the same as Eq. 4 in Swensson.[1] Setting $q = 1/M$ yields (1-q) = (M-1)/M—which makes Eq. 1d formally identical to the point-by-point relation between the ROC and LROC curves developed by Starr, et al[6] for M discrete-location alternatives, or for gross localization to within one of M image sub regions. It is also closely related to the standard formulations used to analyze choice accuracy in multiple-alternative forced-choice (MAFC) tasks.[7,8,9] Unlike those "discrete M" models, however, this extended model for detection and imprecise localization does not need to represent an image as being composed of M or M – 1 orthogonal and identically-distributed samples of "noise." Instead, it assumes only that the perceived-likelihood distribution for the most suspicious *non-target* location on an image does not depend on whether or not an actual target is also present. The value of q is not estimated by the fitting procedure, but must be specified *a priori*.

1.2. Fitting of Incomplete Localization Data or the Constrained ROC Curve

In the extended fitting procedure, a user can also determine how many of the lowest rating categories should be treated as if they contain no information about the observer's localization of lesions. The index *noloc* may be set to any specified integer from zero to the total number of rating categories (*ncat*). If *noloc* = 0, the procedure assumes that every image received a localization that was scored as correct or incorrect, like the original model for complete localization.[1] Otherwise, for *noloc* ≥ 1, this procedure pools together the frequencies of both correct and incorrect localizations within the lowest *noloc* rating categories for the images that actually contained targets, and it fits only these summed image frequencies (the ROC data) for those *noloc* rating categories. But the procedure uses both the correct and incorrect target localizations (the LROC data) within the highest (*ncat* – *noloc*) rating categories. When *noloc* = *ncat* this extended procedure pools the correct and incorrect localizations within *every* rating category, and it fits only the ROC data by the constrained ROC formulation given in Eqs. 1a and 1b. Of course, once this ROC curve is fitted (μ and σ estimated), the predicted LROC curve can also be calculated by using either Eq. 1c or Eq. 1d.

As an additional option in the extended fitting procedure, the images that contain targets may be stratified into $T > 1$ separate classes that sample different types of targets. Then the procedure concurrently fits T separate pairs of ROC and LROC curves, using two parameters (μ and σ) to fit the data from each image class but a single set of likelihood cutoffs for the boundaries between the ordinal rating categories. Unless q is defaulted to zero, a separate value of q must be specified (a priori) for each class of images. The specified value for *noloc* is applied to all T classes of images; if *noloc = ncat*, then the procedure fits T separate (constrained) ROC curves to the rating ROC data alone. The maximum-likelihood procedure that performs this extended analysis of incomplete and imprecise (I&I) localization data also obtains the variance-covariance matrix for the estimated parameters, which permits calculations of standard errors for indices of accuracy like A_z that are specified functions of those parameters. The current software runs on a PC with Windows 95 or NT, and is available on request.

2. METHODS

We compared estimates of A_z and their standard errors for fits of: 1) the usual ROC curve, 2) the constrained ROC curve and 3) the extended I&I model, applied to rating data from a previous observer study in which the localization of lesions was both imprecise and incomplete. The pairwise comparisons of these fits could be used to distinguish between effects produced by: a) the particular formulation of the ROC curve (usual ROC vs. constrained ROC) and b) the available information about an observer's ability to localize the actual lesions (constrained ROC vs. I&I procedure).

2.1 Database of Case Interpretations

The database of chest-film interpretations came from a previous study[10] in which radiologists read a set of 250 cases, both as the original films (8 readers) and on a high-resolution workstation (7 readers). These cases consisted of 175 posterioanterior chest radiographs without nodules and 75 containing actual pulmonary nodules that two radiologist investigators had independently judged to be either "subtle" (n=39) or "typical" (n=36) cases. A reader assigned each case to one of five ordinal rating categories, according to the judged likelihood that an actual nodule was present. For those cases assigned positive ratings (2 to 5), the reader also grossly localized the suspected nodule to one of seven regions of the lung fields (upper, middle or lower regions on the left or right, or retrocardiac). Table 1 also shows the frequency distributions of actual nodule locations, and of the localizations for readers' false-positive reports on the 175 cases without nodules (a mean of 60/175 = 34% false-positive reports). The readers were not required to indicate any locations for possible nodules on the cases they regarded as "negative," and assigned to rating Category 1.

Table 1
Distributions of 75 Actual Nodules (Number and Percent) Across the Seven Lung-Field Regions and Unweighted-Mean Percentages of Readers' False-Positive Localizations in Each Region

Distribution	R. Upper	R. Mid.	R. Lower	L. Upper	L. Mid.	L. Lower	Retroc.	Total
Actual Nodules: Nbr. (%)	10 (13)	14 (19)	18 (24)	6 (8)	13 (17)	12 (16)	2 (3)	75 (100%)
Region % for False-Positives	12.6%	24.9%	19.4%	7.8%	14.6%	14.8%	6.1%	100%

2.2 Scoring for Correct Localization and Estimation of q

Because the individual readers may have drawn different boundaries between the upper, middle and lower lung fields, different readers who found the same nodules may have localized them in two different adjacent regions of the same lung field. Our extended procedure that fits localization data assumes a "generous" scoring for correct vs. incorrect localization of the targets, in the sense that an incorrect localization may be erroneously scored as correct (with specified probability q), but a report of the actual target is presumably never mistaken for an incorrect localization. Accordingly, the present data analysis reviewed all the localization judgments made in the 15 separate interpretations of each nodule case, and identified any cases in which the readers specified regions of the left or right lung-field adjacent to those that had been designated as the actual-nodule locations. Among the 75 cases that contained actual nodules, two or more readers had reported the same adjacent region in 19 cases (5 or more readers in 12 of these cases). Consequently, those 19 cases were "double scored" as correct localizations if a reader had reported the nodule's regional location as either the designated region or that single adjacent region. Table 2 shows an example of one reader's scored rating data for: a) cases without nodules, b) cases with subtle nodules and c) cases with typical nodules.

Table 2

Example of ROC and LROC Data from Reader 2 with Chest Films: Number of Cases in (and Cumulative Fractions of Cases in or Above) Each Rating Category

Rating Category	175 Cases with No Nodules	39 Cases with Subtle Nodules			36 Cases with Typical Nodules		
		All TPs.	TP&CL	TP &IL	All TPs.	TP&CL	TP&IL
1	117 (1.00)	5 (1.00)	—	—	6 (1.00)	—	—
2	23 (.331)	5 (.872)	2 (.718)	3 (.154)	0 (.833)	0 (.833)	0 (0.0)
3	16 (.171)	9 (.744)	8 (.667)	1 (.077)	0 (.833)	0 (.833)	0 (0.0)
4	6 (.080)	5 (.513)	5 (.513)	0 (.051)	1 (.833)	1 (.833)	0 (0.0)
5	8 (.046)	15 (.385)	13 (.333)	2 (.051)	29 (.806)	29 (.806)	0 (0.0)

For each of the 15 combinations of readers and conditions, the analysis calculated a separate value of q from the summed product:

$$q = \sum_{i=1}^{7} \pi_i p_i,$$ (3)

where π_i is the proportion of actual nodules designated in region i and p_i is that reader's proportion of false-positive localizations within the same region on the 175 cases without actual nodules. As seen in Table 1, the distribution of readers' localizations for false positives roughly matched the regional distribution of actual nodules. For this reason, the 15 values of q varied only over the narrow range between 0.14 and 0.19.

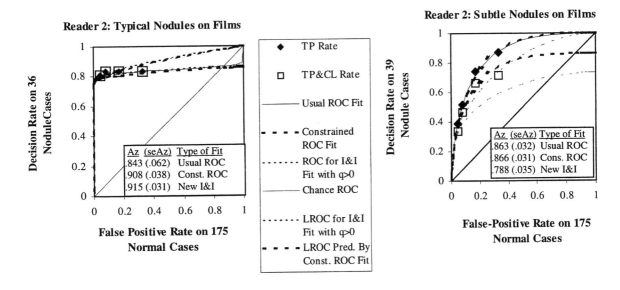

Fig. 1. Measured and fitted ROC and LROC curves for the data presented in Table 2. For typical nodules (left panel), the usual ROC curve fit to these data almost overlies the two predicted LROC curves (adjusted for $q=0.174$) obtained by separately fitting the constrained ROC formulation with or without the localization data. That extrapolated fit of the usual ROC formulation hooks sharply upward as the false-positive probability approaches 1.0. For subtle nodules (right panel), however, both the usual and constrained ROC formulations produced nearly identical fits of the ROC data. But the two incorrect localizations of subtle nodules made with high confidence (Category 5) substantially lowered the ROC and LROC curves (and A_z) estimated by the I&I procedure, forcing it to fit ROC and LROC curves that increased much more gradually than was indicated by the rating data alone.

2.3. Fitting of Data

Four separate analyses were performed on each of the 15 sets of rating and localization data like those seen in Table 2. Each such analysis provided 29 separate fits for either the subtle or the typical nodule cases in these 15 sets of data, including an estimate of A_z and its standard error. (One reader had perfect performance for typical nodules on the workstation; all 36 cases were rated in Category 5 and had correctly localized nodules.) Three of the analyses applied our newly developed software procedures that can be used for image ratings with incomplete and imprecise localization data (I&I). The most complete analysis of these data fitted the new I&I procedure with a prior estimate of q obtained from Eq. 3 for each reader and condition. An additional fit of this I&I procedure was also performed with $q = 0$, in order to evaluate whether or not the estimates of A_z were sensitive to the precise values specified for q. A third analysis used the option *noloc = ncat* to ignore all localization data and fit only the pooled category frequencies for a reader's rating ROC curve. This analysis can determine whether differences in A_z between fits of the usual ROC formulation and fits of the complete I&I model should be attributed to effects of: a) the constrained ROC formulation or b) the inclusion of additional statistical information about accuracy of nodule localization. Since all three of these analyses by the new software procedures estimated the two parameters (μ and σ) in Eqs. 1a–1c, each analysis specified *both an ROC curve and an LROC curve* for the reader's subtle cases or typical cases within a given condition.

An entirely separate analysis fitted the usual formulation for the ROC curve (Eqs. 2a and 2b) to the rating ROC data for subtle and typical cases. This analysis applied an extension of the usual ROC fitting procedure[5] that assumes a different normal distribution for each class of sampled images, but a single set of category boundaries for the ratings of all images. (Essentially identical estimates of the distribution parameters and their standard errors were obtained when the usual ROC formulation was separately fitted to the data for subtle cases and for typical cases, which estimated separate category boundaries for the ratings of those cases.) Figure 1 plots the ROC and LROC data shown in Table 2 for typical-nodule cases (left panel) and for subtle-nodule cases (right panel), together with the predicted curves fitted by three of these analyses.

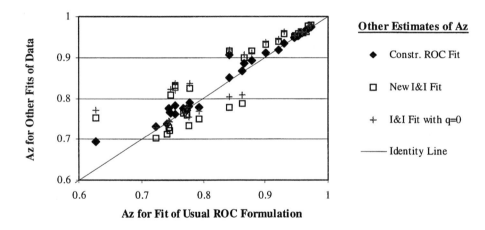

Fig. 2   Estimates of A_z from 29 Fits of the Usual ROC Formulation Compared to Those from the Constrained ROC Formulation Fitted in Each of the Three Other Data Analyses.

3. RESULTS

Figure 2 compares the 29 estimates of A_z obtained by fitting the usual ROC formulation to those (constrained ROC) values that the extended procedures fitted within each of the three other analyses: a) the rating data alone, b) ratings augmented by the incomplete and imprecise localization data ($q > 0$) and c) ratings with the incomplete localization data treated as precise ($q = 0$). The filled diamond-shaped points in Fig. 2 plot the values of A_z estimated when the extended procedure's analysis fit only the image ratings (ROC data) using the constrained formulation of Eqs. 1a and 1b. In all but two of these 29 comparisons, the estimates of A_z were quite similar for both the usual and constrained ROC fits (within 0.02

of the identity line). In those two cases, however, the values of A_z estimated by the constrained fits were more than 0.06 higher than those from the usual ROC fits, because of pronounced upward "hooks" in the two extrapolated ROC curves fitted with the usual formulation (e.g., see right panel in Fig. 1).

The open square data points in Fig. 2 plot the values of A_z estimated by the new I&I fitting procedure with specified q, against those from the usual ROC fits. These I&I estimates of A_z utilize the (incomplete and imprecise) information from a reader's correct and incorrect localization of the nodules within each set of cases. Comparisons between the open and filled points in Fig. 2 show that this additional information about nodule localization often either increased or decreased the estimate of A_z (relative to A_z for the constrained-ROC fit), sometimes rather substantially. When the incomplete reports of nodule locations were treated as precisely scored (by setting $q = 0$), the analysis consistently estimated slightly higher values for A_z (plotted as the crosses in Fig. 2). Most of these differences were quite small, however, suggesting that this I&I analysis may prove to be fairly robust to errors as large as 0.15–0.20 in the values specified for q.

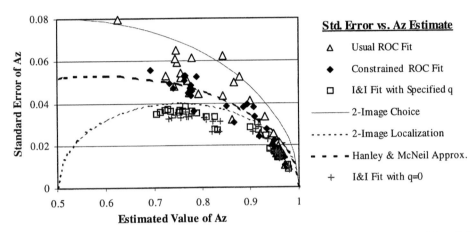

Fig. 3 Standard Errors of A_z Plotted as Functions of their Estimated Values in 29 Separate Fits from Each of Four Different Analyses. The heavy broken curve was suggested by Hanley and McNeil[11] to approximate the functional relation between A_z and its standard error for the usual ROC formulation; it assumes a continuous rating scale and negative-exponential distributions in Eqs. 2a and 2b. The other two curves show upper-bound functions that would relate the standard error of A_z to its different binomial estimates (obtained without any ratings of images) in forced-choice tasks with 36 pairs of target and non-target images. The solid curve assumes that the estimate of A_z is the fraction of pairs in which the target's image was correctly chosen; the thin broken curve uses the localization model's result that $A_z = 0.5 + 0.5P_{T\&CL}$, where $P_{T\&CL}$ is the (binomial) fraction of pairs having not only a correct choice of the target's image but also a correct and precise localization of the actual target.[1,2]

Each of the four analyses also obtained the standard errors for estimates of A_z in their 29 separate fits. Figure 3 plots these standard errors against the estimated value of A_z for each analysis, together with continuous curves that serve to approximate or bound those functional relations. The estimates of A_z from the usual ROC fits always had standard errors that were greater than or equal to those obtained in corresponding fits of the constrained ROC curves. These largest values of $se(A_z)$ for the usual ROC fits were associated with low estimates of the "shape" parameter B, as for the example of typical-nodule cases shown in Fig. 1 ($A_z = 0.843$, $se(A_z) = 0.062$, $B = 0.086$). In 28 of the 29 fits, however, the I&I procedure that included the information about nodule localization estimated A_z with a smaller standard error than did either of the two procedures that ignored localizations and fitted only the ROC data. The single exception occurred in fitting the subtle-nodule data presented in Fig. 1 and Table 2; in that set of data, $se(A_z)$ was slightly higher for the I&I fit than for those of either the constrained ROC or the usual ROC.

Figure 4 shows direct comparisons between pairs of these different statistical fits for relative precision of their A_z estimates. It plots the 29 squared ratios of $se(A_z)$, against the 29 mean estimates of A_z, for three separate paired comparisons of the different fitting procedures: 1) the usual ROC vs. constrained ROC, 2) the constrained ROC vs. I&I analysis with $q > 0$ and 3) the usual ROC vs. I&I analysis with $q > 0$. The squared ratios of $se(A_z)$ are greater than 1.0 for nearly all data points in Fig. 4, because the I&I fit provides the denominator of that ratio in each of its two paired comparisons and the constrained ROC fit provides the denominator in its comparison to the usual ROC fit. This reflects the highly consistent ordering of $se(A_z)$ for these three fitting procedures, as seen in Fig. 3. The ordinate of Fig. 4 gives the relative statistical precision of the two different estimates, which predicts the relative sizes of the image samples required by the two separate procedures in order to achieve an equal precision in estimating A_z. For many of the comparisons in Fig. 4, the I&I procedure estimated A_z with more than twice the statistical precision of procedures that ignored the localization data, particularly those that fit the usual, unconstrained ROC formulation.

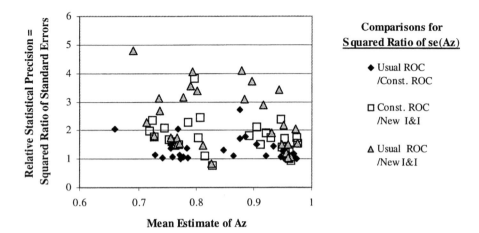

Fig. 4 Comparisons Between Different Pairs of the Fitting Procedures for Statistical Precision in Estimating A_z. The squared ratio of se(A_z) for two given procedures is plotted against their mean A_z for each of the 29 sets of subtle or typical nodule cases. Since the smaller se(A_z) implies better precision, the ratios greater than 1.0 (as most are) indicate a greater statistical precision found for that procedure used in the denominator. This denominator was se(A_z) from the fitted I&I procedure in both of its two types of paired comparisons, and se(A_z) from the fitted constrained ROC in its comparisons with the usual ROC fits.

4. Discussion

As previously found for the concurrent fits of image ratings combined with complete and precise localization data,[1,2] the present results indicate that information from the localization of targets can substantially increase the statistical precision for estimates of detection accuracy (A_z), even when that localization data is incomplete (no localization on many images) and imprecise (a localization may be erroneously scored as "correct"). The new fitting procedures described in this paper can estimate A_z from data for image-ratings alone (by fitting a constrained ROC formulation), or from the ratings of images combined with localization data that are incomplete or imprecise, or both (I&I). The present results suggest that fits of the constrained ROC formulation may provide better (and more precise) estimates of A_z than fits of the usual ROC formulation, particularly when the usual fit would yield an ROC curve that hooks upward at high false-positive rates. When localization data were used in the I&I fitting procedure, the estimated values of A_z sometimes increased and sometimes decreased (relative to those based only on the ratings of images), but they had smaller standard errors in 28 of the 29 separate comparisons. Compared to the usual ROC fits, the I&I fits in many of these comparisons (14 of 29) decreased se(A_z) as much as would twofold to sixfold increases in the case-sample sizes.

There may be problems confronted when attempting to include localization data in the analyses of observer performance, however, because an investigator must be able to score those reports as either "correct" or "incorrect" localizations of the actual targets. The present I&I fitting procedure can accommodate errors in scoring reports of normal findings as correct localizations (assumed to occur with probability q), although it does require having some reasonable way to specify or approximate the value of q. But this I&I model assumes that no reports of the actual targets ever get mistakenly scored as "incorrect localizations," all of which are treated as reports of normal findings that the reader found to be unusually suspicious. Consequently, the fits of this I&I procedure will be quite sensitive to any incorrect localizations made with high degrees of confidence on images that contain actual targets, particularly when many of these target images receive no localization reports (e.g., see data for subtle nodules in Fig. 1 and Table 2).

For most analyses of observer performance that seek to include localization data, a reasonable strategy might be to fit each set of data both with and without the localization data—i.e., not only fitting the appropriate I&I procedure, but also fitting the constrained ROC curve to the rating data alone. There would be no problem encountered for the sets of image interpretation in which both procedures obtained similar estimates, and the I&I fit would generally provide the smaller standard errors of measurement. Any substantial disagreement between estimates from those separate fits would alert the investigator that the given set of data warrants some additional consideration. Such disagreements need not reflect any problems in either the realized image ratings or in the realized localization data, however, because each type of data would be subject to its own independent sources of sampling errors. But to the extent that localization data provides additional valid information about performance accuracy, its inclusion in the analysis would often alter the estimates obtained from an analysis of the rating data alone.

Acknowledgements

Support for this work was provided by NIH Grants CA66594, CA67947 and CA62800.

References

1. R. G. Swensson, "Unified measurement of observer performance in detecting and localizing target objects on images," *Med. Phy.*, **23**, pp. 1709–1725, 1996.

2. R. G. Swensson, "Using localization data from image interpretations to improve statistical estimates of detection accuracy," Submitted for Publication.

3. D. D Dorfman and E. Alf, "Maximum-likelihood estimation of parameters of signal-detection theory and determination of confidence intervals—rating-method data," *J. Math. Psychol.*, **6**, pp.487–496, 1969

4. C. E. Metz, "Some pratical issues of experimental design and data analysis in radiological ROC studies," *Invest. Radiol.*, **24**, pp. 234–245, 1989.

5. M. F. Kijewski, R. G. Swensson and P. F. Judy, "Analysis of rating data from multiple-alternative tasks," *J. Math. Psychol.*, **33**, pp. 428–451, 1989.

6. S. J. Starr, C. E. Metz, L. B. Lusted and D. J. Goodenough, "Visual detection and localization of radiographic images," *Radiology*. **116**, pp. 533–538, 1975.

7. D. M. Green and J. A. Swets, *Signal detection theory and psychophysics*, Wiley, New York, 1966; Reprinted by Peninsula Publishing, Los Altos, CA, 1988.

8. P. A. Elliot, "Tables of d'," in J. A. Swets (ed.) *Signal detection and recognition by human observers*, Wiley, New York, pp. 651–684, 1964; reprinted by Peninsula Publishing, Los Altos, CA, 1988.

9. A. E. Burgess, "Comparison of receiver operating characteristic and forced choice observer performance measurement methods," *Med. Phy.*, **22**, pp. 643–655, 1995.

10. B. S. Slasky, D. Gur, W. F. Good, M. A. Costa-Greco, K. M. Harris, L. A. Cooperstein and H. E. Rockette, "Receiver operating characteristic analysis of chest image interpretation with conventional, laser-printed, and high-resolution workstation images," *Radiology*, **174**, pp.775–780, 1990.

11. J. A. Hanley and B. J. McNeil, "The meaning and use of the area under a receiver operating characteristic curve," *Radiology*, **143**, pp. 29–36, 1982.

The Differential Receiver Operating Characteristic (DROC) Method: Rationale and Results of Recent Experiments

Dev P. Chakraborty, Nelson Scott Howard and Harold Kundel
University of Pennsylvania, Department of Radiology,
3400 Spruce Street, Philadelphia, PA 19104, USA

ABSTRACT

The Differential Receiver Operating Characteristic (DROC) method has been recently proposed as a method of more sensitively determining which of two modalities has a higher A_z value. This method is unlike the Receiver Operating Characteristic (ROC) method, which employs a single image interpretation strategy. The DROC experiment requires the reader to interpret pairs of images of the same patient, one from each modality termed A and B. This study reports on methodological improvements that we have made as well as experiments that we have conducted since this method was last proposed.

The original B-modality image set consisted of 60 digitized normal mammograms. We simulated abnormal images from these original images by superimposing speck-like patterns resembling clustered microcalcifications. Applying a wavelet compression-decompression program to these two sets of images yielded the corresponding A-modality image sets. An image creation and display program was written with a user-friendly interface. Five readers interpreted the images in alternating ROC and DROC sessions. In the ROC sessions the diagnosis (abnormal/normal) and associated confidence level (0-100) was indicated for each image. In the DROC-sessions, two decisions and associated confidence levels were indicated for each image pair: the diagnosis (abnormal/normal) and a preference (A/B) for the modality that yielded the higher confidence level for the diagnosis decision.

It was found that both DROC and ROC showed that $A_z(A) < A_z(B)$, demonstrating that the observers could readily detect the degradation introduced by the compression. In addition, the DROC critical ratio was larger than the corresponding ROC critical ratio for all observers. This confirmed the earlier published results, which used a noise-addition processing and a non-clinical simulation. The combined experiments continue to indicate that DROC has the potential advantage over ROC of increased sensitivity to image quality differences. Issues of bias and their effect on ROC and DROC readings are discussed and suggestions are made for further improvements to DROC methodology. The significance of the increased sensitivity potentially offered by DROC may transform future observer performance studies. Fewer cases and readers may be needed to conduct DROC studies with equivalent power to ROC studies. Thus, DROC would enable more convenient testing of imaging modalities, allowing design engineers to more quickly optimize imaging variables.

Key Words: Differential Receiver Operating Characteristic (DROC), ROC, Observer Performance, Evaluation Methodology

1. INTRODUCTION

Receiver Operating Characteristic (ROC) methodology[1,2,3,4] is widely used in diagnostic radiology to determine which of two imaging modalities is superior for a specified diagnostic task. In the ROC method one first determines A_z, the area under the ROC curve, for each modality. The modality with the larger A_z value is deemed to be superior. Frequently however, the experimenter's primary interest is in the *difference* in A_z values between two modalities, not in the *absolute* values. For such problems an alternative method is desirable, especially if it is more sensitive to image quality differences. The increased sensitivity could be used to detect smaller differences in A_z values, or to detect a specified difference with fewer numbers of images and readers. This is often required in optimization studies.

The Differential Receiver Operating Characteristic (DROC) method has recently[5,6] been proposed in this context. It involves viewing pairs of images of the same patient, one from each modality. The observer's tasks are to (a) make a diagnosis, abnormal or normal and (b) select the modality yielding greater confidence in the diagnosis. Our previous study involved a "noise-addition" processing on images obtained from ACR phantoms. In that study we showed that the DROC method tracked the ROC method, i.e., both indicated the same direction of change. Moreover, we showed that the DROC method was

Part of the SPIE Conference on Image Perception and Performance
San Diego, California • February 1999
SPIE Vol. 3663 • 0277-786X/99/$10.00

more sensitive than the ROC method. Since the publication of the earlier study, some methodological improvements have become apparent. It is clearly desirable to test these with more realistic simulations, different tasks, and different types and levels of processings. In the work to be described we implemented some of the improvements and simulated a more realistic microcalcification detection task. Furthermore, we used a compression algorithm to perform the processing. The aim of this study was to determine if the earlier conclusions were verified with the more realistic simulations.

2. EXPERIMENTAL METHODS

A set of 60 mammograms acquired at our facility provided the starting point for the images. Each image was judged to be normal by the board certified mammographer reading the case. However, some of them did contain native specks (e.g., benign specks) or speck-like artifacts (dust, screen defects, etc). The film images were digitized at 100-micron resolution on a Lumisys LS-100 scanner (LUMISCAN 100, Lumisys Corp., 238 Santa Ana Court, Sunnyvale, CA 94086). The corresponding digital mammograms comprised the *Normal B-modality* images.

We simulated *B-modality Abnormal* images by digitally superimposing computer-generated speck like patterns on the original B-modality images. These patterns resembled clustered microcalcifications seen on real mammograms. They were composed of speck-like objects that were extracted, using 31 x 31 pixel regions-of-interest, from digitized images of American College of Radiology (ACR) phantoms. The phantom images were obtained for a different project[7]. The speck pixel values were 'background subtracted', i.e., a smooth surface was fitted to the exterior region of the speck and this was subtracted from the speck profile. It was critical for the image creation program to allow the user to alter the appearance of the added microcalcification groups. This was enabled in a variety of ways.

First, the user selected the ACR phantom from 6 possible choices. Next, they selected specks out of 18 possible alternatives, derived from the first 3 groups of specks in the phantom (there being 6 specks in each group). Also under program control was a minification factor, which was applied (we used cubic interpolation) to minify the speck before it was digitally added to the image. Finally, we could control a quantity called the speck intensity value. The final digital value was determined by multiplying this number with the pixel value after the minification process. The resulting number was added to the pixel value at the desired location. The resulting control of speck size and speck intensity allowed us to finely tune the difficulty level of the detection task. The targeted A_z was 0.90. The specks were superimposed at random locations within the breast outline. Each cluster contained exactly 5 – 10 specks. Collectively they did not extend beyond a 2 x 2 - cm area. Each speck always appeared brighter than the surround when viewed on the monitor.

We simulated the *A-modality images* by applying a wavelet compression-decompression program (AWARE Technology Inc., 99:1 target compression ratio) to the set of 60 original images and 60 abnormal images. Therefore, a total of 240 images were involved in the study, evenly split between modalities (A and B) and disease condition (Normal vs. Abnormal). Actual images under typical display conditions and intensified speck images are shown in Figs. 1, 2 and 3.

All readings were done on an NT workstation configured around a computer (DELL OptiPlex GX1, 450 MHz, 256 Mbyte RAM, 18 Gbyte SCSI hard disk, Dell Computer Corporation, One Dell Way, Round Rock, TX). A DOME high resolution display controller (MD5-PCI, DOME imaging systems, inc., 400 Fifth Avenue, Waltham, MA) and a BARCO high resolution (2048 x 2560) gray-scale monitor (MGD521, BARCO Inc., Display Systems, 3059 Premiere Parkway Duluth, GA) provided the display. Software was written in IDL (Interactive Data Language, Research Systems, Inc., 4990 Pearl East Circle, Boulder, CO) to display the images under either ROC or DROC conditions. In the ROC condition the viewing order was randomized with respect to modality (A or B), image number (1 of 60 possibilities) and disease condition (normal or abnormal). For each image the following information was elicited from the reader: (a) the diagnosis (normal or abnormal) and the confidence level. The latter was recorded on a 0 – 100 scale using a 'slider' control. Each ROC reading session consisted of 24 images. Following the interpretation of each image, the reader was shown the 'truth' information about the image, i.e., whether or not it was abnormal. If the image was abnormal, the observer was also shown the location of the simulated specks using a box cursor that could be toggled on and off.

Following a ROC session, the next session was in the DROC condition. For example, a normal (abnormal) A-modality image was displayed paired with a normal (abnormal) B-modality image. Normal and abnormal images were never paired together. The following information was elicited: (a) the diagnosis (normal or abnormal) and (b) the preferred image (left or right) that yielded greater confidence in the diagnosis. For each decision the confidence level was also recorded. Note that the responses under (a) are similar to those for the ROC condition, except that they were being elicited for a pair of images of the same

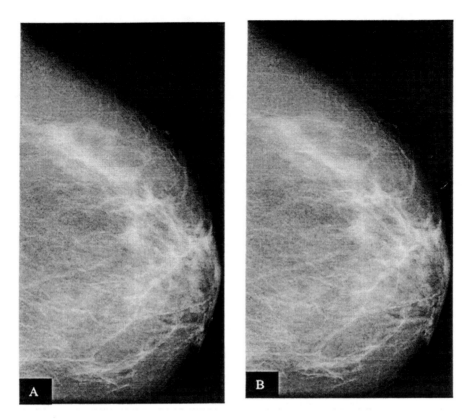

Figure 1: The left image (A) shows a typical normal mammogram. The image shown to the right (B) shows the same image after processing. A wavelet compression-decompression program (AWARE Technology, 99:1) was utilized to form this second modality.

patient. As an example, with reference to Fig. 1, consider the following responses under DROC condition. In (a) the diagnosis normal and confidence level for the normal diagnosis is 90 (high confidence). In (b) the left image is preferred, as it yielded greater confidence in the normal diagnosis and the confidence level for the preference is 50 (moderate confidence that the left image is better). Each DROC reading session consisted of 24 image-pairs. The left vs. right order of presentation of the A- and B- modalities was randomized. In other words, if a particular patient were shown with A-modality on the left and B-modality on the right, in a subsequent (and most likely *different*) DROC session the same patient would be shown with the B-modality on the left and the A-modality on the right. This was done to balance for possible reader bias for a particular side of the monitor. Following each image interpretation, the reader was shown the truth information about the image, as in the ROC condition. Box-cursors to indicate speck locations were shown on both images. In addition the reader was told which modality (A or B) had been chosen.

Each reader had to complete a single session (24 images or image-pairs) in one sitting lasting about 30-min for a DROC session and 15-min for a ROC session. No more that 3 sessions were permitted in a single day. Two-ROC and two-DROC sessions were devoted to training and were not recorded. The recorded study consisted of 10 ROC and 10 DROC sessions and lasted about 10 hours per reader. Readers were encouraged to use a magnifying glass if necessary, but were cautioned to use it equally in providing the differential responses (preference and associated confidence level). We did not want the comparison to be between one modality with a magnifying glass and the other without. Ambient illumination was controlled at 2.0 foot-candles using a rheostat-controlled light source. The observers were not allowed to manipulate window and level on the images, rather these were pre-selected by the author and identical settings were employed between each unprocessed image and its corresponding processed image. If the entire breast was not visible in the display window the observers were allowed to 'rove' the image using standard 'scroll-bar' controls in the user interface. However, the readers were told that the default display did include any relevant abnormality.

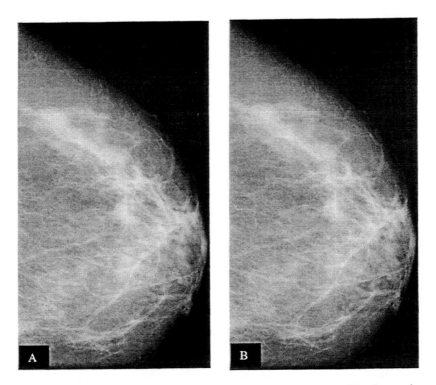

Figure 2: The left image (A) shows a typical abnormal mammogram. The abnormal mammogram was created by adding specks to the image. In the above image, the microcalcifications will not be visible but may be seen more clearly in Figure 3 where the specks have been intensified. The image on the right (B) demonstrates the same image after processing by the wavelet compression-decompression program.

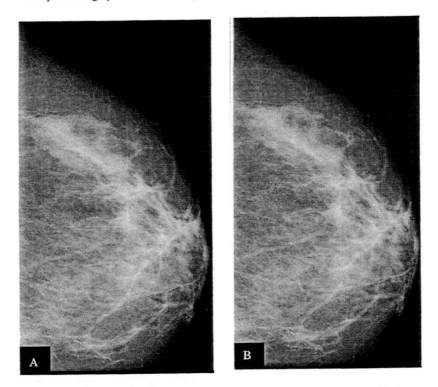

Figure 3: The left image (A) shows an intensified abnormal mammogram. The image shown to the right (B) shows the same image after processing by the wavelet compression-decompression program.

3. ANALYSIS

The reader data saved by the acquisition program was used to generate tables suitable for submission to the CLABROC program[8]. The diagnosis index D1 was defined as D1 = 0 for a normal diagnosis and D1 = 1 for an abnormal diagnosis. The CLABROC program requires the confidence level to be unidirectional from normal to abnormal (or vise-versa), with the ambivalent rating in the middle of the scale. In our case the ambivalent rating was at the '0' end of the scale (which corresponded to no confidence in the diagnosis). Therefore we converted the indicated confidence level D2, which could run from 0 to 100, as follows:

$$X = (2 \bullet D1 - 1) \bullet D2 \quad . \qquad\qquad \text{Eqn. 1}$$

Note that X (which varies from −100 to +100) is unidirectional, with −100 corresponding to high confidence in a normal diagnosis. For the ROC readings the table submitted to the CLABROC program consisted of an image by image record of the ROC confidence levels X_A and X_B, corresponding to the A- and B-modalities, respectively, with the normal images tabulated first followed by the abnormal images. The CLABROC program yielded the A_z values for the two modalities, denoted by A_z (A) and A_z (B), respectively, and the critical ratio CR, which is defined as the difference of the two A_z values divided by the standard deviation of the difference. CR can be thought of as the signal-to-noise-ratio of the ROC analyses. Under the null hypothesis, CR is distributed as a zero-mean unit-standard-deviation Gaussian random variable. A high value of CR indicates high confidence that the modalities are different, and CR can be converted to a significance probability (p-value) by consulting standard statistical tables on integrals of the normal distribution. For example, CR = 1.96 yields a p-value of 0.05 under a two-tailed test of the null hypothesis.

For the DROC analysis, the diagnosis index D1 was also defined as D1 = 0 for a normal diagnosis and D1 = 1 for an abnormal diagnosis. The indicated confidence level D2, which varied from 0 to 100, was converted similarly,

$$Y = (2 \bullet D1 - 1) \bullet D2 \quad . \qquad\qquad \text{Eqn. 2}$$

Note that Y applies to the paired-image DROC presentation, whereas X applies to the single image ROC presentations. In both cases they refer to the detection task (i.e., is the patient abnormal?).

The additional DROC responses apply to the preference task. The index D3 was defined as D3 = 0 when the left image was chosen and D3 = 1 when the right image was chosen. The left vs. right order was coded by the logical variable ARHS (A-modality on the right-hand-side) as follows: ARHS = 0 if the A-modality was on the left-hand-side, and ARHS = 1 otherwise. One defines the variable B_A (B minus A) as follows:

$$B\_A = (2 \bullet ARHS - 1) \bullet (1 - 2 \bullet D3) \quad . \qquad\qquad \text{Eqn. 3}$$

Note that B_A has the following properties. B_A = 1 if the B-modality was chosen, i.e., if B > A and B_A = -1 if the A-modality was chosen, i.e., if B < A. The indicated differential confidence level D4, which varied from 0 to 100, was converted to the DROC confidence level Z as follows:

$$Z = (2 \bullet D1 - 1) \bullet D4 \bullet B\_A \quad . \qquad\qquad \text{Eqn. 4}$$

Note that Z varies for −100 (A is strongly preferred to B) to +100 (B is strongly preferred to A) and is unidirectional. Table 1 shows a few examples of the scoring of the data.

First, only the data with ARHS = 0 were analyzed. For the DROC readings the table submitted to the CLABROC program consisted of an image by image record of Y and Z with the normal images tabulated first followed by the abnormal images. The CLABROC analysis yielded A_z values for the two "modalities" Y and Z, denoted by A_z (Y) and A_z (Z) respectively. The CLABROC critical ratio output is ignored in the DROC analysis. The quantity of interest is A_z (Z). This is the area under the DROC curve. The critical ratio is calculated from

$$CR_{DROC} = \frac{A_z - 0.5}{\sigma(A_z)} \qquad\qquad \text{Eqn.5}$$

TABLE 1: Illustrating the scoring of the DROC responses. The quantity ARHS = 1 if the A-modality was on the right hand side, and 0 otherwise. D1 is the diagnosis, = 1 for abnormal and = 0 otherwise. D2 is the confidence level of the diagnosis, = 0 for no confidence and = 100 for high confidence. D3 is the preference decision, = 1 if the right hand side image was preferred and = 0 otherwise. D4 is the confidence level of the preference. Y is the decision variable corresponding to the diagnosis. B_A is = 1 if B was preferred to A, and = -1 otherwise. Finally, Z is the decision variable corresponding to the preference task. See Eqns. 1 – 4.

Truth	ARHS	D1	D2	D3	D4	B_A	Y	Z
Normal	1	0	100	0	100	1	-100	-100
Normal	0	0	100	1	100	1	-100	-100
Abnormal	1	1	100	0	100	1	100	100
Abnormal	0	1	100	1	100	1	100	100

where the denominator, the standard deviation of A_z (Z), is available from the CLABROC output. The analysis was repeated for the other value ARHS = 1. The two CR_{DROC} values corresponding to ARHS = 0 and ARHS = 1 were averaged to minimize reader bias for a side of the display.

4. RESULTS

While the target compression ratio was 99 (the present limit of the AWARE program) the actual compression ratio obtained was about 120-140. Table 2 summarizes the results of this study. The column labeled SNR is the relative signal-to-noise-ratio of the specks. For the initial task that all readers completed, SNR = 100 in arbitrary units. For the more difficult task (SNR = 81), all the speck-intensity values (see Methods Section) were uniformly decreased by 19%. The next two columns list the A_z values of the two modalities. Listed next are the ROC area correlations between A and B modalities (corr-ROC) and the corresponding correlation between overall and differential tasks (corr-DROC). Finally we list the critical ratios for the two methods.

Note that for each observer we obtained critical ratios with the same sign under both ROC and DROC conditions. This implies that the DROC method is yielding the same direction of change as the ROC method (namely, the B modality is superior). A negative CR would imply that the A-Modality (the compressed-decompressed) was superior. The changes in ROC areas are large, as are the corresponding critical ratios. The DROC critical ratio in each case was larger than the corresponding ROC value. The corresponding p-values for incorrectly rejecting the null hypothesis that the two modalities are identical would be astronomically small for readers A, B and D and E.

TABLE 2: Summary results from the ROC/DROC studies. SNR is the relative signal-to-noise-ratio of the specks. The next two columns list the A_z values of the two modalities. Listed next are the ROC area correlations between A and B modalities (corr-ROC) and the corresponding correlation between overall and differential tasks (corr-DROC). Finally we list the critical ratios for the two methods.

Reader	SNR (AU)	A_z(A)	A_z(B)	corr-ROC	corr-DROC	CR-ROC	CR-DROC
A	100	0.9436	0.8483	0.246	0.397	2.55	24.22
B	100	0.9705	0.8358	0.169	0.346	3.64	23.98
C	100	0.9465	0.7116	0.172	0.389	4.78	6.50
D	100	0.9125	0.7798	0.380	0.211	3.15	13.01
E	100	0.9621	0.7906	0.226	0.240	4.15	10.51
D	81	0.847	0.6797	0.277	0.496	3.27	7.86

The SNR = 100 detection task was rather easy and the processing applied degraded the detectability sharply. The results for the reader D with a more difficult task (SNR = 81) are as expected. The individual modality ROC areas are smaller. The DROC results are consistent with ROC and the critical ratio is larger.

5. DISCUSSION

Our main interest was not in studying the effects of compression but rather to test the DROC method. The important conclusions are first, that the DROC results are consistent with the ROC results and second, that DROC yielded a larger critical ratio for each observer. These results are consistent with our earlier study, which was conducted using 'added noise' as the processing. In that study the task was more difficult and the processing difference was smaller. The present study is complementary since it is focused on an easier task and a stronger processing. We should note that so far we have conducted 17 ROC/DROC runs (see Refs. 5 and 6) and in no case has the main conclusions (tracking and increased power) been shown to be incorrect. In future we plan to conduct further ROC/DROC studies with different difficulty level tasks, compression ratios and task types (e.g., mass and fiber detection) and processings (e.g., x-ray techniques considered as processings, image processings, etc.). These studies are necessary to fully explore and validate the method.

The time needed for the DROC portion of the study was about twice that for the ROC portion. This is due to the fact that in the DROC sessions we collected twice as many decisions as compared to the ROC readings. A difference in experimental methodology of this study from our previous work is that in the previous study we adopted the discrete-rating strategy, whereas in the present we adopted the continuous-rating paradigm[9,10,11]. The reason for this change is the recommendation that the continuous-rating experiment more accurately captures the reader's confidence level and that fewer data degeneracy problems are likely with this paradigm. No data degeneracy problems were encountered in this study. Another difference is the collection of the overall diagnosis confidence level for possible future use. In the study reported earlier only the diagnosis information was collected.

Readers C, D and E were lay readers that we hired for this project. The readers A and B (two of the authors) were very familiar with the images, the task and the processing. The fact that their DROC critical ratios were unusually large, as compared to the rest of the group, is not surprising. Similar differences in discrimination ability were noticed[12] between persons familiar with the processing (engineers) and others (physicians), with the former more adept at detecting the effect of a processing. Note that a larger DROC area or a larger DROC critical ratio does not imply a larger difference in A_z's between the two modalities. Consider two observers 1 and 2 who have the same ROC performances for the two modalities, i.e., $A_z(A,1) = A_z(A,2)$ and $A_z(B,1) = A_z(B,2)$. In the DROC paired image presentation case-sampling-noise and within-reader-noise sources tend to cancel out more than for the ROC single image mode. This is because stronger case-sampling-noise and within-reader noise-correlations are expected when the images are viewed side-by-side than when they are viewed one-at-a-time. In fact this is the main reason for our claim that DROC is superior to ROC for detecting small differences. To the extent that readers 1 and 2 have different degrees of noise-cancellations (or noise-correlations), their DROC areas and critical ratios are expected to be different. It these correlations were measured it should be possible in future to calculate an actual A_z difference from a DROC study. For now one should simply regard the sign of $(A_d-0.5)$ as that of the difference $A_z(B) - A_z(A)$ and the p-value corresponding to the DROC critical ratio as the probability of incorrectly rejecting the null hypothesis that the two modalities are identical. For a given reader and case sample, the value of the DROC critical ratio is expected to increase as the processing difference increases, as is needed to conduct optimization studies.

In commonly performed preference studies a reader *with no diagnostic ability* can mislead the DROC experimenter simply by choosing the preferred modality for all image pairs. It is important to note that the DROC study is free from this type of bias. This is best seen with reference to the DROC data table introduced in a previous publication, and reproduced here for convenience, see Table 3. The quantity BP is the B-preferred positive pair fraction and BN is the B-preferred negative pair fraction[5]. Table 3 is actually for a 5-rating DROC experiment, but the argument applies equally to the continuous-rating DROC case. Assume that for each image pair the observer gives the highest rating (5) to his preferred modality (B). For the actually positive images this translates to an ordinal rating of 5 and for actually negative images an ordinal rating of 1. Therefore, only the cells marked BP_5, BP_1, BN_5 and BN_1 would be populated. Since this reader cannot distinguish between actually positive and actually negative images, we must have on the average, $BP_5 = BN_5$ and $BP_1 = BN_1$. Such a data set when submitted to ROCFIT will yield 0.5 for the area under the DROC curve. The reader, in spite of his efforts, is unable to show that the B-modality is superior.

However, an *expert* reader can mislead (consciously or unconsciously) the DROC experimenter. One way is to simply duplicate the rating entered in response to the first question (diagnosis) while each time preferring his favorite modality (B). In this case the diagnosis and preference decision variables Y and Z (see Eqns. 2 and 4) will be *identical* and $A_z = A_d > 0.5$ for an expert reader. This would imply that modality B was actually superior. In the ROC experiment such a reader could

TABLE 3: This table shows the structure of the final DROC ordinal rating data. Note its similarity to a ROC data set. BP_i (BN_i) is the frequency of the events with ordinal rating = i for positive (negative) pairs.

Ordinal Rating	Differential Rating	Truth = Positive Pair	Truth = Negative Pair
5	B>>A	BP_5	BN_5
4	B>A	BP_4	BN_4
3	B=A	BP_3	BN_3
2	B<A	BP_2	BN_2
1	B<<A	BP_1	BN_1
Sum		N_+	N_-

also make modality-B appear to be superior by adopting a degree of randomness when he is responding to images from the other modality (A). Complete randomness would depress the ROC score for modality-A to 0.5. One way to correct for the problem in the DROC case is to determine the extent of such bias by showing *identical* images (e.g., AA or BB) interspersed with the actual DROC pairs (AB or BA). The DROC area A_d calculated for these identical image pairs should ideally be 0.5. The actual value should be converted to a d' index, and this needs to be subtracted from the corresponding d' from the uncorrected A_d quantity. We have plans to run such experiments in the future. Such modality bias is expected to become less of a problem if the processing difference is small. This type of bias would be difficult to avoid when dealing with modalities that are obviously different.

6. ACKNOWLEDGMENTS

The author is grateful to Ms. Colleen Campbell for serving as a reader in this experiment. This work was supported by a grant from the Department of Health and Human Services, National Institutes of Health, National Cancer Institute, RO1-CA75145.

REFERENCES

[1] D. M. Green and J. A. Swets, "Signal Detection Theory and Psychophysics", (R.E. Krieger, Huntington, N.Y. 1974).

[2] J. A. Swets and R. M. Pickett, "Evaluation of Diagnostic Systems: Methods from Signal Detection Theory", (Academic Press, New York, 1982).

[3] C. E. Metz, "ROC Methodology in Radiologic Imaging", *Investigative Radiology,* 21, 720-733, 1986.

[4] Charles Metz, "Some practical issues of experimental design and data analysis in Radiological ROC studies", *Investigative Radiology*, 24:234-245, 1989.

[5] Chakraborty DP, Kundel HL, Nodine C, Narayan TK and Devaraju V: The Differential Receiver Operating Characteristic Method. SPIE Vol. 3338: 234-240, 1998.

[6] Chakraborty DP: A Paired Image Method for Measuring Small Differences in Image Quality. Submitted to Medical Physics. Conditionally accepted.

[7] Chakraborty DP: Physical measures of image quality in mammography. SPIE Proceedings, The Physics of Medical Imaging, 2708:179-193, 1996.

[8] This is available from Professor Charles Metz at the University of Chicago. Available on the web at http://www-radiology.uchicago.edu/sections/.

[9] Charles Metz, J. H. Shen, B. A. Herman: "New methods for estimating a binormal ROC curve from continuously distributed test results". Presented at the 1990 Joint Statistical Meeting of the American Statistical Society and the Biometrics Society, Anaheim, Calif., August 1990.

[10] Howard Rockette, David Gur, and Charles Metz. The use of continuous and discrete confidence judgments in receiver Operating Characteristic Studies of Diagnostic Imaging Techniques. Invest Radiol 1992; 27:169-172.

[11] King JL. Britton CA. Gur D. Rockette HE. Davis PL. On the validity of the continuous and discrete confidence rating scales in receiver operating characteristic studies. Investigative Radiology, 28(10):962-3, 1993 Oct.

[12] Good WF. Maitz GS. Gur D. Joint photographic experts group (JPEG) compatible data compression of mammograms. Journal of Digital Imaging. 7(3):123-32, 1994 Aug.

Monte Carlo Validation of a Multireader Method for Receiver Operating Characteristic Discrete Rating Data: Split Plot Experimental Design

Donald D. Dorfman,[a,b] Kevin S. Berbaum,[a,b] Russell V. Lenth,[c] Yeh-Fong Chen [c]

[a]Department of Radiology, [b]Department of Psychology, and [c]Department of Statistics and Actuarial Science, The University of Iowa, Iowa City, Iowa.

ABSTRACT

The major purpose of this paper was to evaluate the Dorfman/Berbaum/Metz[1] (DBM) method for analyzing multireader receiver operating characteristic (ROC) discrete rating data on reader split-plot and case split-plot designs. It is not always appropriate or practical for readers to interpret imaging studies of the same patients in all modalities. In split plot designs, either a different sample of readers is assigned to each modality or a different sample of cases is assigned to each modality. For each type of split-plot design, a series of null-case Monte Carlo simulations were conducted. The results suggest that the DBM method provides trustworthy alpha levels with discrete ratings when ROC area is not too large, and case and reader sample sizes are not too small. In other situations, the test tends to be somewhat conservative. Our Monte Carlo simulations show that the DBM multireader method can be validly extended to the reader-split and case-split plot designs.

Keywords: Receiver operating characteristic curve (ROC); Diagnostic radiology; Decision theory, Analysis of variance.

1. INTRODUCTION

The major purpose of this paper was to evaluate the Dorfman/Berbaum/Metz[1] (DBM) method for analyzing multireader receiver operating characteristic (ROC) discrete rating data on reader-split and case-split designs. The method involves analysis of variance of pseudovalues computed by the Quenouille-Tukey jackknife. The basic data for the analysis are pseudovalues of ROC parameters computed by jackknifing cases separately for each observer. The problem of multireader ROC analysis is of considerable importance in the evaluation of diagnostic imaging systems. Recently, Obuchowski and Zepp[2] reviewed the major papers on prospective studies of image interpretation published in the *American Journal of Roentgenology* in the first four months of the years 1990 and 1995. They discovered an important trend: *"In the 1990 literature, we noted eight multiple-reader and 18 single-reader studies; in contrast, in the 1995 literature, we found 29 multiple-reader and eight single-reader studies. This trend reflects an increased awareness of the importance of multiple-reader studies."*

A principal advantage of the fully crossed factorial design analyzed by Dorfman, Berbaum, Metz[1] is that it provides good precision for comparing modalities because between-reader variability is excluded from the experimental error. In the factorial design, only within-reader variation enters the experimental error, since any two modalities can be compared directly for each reader. It is not always appropriate or practical for readers to interpret imaging studies of the same patients in all modalities. For instance, when it is rare for readers to be expert in both modalities being compared, it is better to assign different readers to each modality. Also, when an interpretation of a case in one modality can affect interpretation of that case in another modality, it is appropriate for each same reader to interpret different cases in each

Part of the SPIE Conference on Image Perception and Performance
San Diego, California • February 1999
SPIE Vol. 3663 • 0277-786X/99/$10.00

91

modality. Under these circumstances, split-plot designs offer solutions. In split plot designs, either a different sample of readers is assigned to each modality or a different sample of cases is assigned to each modality. In our adaptation of the reader split-plot design, it is assumed that readers, called blocks, are a random sample from some population and that each reader is tested under one of the two modalities. To facilitate comparison between the factorial and reader split-plot designs, we assume that there are n different readers in each modality, whereas in the factorial design, the same n readers are tested in both modalities. Similarly, in the case split-plot design we assume that there are c different cases in each modality, whereas in the factorial design the same c cases are tested in each modality.

2. METHODS

The following mixed-effect linear decision model was used for the split-plot on reader design to generate raw data from different magnitudes for the variance components:

$$Y_{ijkt} = \mu_t + \tau_{it} + R(\tau)_{ijt} + C_{kt} + (\tau C)_{ikt} + \varepsilon_{(ijkt)} \ ,$$

in which $\mu_t = 0$ if truth value (t) is negative or $\mu_t = a/b$ if truth value (t) is positive, where a and b are the population "location" and "scale" parameters, respectively, of the mean binormal ROC curve, τ_{it} is the fixed effect of modality i for truth value t, $R(\tau)_{ijt}$ is the random effect of reader j nested within modality i for truth value t, C_{kt} is the random effect of case k for truth value t, $(\tau C)_{ikt}$ is the random modality by case interaction effect for modality i, case k for truth value t, and $\varepsilon_{(ijkt)}$ is the random error associated with one reading defined by modality i, reader j, case k for truth value t.

The population ROC areas, latent variable structures, case-sample sizes and normal/abnormal case-sample ratios studied by Roe and Metz[3] were adapted for these simulations. Two changes were instituted for the split-plot on readers design. First, the variance component for reader-case interaction in the factorial design was combined with the residual in the split-plot on readers design. Second, the reader component of variance and the treatment by reader component of variance of the factorial design were summed to produce the readers nested within treatments component of variance in the split-plot on readers design.

Table 1 presents the analysis of variance for the split-plot design on readers using unrestricted parameterization. The lower part of Table 1 gives rules for selecting error terms to test treatment effects.

Table 1: Split Plot on Readers Analysis of Variance: Unrestricted Parameterization

Source	df	Expected Mean Square
Treatments (T)	1	$rc\sigma^2_\tau + c\sigma^2_{R(\tau)} + r\sigma^2_{\tau C} + \sigma^2_{R(\tau)C}$
Readers (Treatments)(R(T))	2(r−1)	$c\sigma^2_{R(\tau)} + \sigma^2_{R(\tau)C}$
Cases (C)	c−1	$2r\sigma^2_C + r\sigma^2_{\tau C} + \sigma^2_{R(\tau)C}$
T × C	c−1	$r\sigma^2_{\tau C} + \sigma^2_{R(\tau)C}$
R(T) × C	2(r−1)(c−1)	$\sigma^2_{R(\tau)C}$

Rules for Selecting Error Term to Test for Treatment Effects:

(i)   If $MS_{R(\tau)} / MS_{R(\tau) \times C} \le 1$, and $MS_{\tau C} / MS_{R(\tau) \times C} \le 1$, use $MS_{R(\tau) \times C}$;

(ii) If $MS_{R(\tau)} / MS_{R(\tau) \times C} \le 1$, and $MS_{\tau C} / MS_{R(\tau) \times C} > 1$, use $MS_{\tau C}$;

(iii) If $MS_{R(\tau)} / MS_{R(\tau) \times C} > 1$, and $MS_{\tau C} / MS_{R(\tau) \times C} \le 1$, use $MS_{R(\tau)}$;

(iv) If $MS_{R(\tau)} / MS_{R(\tau) \times C} > 1$, and $MS_{\tau C} / MS_{R(\tau) \times C} > 1$, use Satterthwaite error term.

The following mixed-effect linear decision model was used for the split-plot on cases design to generate raw data from different magnitudes for the variance components:

$$Y_{ijkt} = \mu_t + \tau_{it} + C(\tau)_{ikt} + R_{jt} + (\tau R)_{ijt} + \varepsilon_{(ijkt)} \quad ,$$

in which $\mu_t = 0$ if truth value (t) is negative or $\mu_t = a/b$ if truth value (t) is positive, where a and b are the population "location" and "scale" parameters, respectively, of the mean binormal ROC curve, τ_{it} is the fixed effect of modality i for truth value t, $C(\tau)_{ikt}$ is the random effect of case k nested within modality i for truth value t, R_{jt} is the random effect of reader j for truth value t, $(\tau R)_{ijt}$ is the random modality by reader interaction effect for modality i, reader j for truth value t, and $\varepsilon_{(ijkt)}$ is the random error associated with one reading defined by modality i, reader j, case k for truth value t.

Two changes were instituted for the split-plot on cases design. First, the variance components for cases and treatment by cases of the factorial design were combined to produce the component of variance for cases nested within treatments. Second, the reader-by-case interaction and the residual of the factorial design were summed to produce the residual component of variance for the split-plot on cases design.

Table 2 presents the analysis of variance for the split-plot design on cases using unrestricted parameterization. The lower part of Table 2 gives rules for selecting error terms to test treatment effects.

Table 2: Split Plot on Cases Analysis of Variance: Unrestricted Parameterization

Source	df	Expected Mean Square						
Treatments (T)	1	$cr\sigma^2_\tau$	$+$	$r\sigma^2_{C(\tau)}$		$+$	$c\sigma^2_{\tau R}$	$+$ $\sigma^2_{C(\tau)R}$
Case (Treatments)(C(T))	$2(c-1)$			$r\sigma^2_{C(\tau)}$				$+$ $\sigma^2_{C(\tau)R}$
Reader (R)	$r-1$				$2c\sigma^2_R$	$+$	$c\sigma^2_{\tau R}$	$+$ $\sigma^2_{C(\tau)R}$
$T \times R$	$r-1$						$c\sigma^2_{\tau R}$	$+$ $\sigma^2_{C(\tau)R}$
$C(T) \times R$	$2(r-1)(c-1)$							$\sigma^2_{C(\tau)R}$

Rules for Selecting Error Term to Test for Treatment Effects:

(i)   If $MS_{C(\tau)} / MS_{C(\tau) \times R} \le 1$, and $MS_{\tau R} / MS_{C(\tau) \times R} \le 1$, use $MS_{C(\tau) \times R}$;

(ii) If $MS_{C(\tau)} / MS_{C(\tau) \times R} \le 1$, and $MS_{\tau R} / MS_{C(\tau) \times R} > 1$, use $MS_{\tau R}$;

(iii) If $MS_{C(\tau)} / MS_{C(\tau) \times R} > 1$, and $MS_{\tau R} / MS_{C(\tau) \times R} \le 1$, use $MS_{C(\tau)}$;

(iv) If $MS_{C(\tau)} / MS_{C(\tau) \times R} > 1$, and $MS_{\tau R} / MS_{C(\tau) \times R} > 1$, use Satterthwaite error term.

For each type of split plot design, a series of null-case Monte Carlo simulations were conducted with two modalities. For the split-plot design on readers, 3, 5, and 10 different hypothetical readers were nested within each modality, and 10+/90−, 25+/25−, 50+/50−, and 100+/100−cases were crossed with modalities. For the split-plot design on cases, 10+/90−, 25+/25−, 50+/50−, and 100+/100−cases were nested within each modality, and 3, 5, and 10 hypothetical readers were crossed with modalities.

Our series of null-case computer simulations were conducted to examine the relation between the nominal type I error rate and the empirical type I error rate with five-category discrete rating data as recommended by Swets and Pickett.[4] Two thousand samples were generated for each condition. In the computer simulation, a continuous decision variable was generated by assuming a linear mixed model for the decision variable comparable to the linear mixed model for the jackknife pseudovalues. Roe and Metz[3] and Dorfman, Berbaum, Lenth et al.[5] used the equal-variance binormal model ($b = 1$) . Therefore, in all of the Monte Carlo simulations that follow, we also used the equal-variance binormal model to facilitate comparison between our results and their results.

The null hypothesis was true in all simulations, and the population ROC curves were the same for both modalities. Three binormal population ROC curves with A_z values of .702, .855, and .961, corresponding to μ_{pos} = 0.75, 1.5, and 2.5, were included in the study. The magnitudes of the decision-variable variance components were chosen to be the same for actually-positive and actually-negative cases. The decision thresholds were set at 0.25, 0.75, 1.25, and 1.75 corresponding to false-positive fractions of 0.40, 0.23, 0.11, and 0.04. The decision thresholds serve mathematically as the values of the category boundaries for the continuous random decision variable. The decision thresholds were chosen to mirror the moderate conservatism often observed in radiologic image interpretation.

3. RESULTS

For equal allocation ratios, small (A_z=0.702) and moderate ROC area (A_z=0.855), empirical Type I error rate closely matched nominal alpha level; however, for very large ROC area (A_z=0.961), empirical Type I error rate was somewhat smaller than nominal alpha level. For the most part, these findings are consistent with those reported by Roe and Metz,[3] and by Dorfman, Berbaum, Lenth, et al.[5]

Figures 1, 2, and 3 present the results for areas of .702, .855, and .961, respectively, with the upper panel representing the split-plot design on readers and the lower panel representing the split-plot design on cases. To facilitate comparison with Monte Carlo studies based on the factorial design, we used the same labels for the variance structures as those employed by Roe and Metz,[3] and Dorfman, Berbaum, Lenth et al.[5] In these figures, the 95% probability band about the nominal alpha level is shown as the band between the two horizontal lines at 0.040 and 0.060 for α = 0.05. The boundaries we selected are standard critical values for 95% probability bands for a binomially distributed random variable derived from the normal approximation to the binomial distribution when the sample size n is large and the binomial probability p is known.[6] The boundaries define a 5% rejection region for the null hypothesis that alpha is a specified value, and that empirical Type I error rate follows a binomial distribution with parameters n = 2000 and p = 0.05.

In this paper, we focus on equal allocation ratios. The split-plot design on readers appears to perform somewhat better than the split-plot design on cases. The top panel of Figures 1 and 2 (A_z = 0.702 and 0.855, split-plot on readers) shows that the Monte Carlo data points fell, for the most part, within the 95% probability band when the number of cases was at least a hundred (50+/50−), or the number of readers per modality was at least ten. With fewer than a hundred cases and fewer than ten readers per modality, the statistical test was slightly conservative. The bottom panel of Figures 1 and 2 (A_z = 0.702 and 0.855, split-plot on cases) shows that the Monte Carlo data points fell, for the most part, within the 95% probability band when there are ten readers. With fewer than ten readers, the statistical test was slightly conservative.

Figure 3 (A_z = 0.961) shows that the Monte Carlo data points almost always fell outside the 95% probability band. For both split-plot designs, 200 cases was sufficient to keep the points either within the band or close to it. With 100 cases, the test was somewhat conservative; with 50 cases, the test was quite conservative.

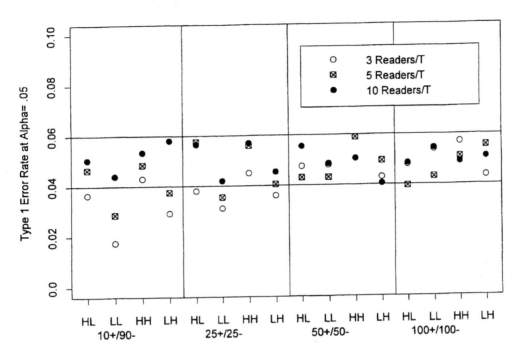

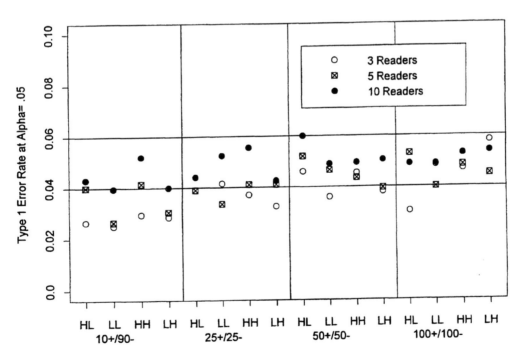

Figure 1: Split-plot results on readers (top) and cases (bottom) for A_z=.702, and nominal α=.05.

Split-plot Design(on readers) for Az=.855

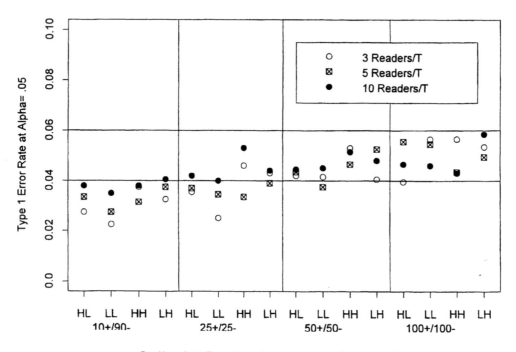

Split-plot Design (on cases) for Az=0.855

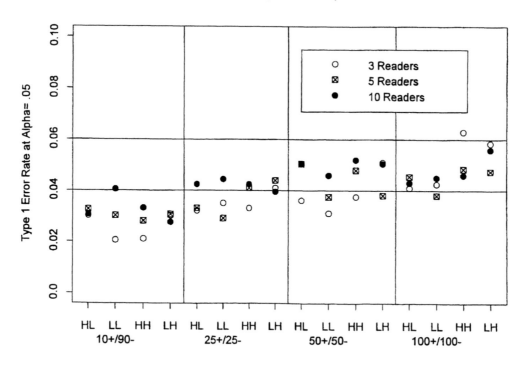

Figure 2: Split-plot results on readers (top) and cases (bottom) for A_z=.855, and nominal α=.05.

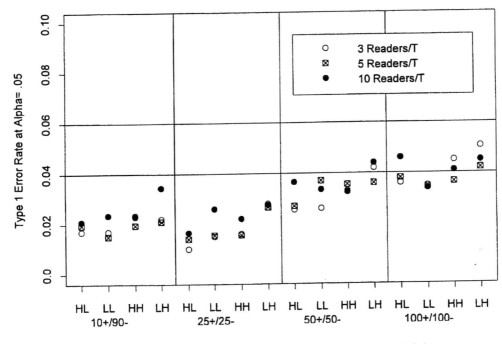

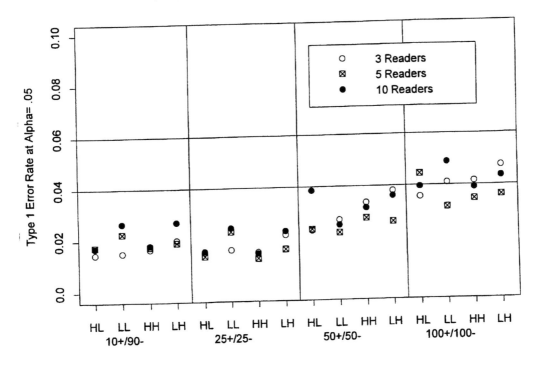

Figure 3: Split-plot results on readers (top) and cases (bottom) for A_z=.961, and nominal α=.05.

4. DISCUSSION

Our Monte Carlo simulations show that the DBM multireader method can be validly extended to the reader-split and case-split plot designs. The results suggest that the DBM method provides trustworthy alpha levels with discrete ratings when ROC area is not too large, and case and reader sample sizes are not too small. In other situations, the test tends to be conservative. A statistical test is conservative if the empirical Type I error rate level is smaller than the nominal alpha level. If one rejects the null hypothesis at a specified nominal alpha level, a conservative statistical test is preferred to a liberal test because it has a lower Type I error rate. The Monte Carlo data showed that the statistical test generally becomes more conservative with large area and decreasing case sample size.

In our previous Monte Carlo validation of the DBM multireader method in a fully crossed factorial design as well as in these reader and case split-plot studies, we used discrete rating scales. Pseudo-continuous rating scales have been recommended over discrete scales for routine use in ROC studies in diagnostic radiology primarily because it was concluded that pseudo-continuous rating scales were less likely to yield binormal degenerate data sets than discrete rating scales.[7,8] Binormal degenerate data sets are no longer an issue in ROC analysis.[9-11] Moreover, the empirical evidence suggests that discrete and pseudo-continuous scales can often be used interchangeably in image evaluation studies when the investigator is interested in ROC area because they produce virtually the same results.[7] If, however, the experimenter is interested in the operating points as well ROC area, then discrete rating scales should be used.[5] Sensitivity and specificity are determined by the location of the operating points on the ROC curve as well as by the discriminability of the underlying distributions of normal and abnormal cases on the latent decision dimension. The operating points are determined by decision thresholds, and in clinical trials, these decision thresholds are, in fact, action thresholds. For instance, in the American College of Radiology Breast Imaging Reporting and Data System (BI-RADS), "probably benign finding" translates into the course of action "short interval followup suggested," "suspicious abnormality" translates into the course of action "biopsy should be considered," and "highly suggestive of malignancy" translates into "appropriate action should be taken".[12] Some diagnostic imaging systems may lead to more conservative or liberal actions than others. For example, a concern with algorithms for computer-aided diagnosis (CAD) is that they seem to give too many false positives.[13] If the radiologist's decision thresholds are changed by the rate of CAD false positives, changes in sensitivity and specificity would occur, but would not be observed with LABROC-type algorithms that sort pseudo-continuous rating data into discrete uniformly distributed categories.[14,15] Because the category boundaries defined by such algorithms do not correspond to the decision thresholds used by the observers both within and between modalities, conclusions about radiologist performance might be drawn based solely on the ROC area, while inappropriately ignoring the differences in true and false positive fractions associated with the observers' operating points.[5]

5. CONCLUSIONS

Our Monte Carlo simulations show that the DBM multireader method can be validly extended to reader-split and case-split plot designs.

6. ACKNOWLEDGMENTS

Supported in part by National Institutes of Health grants R01 CA 62362 (D.D.D., K.S.B., R.V.L., Y-F.C.), and R01 CA 42453 (D.D.D and K.S.B.) and in part by US Army Medical Research and Materiel Command grant DAMD17-96-1-6254 (D.D.D., K.S.B., R.V.L.).

7. REFERENCES

1. Dorfman DD, Berbaum KS, Metz CE. Receiver operating characteristic rating analysis: generalization to the population of readers and patients with the jackknife method. Invest Radiol 1992; 27:723-731.
2. Obuchowski NA, Zepp RC. Simple steps for improving multiple-reader studies in radiology. AJR 1996; 166:517-521.
3. Roe CA, Metz CE. The Dorfman-Berbaum-Metz method for statistical analysis of multi-reader, multi-modality ROC data: Validation by computer simulation. Acad Radiol 1997; 4:298-303.
4. Swets JA, Pickett RM. Evaluation of Diagnostic Systems: Methods from Signal Detection Theory. New York, NY: Academic Press, 1982.
5. DD Dorfman, KS Berbaum, RV Lenth, Y-F Chen, BA Donaghy. Monte Carlo validation of a multireader method for receiver operating characteristic discrete rating data: Factorial experimental design. Academic Radiology 1998;5:591-602.
6. Snedecor GW, Cochran WG. Statistical Methods. (Eighth Edition). Ames, IA: Iowa State University, 1989.
7. Rockette HE, Gur D, Metz CE. The use of continuous and discrete confidence judgments in receiver operating characteristic studies of diagnostic imaging techniques. Invest Radiol 1992; 27:169-172.
8. King JL, Britton CA, Gur D, Rockette HE, Davis PL. On the validity of the continuous and discrete confidence rating scales in receiver operating characteristic studies. Invest Radiol 1993; 28:962-963.
9. Dorfman DD, Berbaum KS. Degeneracy and discrete ROC rating data. Acad Radiol 1995; 2:907-915.
10. Dorfman DD, Berbaum KS, Metz CE, Lenth RV, Hanley JA, Abu-Dagga H. Proper receiver operating characteristic analysis: The bigamma model. Acad Radiol 1997; 4:138-149.
11. Pan X, Metz CE. The "proper" binormal model: Parametric receiver operating characteristic curve estimation with degenerate data. Acad Radiol 1997; 4:380-389.
12. Breast imaging - reporting and data system (BI-RADS). Reston, VA.: American College of Radiology, 1993.
13. Yoshida H, Doi K, Nishikawa RM, Giger ML, Schmidt RA. An improved computer-assisted diagnostic scheme using wavelet transform for detecting clustered microcalcifications in digital mammograms. Acad Radiol 1996; 3:621-7.
14. Metz CE, Shen JH, Herman BA. New methods for estimating a binormal ROC curve from continuously-distributed test results. Presented at the 1990 Joint Statistical Meetings of the American Statistical Association and the Biometric Society, Anaheim, CA, August, 1990.
15. Vittitoe NF, Baker JA, Floyd CE Jr. Fractal texture analysis in computer-aided diagnosis of solitary pulmonary nodules. Acad Radiol 1997;4:96-101.

Gains in Accuracy from Averaging Ratings of Abnormality

Richard G. Swensson*, Jill L. King, David Gur, Walter F. Good

Department of Radiology, University of Pittsburgh, Pittsburgh, PA 15261

ABSTRACT

Six radiologists used continuous scales to rate 529 chest-film cases for likelihood of five separate types of abnormalities (interstitial disease, nodules, pneumothorax, alveolar infiltrates and rib fractures) in each of six replicated readings, yielding 36 separate ratings of each case for the five abnormalities. Analyses for each type of abnormality estimated the relative gains in accuracy (area below the ROC curve) obtained by averaging the case-ratings across: a) six independent replications by each reader (30% gain), b) six different readers within each replication (39% gain) or c) all 36 readings (58% gain). Although accuracy differed among both readers and abnormalities, ROC curves for the median ratings showed similar relative gains in accuracy. From a latent-variable model for these gains, we estimate that about 51% of a reader's total decision variance consisted of random (within-reader) errors that were uncorrelated between replications, another 14% came from that reader's consistent (but idiosyncratic) responses to different cases, and only about 35% could be attributed to systematic variations among the sampled cases that were consistent across different readers.

Keywords: observer variability, accuracy, between-reader, within-reader effects, ROC analysis

1. INTRODUCTION

Observer performance with medical images is often measured by Receiver Operating Characteristic (ROC) curves obtained when readers are asked to rate both normal and abnormal images for likelihood of abnormality. Performance accuracy depends on the individual reader, as well as on the samples of normal and abnormal cases, and is typically estimated by the area below the fitted ROC curve (A_z). The standard procedure for fitting binormal ROC curves assumes that a reader's ratings are determined by an underlying latent variable that is normally distributed with different parameters for the normal and abnormal cases.[1,2] Estimates of performance accuracy (like A_z) vary, both between readers and between a reader's own replicated decisions, presumably because the human observer contributes some additional perceptual variation to the latent variable realized for different cases. These observer effects are generally assumed to include both: a) random sources of variation within each reader and b) idiosyncratic case interpretations that differ between readers.[3,4,5]

One implication of observer variations in different ratings of the cases is a potential for improving the accuracy of classifications by reducing the magnitude of those variations.[6,7] Since all unsystematic variations are reduced by averaging, a suitable non-linear averaging of the different ratings assigned to an individual case should increase the accuracy for an ROC curve that is generated from such averaged ratings. A within-reader average (WR) of the ratings an individual observer assigns to a particular case in replicated readings will reduce any inconsistent rating variations produced by random sources of variation within that observer—i.e., internal "observer noise." For this reason, sets of these WR ratings should generate an ROC curve that provides more accurate differentiation between the abnormal and normal cases (a larger A_z) than the ROC curves from a reader's single ratings of those cases.

A between-reader average (BR) of the ratings that different individual readers assigned to a particular case serves to reduce, not only the inconsistent variations from WR sources, but also any other variations in ratings that might represent consistently different interpretations by those individual readers. To the extent that even readers of equal ability will differ idiosyncratically in evaluating specific cases, then the BR ratings from n different readers would generally retain even less unsystematic variation across cases than the WR ratings from n replicated readings by the same observer. Consequently, an ROC curve generated from BR ratings (of n readers) should distinguish more accurately between the abnormal and normal cases than an ROC curve from WR ratings (of n replications). The following section presents an orthogonal-components model for the observer variance that quantifies the expected gains in measured performance accuracy (A_z) from different ways of averaging the case ratings. We tested those predictions, and estimated the relative-variance components, using reader performance data collected in a large previous study of chest-film cases evaluated for five separate types of abnormalities.

Correspondence: Email: rswensson@radserv.arad.upmc.edu; Telephone: 412 648-3148; Fax: 412 648-9127

100

Part of the SPIE Conference on Image Perception and Performance
San Diego, California • February 1999
SPIE Vol. 3663 • 0277-786X/99/$10.00

2. OBSERVER MODEL FOR TOTAL RATING VARIANCE

The standard ROC analysis represents an observer's latent variable (X_i) for the ratings of normal or abnormal cases as being sampled from different normal distributions with respective means and standard deviations (μ_n, σ_n) or (μ_a, σ_a). In this general binormal model, the area below the ROC curve is given by $A_z = \Phi(Z_a)$, the lower-tail area of the cumulative standard normal distribution with Z_a defined as:

$$Z_a \equiv \frac{\mu_a - \mu_n}{\sqrt{\sigma_a^2 + \sigma_n^2}} = \frac{A}{\sqrt{1 + B^2}}, \tag{1}$$

where $A \equiv (\mu_a - \mu_n)/\sigma_a$ and $B \equiv \sigma_n/\sigma_a$ are the two scale-independent binormal parameters estimated by the maximum-likelihood fitting procedure.[1,2] For values of Z_a equal to 0.0, 0.25, 0.5, 1.0, 1.5 and 2.0, corresponding values of the index A_z are 0.50, 0.599, 0.691, 0.841, 0.933 and 0.977. In multi-task interpretations,[8] observers rate all cases for several different types of abnormalities that may be either present or absent, but the ratings for each separate type of abnormality are generally assumed to be independent and are fitted by separate ROC analyses that estimate different parameters (including Z_a and A_z) for each type of abnormality.

To include explicit observer effects in this binormal model, the normal rating variable for a given type of abnormality may be expanded as a sum of assumed orthogonal components, $X_{i,j,k,m} = \mu_{i,k} + c_{i,j} + r_{i,j,k} + e_{i,j,k,m}$, where $X_{i,j,k,m}$ represents the realized value obtained by Reader k for individual Case j within case-sample i ($i = a$ or n) in any single interpretation m. This is similar to the model proposed by Metz and Shen.[6] The component $c_{i,j}$ is a deviation associated with a particular individual case (the jth case in sample i), which remains constant whenever that case gets evaluated by any reader for the specific abnormality in question. It is assumed to be normally distributed with zero mean and standard deviation σ_i across the cases within sample i. The term $r_{i,j,k}$ represents an idiosyncratic deviation that Reader k adds for this particular individual case, assumed to be normally distributed across the cases with zero mean and standard deviation $\sigma r_{i,k}$. The term $e_{i,j,k,m}$ represents a random (within-reader) deviation that Reader k adds to the realized variable for each rating judgment, and is assumed to be normally distributed with zero mean and standard deviation $\sigma e_{i,k}$. In this expanded binormal model, the rating variable for Reader k has variances $\sigma_{n,k}^2 \equiv \sigma_{n,c}^2 + \sigma r_{n,k}^2 + \sigma e_{n,k}^2$ and $\sigma_{a,k}^2 \equiv \sigma_{a,c}^2 + \sigma r_{a,k}^2 + \sigma e_{a,k}^2$ for the respective samples of normal and abnormal cases.

Since the linear scale of measurement is always arbitrary, it is convenient to set $\mu_{n,k} = 0$ and $\mu_{a,k} = 1.0$ (assuming that $Z_a > 0$), so that $\sigma_{n,k} = B_k/A_k$ and $\sigma_{a,k} = 1/A_k$. Then the accuracy index of Eq. 1 can be written for Reader k as:

$$Z_k = \frac{\mu_{a,k} - \mu_{n,k}}{\sqrt{\sigma_{n,k}^2 + \sigma_{a,k}^2}} = \frac{1}{\sqrt{\sigma_c^2 + \sigma_{r,k}^2 + \sigma_{e,k}^2}}, \text{ where } \sigma_c^2 = \sigma_{n,c}^2 + \sigma_{a,c}^2,$$

$$\sigma_{r,k}^2 = \sigma r_{n,k}^2 + \sigma r_{a,k}^2 \text{ and } \sigma_{e,k}^2 = \sigma e_{n,k}^2 + \sigma e_{a,k}^2. \tag{2}$$

The squared reciprocal value of Z_k estimates the *total variance* in the latent rating variable across these case samples for Reader k.

2.1 Gains in Accuracy from Averaging Ratings of Cases

Consider an experiment in which each of K individual readers performed M separate replicated readings in which they independently rated the same samples of normal and abnormal cases. The ratings assigned to each individual case could then be averaged: a) *within-readers* (WR[k]), across the M separate replications by a single reader k, b) *between-readers* (BR[m]), across the K separate readers for a single replication m, or c) *both between and within readers* (WxB), across all the MK separate readings of each case. Each process of averaging would serve to reduce the amount of variability from all the unsystematic components of those particular quantities being averaged. Since the averaged values for individual cases would have a reduced variability within both the normal and abnormal samples (compared to the original values), the resulting ROC curve would yield a higher level of accuracy for differentiating between these two case samples. If one could measure and average the actual values of each reader's latent rating variable for the individual cases, then the variance of each unsystematic component would decrease in proportion to the number of values being averaged.

For the WR means obtained from an individual Reader k, Eq. 2 would then become:

$$Z(\text{WR}[k]) = [\sigma_c^2 + \sigma_{r,k}^2 + \sigma_{e,k}^2 / M]^{-1/2} = Z_k \left[1 - \left(\frac{M-1}{M}\right) \frac{\sigma_{e,k}^2}{\sigma_c^2 + \sigma_{r,k}^2 + \sigma_{e,k}^2}\right]^{-1/2}. \tag{3}$$

Equation 3 shows that the expected gain in this linear index of accuracy from averaging M replicated readings is proportional to Z_k, and it depends on the fraction of the total rating variance contributed by the random *within-reader* variations. This same formal representation and interpretation of the variance components is maintained for the average of readers by taking appropriate (reciprocal root mean squared) averages of these $Z(WR[k])$ and Z_k values across all the K different readers:

$$\overline{Z}(\text{WR}) \equiv \left[\frac{1}{K} \sum_k \frac{1}{Z(\text{WR}[k])^2} \right]^{-1/2}$$

$$= [\sigma_c^2 + \overline{\sigma}_r^2 + \overline{\sigma}_e^2 / M]^{-1/2} = \overline{Z} \left[1 - \left(\frac{M-1}{M} \right) \frac{\overline{\sigma}_e^2}{\sigma_c^2 + \overline{\sigma}_r^2 + \overline{\sigma}_e^2} \right]^{-1/2} , \qquad (4)$$

$$\text{where } \overline{\sigma}_r^2 \equiv \sum_k \sigma_{r,k}^2 / K, \quad \overline{\sigma}_e^2 \equiv \sum_k \sigma_{e,k}^2 / K \quad \text{and} \quad \overline{Z} \equiv \left[\frac{1}{KM} \sum_{k,m} \frac{1}{Z_{k,m}^2} \right]^{-1/2}$$

The same definitions and notation can also be used to express the expected effects from the two other procedures for averaging these ratings, the BR means across K different readers and the WxR means across all KM separate readings of each individual case. For these averaging procedures Eq. 2 becomes:

$$Z(\text{BR}[m]) = \left[\sigma_c^2 + \frac{\overline{\sigma}_r^2 + \overline{\sigma}_e^2}{K} \right]^{-1/2} = \overline{Z} \left[1 - \left(\frac{K-1}{K} \right) \frac{\overline{\sigma}_r^2 + \overline{\sigma}_e^2}{\sigma_c^2 + \overline{\sigma}_r^2 + \overline{\sigma}_e^2} \right]^{-1/2} \qquad (5)$$

$$\text{and} \quad Z(\text{WxB}) = \left[\sigma_c^2 + \frac{\overline{\sigma}_r^2}{K} + \frac{\overline{\sigma}_e^2}{KM} \right]^{-1/2} = \overline{Z} \left[\frac{\overline{Z}^2}{\overline{Z}^2(\text{BR})} + \frac{1}{K} \left(\frac{\overline{Z}^2}{\overline{Z}^2(\text{WR})} - 1 \right) \right]^{-1/2} \qquad (6)$$

Equation 5 shows that, just as for $Z(\text{WR}[k])$, the gain measured for $Z(\text{BR}[m])$ is proportional to the overall level of accuracy in the original readings; but it depends on the fraction of the total rating variance contributed by *all* types of reader variations, both consistent (idiosyncratic) effects and inconsistent (random) effects. The complementary fraction of that total rating variance (from only the component σ_c^2) can be attributed to variations in perceived likelihood of abnormality among the sampled normal and abnormal cases that remain consistent for all readers. Equation 6 shows that the gain for WxB averaging should be larger than (but predicted by) the two relative gains measured for the separate WR and BR procedures.

Equations 4 and 5 can also be used to partition the total variance in the assumed latent rating variables into the estimated fractions that can be attributed to the three orthogonal components. Each fraction of the total variance in an average of the readers is calculated from the estimated relative gain in accuracy for $Z(\text{WR})$, for $Z(\text{BR})$ or for both. From $Z(\text{WR})/Z$, Eq. 7 estimates the fraction of random variance that was inconsistent across the same observer's replicated readings of a given case. From $Z(\text{BR})/Z$, Eq. 8 estimates the fraction of total variance attributable to those variations in perceived abnormality among the normal and abnormal cases that remained consistent across all the different readers. The remaining fraction (given directly by Eq. 9) estimates the relative amount of total variance attributable to idiosyncratic effects that remained consistent across each observer's replicated ratings of the cases, but were inconsistent from one reader to another.

$$\frac{\overline{\sigma}_e^2}{\sigma_c^2 + \overline{\sigma}_r^2 + \overline{\sigma}_e^2} = \frac{M}{M-1} \left(1 - \frac{Z^2}{Z^2(\text{WR})} \right) \qquad (7)$$

$$\frac{\sigma_c^2}{\sigma_c^2 + \overline{\sigma}_r^2 + \overline{\sigma}_e^2} = 1 - \frac{K}{K-1} \left(1 - \frac{Z^2}{Z^2(\text{BR})} \right) \qquad (8)$$

$$\frac{\overline{\sigma}_r^2}{\sigma_c^2 + \overline{\sigma}_r^2 + \overline{\sigma}_e^2} = \frac{K}{K-1} \left(1 - \frac{Z^2}{Z^2(\text{BR})} \right) - \frac{M}{M-1} \left(1 - \frac{Z^2}{Z^2(\text{WR})} \right) \qquad (9)$$

2.2 Median-Averaging of Ordinal Ratings

Of course, one cannot actually average the values of an observer's latent perceptual variable, but only the judgments made explicit in the ratings assigned to the individual cases. Whether those explicit judgments are made on a continuous rating scale or grouped into discrete categories, however, the maximum-likelihood fitting procedure only requires the same *orderings of cases* in the assigned ratings as in the (presumed-binormal) latent values. The estimated binormal parameters remain unaffected by any positive monotonic transformation of the underlying linear variable onto this output scale. The median provides an appropriate statistic for averaging across the separate ordinal ratings of a given case, because it is unaffected by any non-linear (but monotonic) mapping from the assumed-normal variable to the observable scale of ratings. But the median has less statistical efficiency than the mean for reducing any uncorrelated errors present in normal samples. The statistical efficiency of the median (relative to the mean) decreases slightly with the number of sampled values, from 0.743 (median of 3) to an asymptote of 0.637.[9]

This consideration suggests that, whenever Eqs. 3-9 are applied to median-averaged ratings, the values of M, K and MK should each be multiplied by some efficiency factor less than unity. That modification would maintain the same proportional forms for the expected gains (Eqs.3–6), but it would change the estimated fractional components of the total rating variance (Eqs. 7–9) and the prediction for Z(WxB) in Eq. 6. For the BR medians of ratings across different readers, the above equations assume that all the readers used similar non-linear mappings from their latent rating variables to the output rating scale.

3. METHODS

3.1 Database of Chest-Film Readings

A previous large-scale observer study collected rating data from six radiologists who read a series of 529 chest film cases (124 normal, 405 abnormal) in each of six separate conditions. These films contained a total of 602 abnormal findings, representing five different types of clinical abnormalities: interstitial disease (n = 149), pulmonary nodules (n = 181), pneumothorax (n = 119), alveolar infiltrates (n = 77) and rib fractures (n = 76). Although most of the 405 abnormal cases contained only a single lesion (253 cases), 111 cases contained two separate abnormalities and 41 cases contained more than two different lesions. Each abnormal finding had been verified using positive follow-up information from the patient's primary medical records (surgical reports, biopsies, laboratory results or other imaging studies like chest CT), and from the patient's clinical status. For the 124 normal cases, information from negative follow-up examinations (radiological or physical) was used to verify that these patients had subsequently remained disease-free over sufficient time-intervals for the relevant types of abnormalities. Similar information verified the absence of any additional lesions in cases found to be actually positive for the specific abnormalities.

The chest films were digitized at 100 μm resolution with a dynamic range of 12 bits, subjected to varying amounts of image compression (6 levels, from 1:1 to 1:60), and then printed at full size on films by a laser printer that reproduced the same contrast response as the original films. In every reading of an individual case, radiologists gave separate ratings of likelihood for each of the five different types of abnormalities. These judgments were made by adjusting the position of a pointer on a continuous, unmarked ordinal scale, recorded as 100 digital units. Previous ROC analyses of these rating data found no evidence for any systematic changes in detection accuracy (A_z) across the six different levels of image compression for any of the five types of abnormalities. Consequently, the present analyses of these data treat an observer's ratings of abnormality in the separate image-compression conditions simply as six independently replicated readings of the same 529 chest films.

3.2 Data Analyses and Median Ratings

Independent data analyses were performed for each of the five different types of abnormalities that the readers had separately evaluated and rated on each case. For each abnormality, the six different readers and six reading conditions had produced a total of 36 sets of ratings on the 529 cases. An additional 13 sets of data were obtained by taking the medians across separate ratings of the given abnormality for each individual case. Six within-reader (WR) sets took medians of each reader's ratings across the six separate replications, six between-reader (BR) sets took medians across the six readers within each replication and one overall (WxB) set of data took the median of all 36 ratings. All statistical analyses of the ROC curves for these sets of rating data used a maximum-likelihood procedure[10] called "LABROC," which assumes an underlying binomial ROC curve and fits ratings that are measured on a continuous scale. For each of the five abnormalities, separate analyses estimated 36 values of $Z_{k,m}$ from the sets of single-rating data, and the different values of Z(WR[k]), Z(BR[m]) and Z(WxB) from the sets of median-rating data. For one reader, the LABROC procedure was unable to fit the WR median ratings of pneumothorax because that performance was too accurate (the single-rating A_z was 0.964). All statistical averaging of estimated quantities applied the reciprocal procedure defined in Eq. 4. That procedure obtained the six values of Z_k, six values of Z_m and values of Z, Z(WR) and Z(BR) for each separate type of abnormality, as well as their average values across the five types of abnormalities.

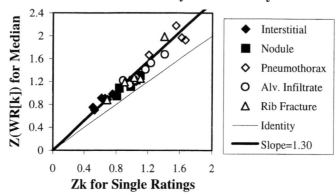

Fig. 1 Gains in Accuracy from within-reader medians of ratings for five types of abnormalities by six individual readers.

4. RESULTS

4.1 Gains in Accuracy

Figure 1 shows the relative gains in accuracy obtained from within-reader averaging of the ratings assigned to each of the five types of abnormalities; it plots $Z(WR[k])$, a reader's median-rating accuracy, against the averaged accuracy of that reader's single ratings (Z_k) for each type of abnormality. Although the absolute levels of performance accuracy varied considerably from one reader to another, and across the five different types of abnormalities, the relative gains in accuracy remained quite similar for all readers and abnormalities. The data in Fig. 1 are well described by a single proportional line with slope 1.30 (30% relative grain), which is the ratio of $Z(WR[k])$, when averaged across both readers and abnormalities, to the similar average for Z_k. According to Eq. 3, this constant relative gain of 30% for the WR medians implies that all six readers had about the same relative amounts of inconsistent (intra-reader) variations in their ratings, regardless of the measured performance accuracy—either its absolute level or relative to other readers. This "observer noise" component of random variation must have been scaled from one type of abnormality to another (along with the total variation in sampled cases), because it remained a constant fraction of the total variance in each reader's underlying rating variable.

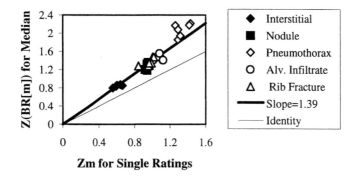

Fig. 2 Gains in Accuracy from Between-Reader Median Ratings of Five Abnormalities within Six Separate Conditions.

Figure 2 shows the relative gains in accuracy obtained from the between-reader medians of ratings for each type of abnormality; the 30 data points plot $Z(BR[m])$ against Z_m within each of the six replicated conditions for all five abnormalities. In the absence of systematic reader variations in accuracy, Fig. 2 more clearly shows the large differences in performance accuracy for the different types of abnormalities in these case samples. Detection accuracy was lowest for cases with interstitial disease, highest for cases of pneumothorax and intermediate for those with nodules, alveolar infiltrates and rib fractures. The line with slope 1.39 in Fig. 2 represents a ratio of the averaged values for $Z(BR[m])$ to those for Z_m, and it would estimate a single relative gain in accuracy of 39% for the BR median ratings of all five abnormalities. That single value of 39%, however, considerably underestimates the relative gain of 55% obtained for the BR medians when different readers had rated the cases for likelihood of pneumothorax. Together with the data in Fig., 1, this particular result suggests that the case-to-case variations from consistent but idiosyncratic ratings by different readers (reduced in BR medians, but not in WR medians) were somewhat larger when these readers were asked to evaluate the chest-film cases for pneumothorax.

Averaged Gains in Accuracy for Five Abnormalities

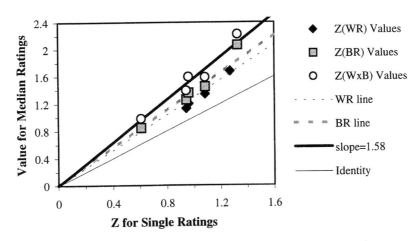

Fig. 3 Averaged Gains in Accuracy from Median Ratings Obtained by the WR, BR and WxB Procedures for the Five Types of Abnormalities

Figure 3 compares the relative gains in accuracy from all three procedures that averaged the ratings of cases, plotting the values of $Z(WR)$, $Z(BR)$ and $Z(WxB)$ against the single-rating value of Z for each of the five types of abnormalities. The slope of 1.58 for the heavy solid line in Fig. 3 is given by the ratio of the averaged values of $Z(WxB)$ to the averaged values of Z. For each of the five types of abnormalities, a single value of 58% closely estimates the relative gain in accuracy obtained by taking a WxB median of all 36 separate ratings of every case. This measured relative gain of 58% is predicted reasonably well by Eq. 6, from the gains estimated for WR medians (30%) and BR medians (39%), provided that K is adjusted (from 6 to 4.09) to compensate for the decreased statistical efficiency of median averaging. The relative gain of 55% predicted with this adjustment is slightly smaller than the measured value of 58%, but Eq. 6 without adjustment predicts an even smaller gain of only 49%.

4.2 Estimated fractions of rating variance

Table 1 presents estimated fractions of the total variance in readers' latent rating variables that could be attributed to each of the model's three orthogonal components for the five different types of abnormalities. These three fractions were calculated (using Eqs. 7–9) from the relative gains in accuracy obtained by the WR and BR averaging of the case ratings for a given abnormality. The median adjustment assumed that a median of ratings was less efficient than a mean would be for reducing the uncorrelated errors in readers' latent variables. This adjustment slightly increased the estimated fractions of random reader variance and it decreased the fractions attributed to the systematic variations in ratings of cases across all readers. The three estimated fractions of total rating variance were fairly similar across the five different abnormalities, about 51% attributed to random effects for the adjusted estimates, about 14% to idiosyncratic reader effects and only about 35%

attributed to case-sample effects. The random variations were largest (63%) in the ratings of interstitial disease, which also had the lowest accuracy (i.e., the largest total variance). Individual readers were then about as inconsistent with their own repeated ratings as with those made by other readers. The ratings of pneumothorax, which had the highest accuracy for most readers, produced both the smallest fraction of variance from consistent case-sample effects (22%) and the largest fraction from idiosyncratic reader effects (21%).

Table 1

Estimated Fractions of Total Rating Variance from Case-Sample Effects, Consistent Reader Effects and Random Errors for the Five Types of Abnormalities

Type of Abnormality	Adjusted for Median*			Not Adjusted for Median*		
	Random	Readers	Cases	Random	Readers	Cases
Interstitial Disease	0.628	0.008	0.365	0.569	0.007	0.424
Nodule	0.403	0.180	0.418	0.365	0.163	0.472
Pneumothorax	0.564	0.211	0.225	0.512	0.191	0.297
Alveolar Infiltrate	0.464	0.124	0.412	0.420	0.113	0.467
Rib Fracture	0.478	0.186	0.336	0.334	0.169	0.397
Mean Values	0.507	0.142	0.351	0.460	0.128	0.412

* Unadjusted estimates were obtained from Eqs. 7–9 as given; estimates adjusted for the decreased efficiency of medians had each value of M and K in Eqs. 7–9 multiplied by 0.682.

5. DISCUSSION

5.1 Accuracy Gains and Observer Inconsistencies

A few previous studies have measured the accuracy gains obtained as a result of averaging judgments made about the same image samples, either from different individual readers,[6,11,12] or from the same observer in independent readings.[7] Those studies invariably found gains in accuracy for the average of ratings (compared to the mean accuracy for single ratings), demonstrating the presence of substantial inconsistent variation in the rating judgments both between and within observers. Other studies have used various procedures to measure the relative amounts of consistent and inconsistent ("internal noise") variations present in an observer's detection decisions about noise-limited visual or auditory stimuli.[13,14,15] Such studies have estimated that, in the latent variable that underlies an observer's decisions or ratings, between 35% and about 60% of the total variance is inconsistent across independently replicated judgments. The smaller estimates of inconsistency tend to come from psychophysical tasks that observers perform relatively efficiently (compared to "ideal" performance),[7,15] whereas more inconsistency seems to be measured when the observer's perceptual efficiency is low—even if the task permits reasonably high levels of performance accuracy.[7,16]

As seen in Table 1 of the present study, the estimated amount of inconsistent rating variation from random intra-reader sources ranged between 40% and 63% across the five different types of abnormalities, with a mean value of 51%. Figure 1 shows that the proportional gains in accuracy (from reducing those inconsistencies in the averaged ratings) remained similar across both readers and abnormalities, despite large changes in the absolute levels of performance accuracy. Total variance in a reader's latent rating variable is defined as an inverse function of the estimated accuracy (see Eq. 2). This means that the similar proportional gains in Fig. 1 produce similar fractions of estimated inconsistent variance for the different readers and for the different types of abnormalities.

5.2 Design Implications for Observer Studies

The estimated relative fractions of total rating variance from the three orthogonal components can have implications for the design of observer performance studies intended to compare alternative display modalities or imaging techniques. In such studies, investigators wish to control and hold constant any sources of variation that might affect the measured performance accuracy, so that even small differences in accuracy can be reliably detected. Variability associated with the particular samples of cases can be controlled by using the same cases for all the modalities or techniques being studied, and variability between different samples of readers can be controlled by using the same readers for all conditions. One can anticipate the statistical gains that may be obtained from using these two control procedures by considering the relative amounts of variance estimated for the orthogonal components of the present observer model. Across the five types of abnormalities rated in these chest-film cases, however, roughly half of the total variance in a reader's decision variable was estimated to be uncontrollable error—coming from intra-reader sources of random variation that were uncorrelated from one time of interpretation to another. This large within-reader variation of about 50% severely limits how much the sensitivity of an observer study could be improved, even by designs that used *both* the same readers and the same case samples in all conditions. Those control procedures could not decrease the standard error for a difference in estimated A_z below about $1/\sqrt{2}$ = 0.71 of what its value would be for the same readers with new samples of cases.

For most types of chest-film abnormalities, the fraction of decision variance attributable to case samples (reproduced by all readers) was more than twice as large as the average amount from idiosyncratic reader effects (not reproduced by different readers). That result suggests that, in comparing performance accuracy between two different conditions, it should be substantially more beneficial to have the same sample of cases rated by different readers in the two conditions than to have the same individual readers rate different case samples—provided, of course, that those different readers were matched for their levels of accuracy. By using the same individual readers in both conditions, however, an investigator automatically controls for possible differences in readers' overall accuracy, as well as for any idiosyncratic variations in interpreting the particular individual cases.

ACKNOWLEDGMENTS

Support for this work was provided by NIH Grants CA66594, CA67947 and CA62800.

REFERENCES

1. D. D Dorfman and E. Alf, "Maximum-likelihood estimation of parameters of signal-detection theory and determination of confidence intervals—rating-method data," *J. Math. Psychol.*, **6**, pp.487–496, 1969.
2. C. E. Metz, "Some pratical issues of experimental design and data analysis in radiological ROC studies," *Invest. Radiol.*, **24**, pp. 234–245, 1989.
3. J. A. Swets and R. M. Pickett, *Evaluation of Diagnostic Systems: Methods from Signal Detection Theory*, New York, Academic Press, 1982.
4. N. A. Obuchowski, "Multireader receiver operating characteristic studies: A comparison of study designs," *Acad. Radiol.*, **2**. pp. 709–716, 1995.
5. C. A. Roe and C. E. Metz, "Variance-component modeling in the analysis of receiver operating characteristic index estimates," *Acad. Radiol.*, **4**, pp. 587–600, 1997.
6. C. E. Metz and J–H. Shen, "Gains in accuracy from replicated readings of diagnostic images: Prediction and assessment in terms of ROC analysis," *Med. Dec. Making*, **12**, pp. 60–75, 1992.
7. R. G. Swensson and P. F. Judy, "Measuring performance efficiency and consistency in visual discriminations with noisy images," *J. Exp. Psychol.: Hum. Percept. Perf.*, **22**, pp. 1393–1415, 1996.
8. R. S. Slasky, D. Gur, W. F. Good, M. A. Costa-Greco, K. M. Harris, L. A. Cooperstein and H. E. Rockette, "Receiver operating characteristic analysis of chest image interpretation with conventional, laser-printed, and high-resolution workstation images," *Radiology*, **174**, pp. 775-780, 1990.
9. M. G. Kendall and A. Stuart, *The Advanced Theory of Statistics: Vol. 2*, Chas. Griffin, London, p. 7, 1973.
10. C.E. Metz, B. A. Herman and J–H. Shen, "Maximum likelihood estimation of receiver operating characteristic (ROC) curves from continuously-distributed data" *Stat. in Med.*, **17**, pp. 1033–1053, 1998.
11. A. Baumstark, R. G. Swensson, S. J. Hessel, D. C. Levin, W. Grossman, J. T. Mann, III and H. L. Abrams, "Evaluating the radiographic assessment of pulmonary venous hypertension in chronic heart disease," *Amer. J. Roent.*, **141**, pp. 877–884, 1984.
12. P. F. Judy and R. G. Swensson, "Display thresholding of images and observer detection performance," *J. Opt. Soc. Amer.*, **A4**, pp. 954–965, 1987.
13. D. M. Green, "Consistency of auditory detection judgments," *Psychol. Rev.*, **71**, pp. 392–407, 1964.
14. M. F. Spiegel and D. M. Green, "Two procedures for estimating internal noise," *J. Acoust. Soc. Amer.*, **70**, pp. 69–73, 1981.
15. A. E. Burgess and B. Colborne, "Visual signal detection: IV. Observer inconsistency," *J. Opt. Soc. Amer.*, **A5**, pp. 617–627, 1988.
16. S. E. Seltzer, P. F. Judy, R. G. Swensson, K. H. Chan, and R. D. Nawfel, "Flattening of the contrast-detail curve for large lesions on liver CT images," *Med. Phy.*, **21**, pp. 481–488, 1994.

Dynamic viewing protocols for diagnostic image comparison

David H. Foos[a], Richard M. Slone[b], Bruce Whiting[b], Kevin Kohm[a],
Susan Young[a], Edward Muka[b], and Dan Hendrickson[b]

[a]Health Imaging Research Laboratory, Eastman Kodak Company, Rochester, NY 14580-2033,
[b]Mallinckrodt Institute of Radiology, Washington University School of Medicine, St. Louis, MO 63110

ABSTRACT

There is an ongoing need to evaluate the impact of various digital image processing and display variables on diagnostic image quality. In most cases, evaluation includes comparison of images, often multiple versions of the same image. In order to improve speed and sensitivity, new protocols were developed to enhance a radiologist's ability to detect subtle changes in images and provide a means to quantify differences in a standard fashion. The protocols make use of the rapid sequential display of registered images on a single high-resolution CRT (a.k.a., flicker) and 2X magnification in order to increase observer sensitivity. The flicker technique was implemented in the form of an image comparison workstation (ICW) that was designed to facilitate the evaluation of different image processing options. The ICW was developed with capabilities to interactively control the rate of flicker between image pairs (up to 5 Hz), the degree of image magnification (1X to 4X), and the selection of the region of interest (ROI). Three specific protocols were developed based on the flicker technique, two forms of forced-choice and a rank-ordering protocol employing a reference set comprised of images with varying degrees of spatial-resolution degradation. All three protocols were exercised as part of an observer study whose goal was to establish visually lossless compression levels for JPEG and a wavelet-transform based algorithm. The results indicate that, for high resolution digitally acquired posteroanterior (PA) chest radiographs presented to observers at 2X magnification on a 2K X 2.5K addressable pixel monochrome display, the visually lossless thresholds for both JPEG and wavelet occur in the range of 2.0 to 1.5 bits-per-pixel ($\approx$10:1). These results are a conservative estimate of the visually lossless threshold because of the sensitive nature of the experimental methodology.

Keywords: Alternative forced-choice, sequential display, rank-order, compression, image quality, visually lossless

1. INTRODUCTION

1.1 PACS Image Compression

Picture archive and communication systems (PACS) must provide rapid delivery of high-quality images to ensure quality patient care. These two requirements pose conflict in bandwidth limited systems because factors that maintain image quality, for example higher spatial resolution and greater bit-depth, result in larger image file sizes, and hence increased storage requirements and transmission time. Although the technology exists to satisfy both requirements, such systems are cost prohibitive to implement. Irreversible (lossy) image compression provides a means for substantially reducing image file size,[1-3] and thus costs by utilizing available network bandwidth more efficiently. Today, there are two varieties of lossy compression algorithms competing for acceptance in the medical imaging community, the block DCT approach, i.e., JPEG,[4] and the family of wavelet transform-based approaches.[5-8] The purpose of this study was to establish a robust method for comparing the relative performance of irreversible image compression algorithms and to use the methodology to establish a conservative bit rate appropriate for the irreversible compression of medical imagery intended for diagnostic interpretation.

1.2 Compression Algorithm / Ratio Selection

Tremendous gains in research efficiency could be realized if there existed a robust, standardized means for measuring image quality automatically from image pixel data. In particular, degradation introduced by irreversible compression lends itself to automated assessment because perceived image quality loss should logically increase as compression ratio, and consequently statistical deviation of the pixel values from the original (i.e., compression distortion), increases. To this end, the image quality performance of compression algorithms is often reported in mathematical terms that quantify the error between the unaltered original image and the compressed-reconstructed version. However, even the ostensibly straightforward problem of quantifying image quality degradation caused by irreversible compression is problematic because numerical metrics do not always correlate well with visual preferences. For example, consider one of the most intuitive and historically most widely

---

[a] Further author information: (Send correspondence to D.H.F.)
D.H.F: email: dfoos@kodak.com

108

Part of the SPIE Conference on Image Perception and Performance
San Diego, California • February 1999
SPIE Vol. 3663 • 0277-786X/99/$10.00

used metrics, mean-squared error (MSE). Although helpful for coarse characterization of image quality performance of compression algorithms, it is well known that MSE does not accurately predict perceived quality,[9,10] especially near thresholds of compression distortion visibility. A variety of more sophisticated numerical metrics that model the human visual system[11] and take into account localized background variations[12,13] have been proposed, however, there is still no single, widely accepted objective metric. Good, et al.[14] discusses the human visual system modeling and computational complexity limitations of various types of metrics reported in the technical literature, including metrics based on signal detection theory and psychovisual-based methods. Girod[10] discusses the challenges of defining a reliable objective measure of image quality because of the complex spatio-temporal response of the human visual system, hence still requiring researchers to include subjective evaluation.

The subjective evaluation of distortion caused by irreversible compression requires special attention for medical imagery; of particular concern is imagery intended for primary diagnosis. The absolute minimum criterion that must be satisfied for the acceptance of lossy compression is that the diagnosis, which a radiologist makes from a compressed version, does not differ from the diagnosis determined from the original image. Diagnostic accuracy is established via studies that require radiologists to evaluate original unaltered images and images that have been compressed and reconstructed or of potential abnormalities. These experiments involve the careful selection of images that exhibit subtle, but verified, pathologies. Images that exhibit subtle disease states are necessary because images that show conspicuous disease would likely be detected correctly regardless of presentation technique. Because subtle effects are difficult to detect, both a large number of images and a large number of observers are required to produce a statistically meaningful result.[15] Moreover, the experimental process of trying to detect subtle details from images can be slow and arduous.

Study methodologies that make use of classical receiver operating characteristic (ROC) analysis,[16,17] can be used to establish the compression ratio corresponding to a diagnostically lossless threshold. The diagnostically lossless threshold is defined as the bit rate, above which, a change in the area under the ROC curve, A_z[18] cannot be detected. Alternative forced-choice (AFC) methods can also be used to establish the diagnostically lossless threshold via A_z[19] but, in addition, can be used to determine a more conservative compression ratio corresponding to a visually lossless threshold.[20-23] A compressed-reconstructed image is considered to be below the visually lossless threshold if it cannot be distinguished from the unaltered original in a blind forced-choice comparison, logically inferring that the image is also diagnostically lossless. Compression ratios that satisfy diagnostically lossless criteria may be substantially higher[24,25] than compression ratios that satisfy visually lossless criteria. This is because an image can exhibit a small amount of perceptible distortion, e.g., contouring or blurring, without adversely impacting diagnostic information content. However, radiologists may still perceive the image as degraded, thus lowering their confidence that compressed imagery will satisfy requirements for primary diagnosis.[26] Hence, we chose to use the visually lossless threshold as the criterion for evaluating JPEG and wavelet compression algorithms, because it supports a modest level of compression efficiency while still maintaining radiologist confidence in the diagnostic quality of the image.

Rank-order methods have also been successfully used for the selection of image compression algorithms.[27,28] These methods can be used to glean additional information about a compression algorithm's image quality performance at points between and beyond diagnostically lossless and visually lossless threshold quality levels. This additional information can prove useful for quantifying the performance of compression algorithms for imagery not intended for primary diagnosis, for example for imagery intended for review on clinical and referral workstation displays.

1.3 Side-by-Side Versus Flicker Comparisons

Experiments that seek to quantify changes in diagnostic image quality require test participants to perform at a minimum, a two-part task. First, observers must detect a difference (signal) among the image choices; for our purposes, the search process assumed to be implicit. Second, observers must classify the nature of the difference, e.g., "image A contains a simulated lung nodule while image B does not", or subjectively score the importance of the difference using some form of psycho-metric scale. The detection portion of the task is tremendously complex. The ability of an observer to detect a difference between two images will depend not only on the observer's domain expertise, but also on numerous physical parameters related to the image formation and display process and the response of the human visual system. Once a difference between two images has been detected, a domain expert can classify or score the diagnostic importance of the difference. The accuracy of the classification or scoring portion of the task is predominantly driven by the domain expertise of the image interpreter.

Alternative forced-choice and rank-order experimental protocol has traditionally been founded on side-by-side presentation of two or more hardcopy images for observers to choose from. It is our assertion that side-by-side presentation implicitly confounds the signal detection portion of the forced-choice experiment task, thus introducing both systematic and random errors. For example, observers are required to remember complex image structure, possibly for as much as several seconds, while reorienting eye position to compare the same region when looking from side-to-side. Consequently, it's possible for different image structure to be visible, but because of image complexity (clutter), coupled with the time delay when looking from side-to-side, not remembered. Hence, two images may, in fact, have perceptible differences, but be recorded in the study as the same. Another inherent problem with side-by-side comparisons has to do with the imperfections associated with the production and presentation of two or more images (e.g., density variations on laser-printed films, light box luminance differences, and errors in luminance and focus calibration on softcopy displays). These types of experimental errors can be randomized, in which case they contribute to a loss in precision. Unattended, they will be manifested as systematic errors. This can also be a problem with ROC experiments that require observers to rate various renderings of the same image, in particular if using a single softcopy system over the course of weeks or months. Even the most carefully calibrated and maintained monitors are subject to luminance, dynamic range, and focus variations over time. The aforementioned problems all logically become more dominant factors as differences among image renderings approach thresholds of detection. Moreover, the process of comparing images exhibiting only a subtle difference, causes the side-by-side comparison process to be tedious.

An alternative to side-by-side presentation is to use the sequential presentation of two images on a single CRT (a.k.a., flicker). Several of the problems with side-by-side comparison can be mitigated or completely eliminated by "flickering" two images, without blanking time, on a single display. The time required to-remember image structures is greatly reduced if an observer is capable of focusing on a specific image area while the test and control image is varied. In addition, the concerns about inconsistencies between two versions of an image caused by imperfect image reproduction are eliminated. Two forced-choice protocols (traditional 2AFC and original revealed forced-choice) that were based on the use of flicker were developed and used for estimating the visually lossless thresholds for digital projection radiographs that were compressed using either JPEG or wavelet algorithms.

The flicker methodology can also be used for subjective rank-order experiments. The flicker methodology facilitates the use of an image-based scale (i.e., a reference set) for rank-ordering as opposed to using a word-based scale (e.g., most similar, somewhat similar, least similar etc.). The control sets were generated by systematically degrading each original image using prescribed amounts of blur (a.k.a., varying degrees of spatial resolution). Although there were many good choices for the control dimension, spatial resolution was chosen for two reasons. First, the image degradation effects caused by loss in spatial resolution (within a single modality) are intuitive, and, as such, provide a reasonable choice for use as a standard reference dimension. Second, there are several practical system design choices for which spatial resolution is the principle physical variable impacting image quality, e.g., acquisition system pixel size, number of addressable softcopy display pixels, etc. The use of spatial resolution as the standard reference for relating image quality losses caused by various factors in the image chain (e.g., noise, image compression, anamorphic sampling, etc.) has precedence in remote sensing. The Generalized Image Quality Equation (GIQE)[29] has been used to predict end-to-end image quality performance for aircraft-based, unmanned aerial vehicle (UAV), and satellite imaging systems.[30] The principle variable in the GIQE model is spatial resolution. The response variable for the model is NIIRS[31] (National Image Interpretability Rating Scale), which is an "image-observables", or task-based metric for image quality that can be used to quantify target readout difficulty.

Because compression is a process that inherently "throws away information", we believe that experiment protocols that are based on flicker presentation are particularly powerful because the compressed-reconstructed images can be directly compared against the original uncompressed versions. We have developed a versatile workstation tool and implemented three protocols on the workstation based on the dynamic, or flicker, presentation of images. This paper describes the results of our experience in using the dynamic viewing protocols to study the effects of irreversible compression on medical image quality.

2. METHODS AND MATERIALS

2.1 Image Comparison Workstation
The flicker capability was implemented in the form of an image comparison workstation (ICW). The ICW was designed as a collaborative project between the Health Imaging Research Laboratory at Eastman Kodak Company (Rochester, NY) and the Mallinckrodt Institute of Radiology at the Washington University School of Medicine (St. Louis, MO). Although designed specifically to evaluate irreversible compression algorithms, the ICW design is flexible and can be used to evaluate differences among a variety of image processing options, as long as the images are registered. It is important to emphasize

that exact image superposition is critical, thus the technique only allows comparison of renderings of the same image, but not different images.

The workstation was developed using commercially available hardware components. The ICW platform was comprised of a Hewlet Packard (Palo Alto, CA) Kayak personal computer equipped with dual 300 MHz Pentium II processors, a Microsoft (Redmond, WA) Windows NT operating system, (2) 9 Gigabyte fast wide SCSI hard drives, and an HP FastRAID option to stripe the disk drives together, 512 Megabytes of RAM, two Dataray (Westminister, CO) 21-inch DR 110 high-resolution monochrome monitors, and two Metheus (Beaverton, OR) P1540 10 bit-per-pixel display driver cards. The Dataray monitors were built with p45 phosphor and a 71 Hz refresh rate. The maximum luminance output was calibrated to 220 Cd/m^2 with a dynamic range of 650:1. The natural response of the monitors to input drive level were periodically measured and, if necessary, appropriately compensated to maintain the desired aim. The desired aim resulted in a displayed image exhibiting the same tonal characteristics as the image when laser printed to film. In addition, the monitors were focused prior to the observer study.

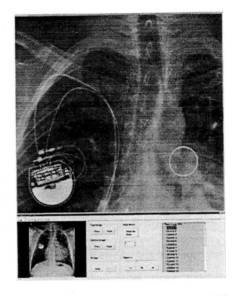

Figure 1. The figure to the right shows a reduced resolution version of how the full screen would appear to a evaluation participant on the Image Comparison Workstation (ICW). The interactive controls for magnification ("zoom in"), region-of-interest selection (white box), and manual or auto rate of flicker are part of the graphical user interface shown just below the image. Notice that the image is displayed at 2X magnification. The figure below shows an exploded view of the graphical user interface. Note that "Control 1" is highlighted indicating that the test image is flickering, or toggling with the first control image, which also turns out to be the original uncompressed version. The observer can vary the control image interactively by either rolling the mouse wheel or by "pointing and clicking on any of the control image choices displayed in the window or by using "Prev", "Next" buttons. The test image continues to flicker with the control image, even as the control image is varied.

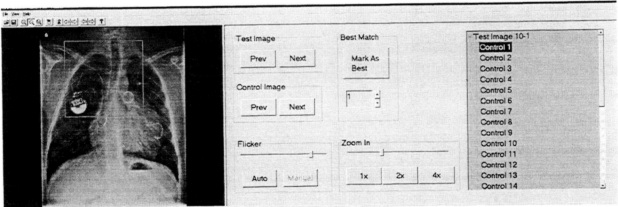

The ICW software was custom developed by the Health Imaging Research Laboratory at Eastman Kodak Company (Rochester, NY). The software GUI (graphical user interface) provided evaluation participants with capabilities to interactively vary the rate of flicker between control and test images (continuously adjustable up to a maximum rate of 5 Hz in automatic mode or manual toggle), interactively vary image magnification (1X, 2X, or 4X), and control over the region of interest (ROI) via moving box or icon. The test participants could also vary the control image via the mouse wheel. For each test image, the evaluation participants could interactively "wheel" through a series of images that had been systematically degraded in spatial resolution. Evaluation participants were provided a mechanism for indicating their responses via the GUI for automatic recording. One version of the graphical user interface is shown in Figure 1.

2.2 Imagery

Twenty digital (2K x 2.5K, 0.2 mm pixel pitch) postero-anterior (PA) chest radiographs were selected for the image compression study. The images were obtained in the outpatient admitting area of Barnes-Jewish Hospital at BJC Health Systems, St. Louis MO, and were acquired using the selenium-based Thoravision System (Philips Medical, Shelton, CT). The images selected for the study included examples of pneumonia, pulmonary nodules, interstitial lung disease, mediastinal masses, catheters, and implanted hardware.

2.3 Image Processing

Each image used in the study was nominally brightness, contrast, and sharpness enhanced for softcopy diagnostic interpretation prior to image compression or spatial resolution degradation processing. The enhancement parameters used were the same as those that had been previously established by BJC for processing Thoravision images for diagnostic interpretation. All images were scaled to 12 bits-per-pixel prior to compression processing. The image chain is shown in Figure 2.

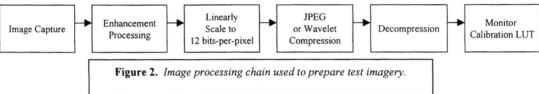

Figure 2. *Image processing chain used to prepare test imagery.*

2.3.1 Test images

The test images were compressed and reconstructed using either 12 bit-per-pixel JPEG or the wavelet/trellis-coded-quantization (wavelet/TCQ) algorithm[32] that was developed by the University of Arizona. All 20 images were compressed to 7 different bit rates (2.0, 1.5, 1.0, 0.75, 0.5, 0.25, and 0.125), then reconstructed.

An Eastman Kodak Company (Rochester, NY) implementation of the 12 bits-per-pixel JPEG algorithm was used. A single quantization table shape generated using tools developed by Kodak and based on the visual optimization techniques developed by Daley[33] was applied to the Thoravision Images for the specific viewing conditions of the study. The software allowed for the specification of a target bit rate, then iterated and converged (typically 3 iterations or less) to the target bit rate to within ±5%. The target bit rates were achieved by scaling the quantization table; the quantization table shape did not change. Entropy coding was done using Global Huffman codes.[4]

The wavelet/TCQ algorithm was made available to the Health Imaging Research Laboratory at Kodak by the JPEG 2000 committee for processing the images to be evaluated in this study. The transform portion of the wavelet/TCQ utilized floating point 9/7 tap symmetric kernels developed by Antonini, et al.[5] A scan algorithm was used to develop sequences of wavelet coefficients for TCQ processing and the quantizer step sizes were determined for the specified target bit rate using a human visual system-based weighting scheme. Entropy coding was performed via arithmetic coding.

2.3.2 Reference images

The control images used for both the forced-choice experiments were the enhanced, but otherwise uncompressed original images.

The rank-order experiment required the generation of a separate set of 15 reference images for each of the 20 unique input images. The reference set was generated using Fourier-based windowing methods. Fourteen reference images, plus the original, were generated representing various prescribed levels of spatial resolution degradation. The reduced resolution images were produced by forward Fourier transformation, windowing to reduce image bandwidth, zero padding to retain the original image scale, and inverse transfomation. Fourteen different windows, or frequency domain filters, were generated. A power window[34] provided sufficient control over the definition of the filter shapes to enable a close approximation of the ideal bandwidth cutoff filter, but allow for the emperical minimization of perceptible ringing or aliasing artifacts associated with Gibbs phenomena. The radial spatial frequency power window is defined as:

$$W(\rho) = \exp\left(-\alpha\rho^n\right),$$

where the parameters (α,n) are specified according to the desired characteristics for the filter to be derived. The values of (a,n), and thus the shape of the power window filter, can be determined by specifying two values for $W(\rho)$, then solving the two equations for the two unknowns α and n. For example, the specification of:

$$\rho 1 = 0.7\rho_{s0} \quad \text{and} \quad 20\log_{10} W1 = -3 \text{ dB};$$
$$\rho 2 = \rho_{s0} \quad \text{and} \quad 20\log_{10} W2 = -21.9 \text{ dB},$$

indicates that the magnitude of the Fourier spectrum drops by 3 dB at 70% of the band-pass, and the magnitude drops by 21.9 dB at the cutoff frequency ρ_{s0}. The solution for the parameters α and n are:

$$\alpha = 2.5 \times 10^{-8} \text{ and } n = 6$$

The spacing of the power-window cutoff frequencies was based on just noticeable differences for the first few reference levels established via a pilot study. The spacing of the power window cutoff frequencies was proportionally decreased to obtain the more degraded reference images in order to span the quality range expected for the compression ratios to be tested. The spatial resolution for the reduced resolution images was defined as the percent of the bandwidth of the original image that is retained. Note that a factor of two change in resolution approximately corresponds to ¼ the number of pixels to cover the same image area. Figure 3 shows plots of the power windows used to generate the reference images. Figure 4 shows a plot of the spatial resolution variation for the reference set images.

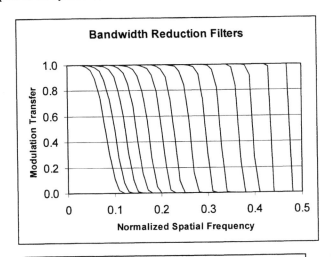

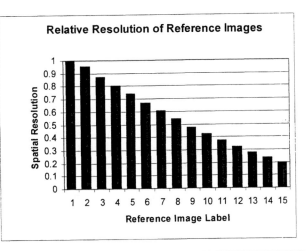

Figure 3. Spatial frequency domain filters used to generate reference images. Transformed images were zero padded to ensure registration of degraded images with originals. The filter shapes were emperically determined to approximate the ideal cutoff filter but minimize effect of Gibbs Phenomena.

Figure 4. Relative spatial resolution of reference set imagery with respect to the original image. The relative spatial resolution corresponds to the percent of the bandwidth in each dimension that is retained relative to the bandwidth of the original image. Downsampling by 2 (about reference image 9) results in an image with only ¼ the number of pixels of the original.

2.4 Evaluation Participants
There were five evaluation participants from the Mallinckrodt Institute of Radiology at the Washington University School of Medicine, three board-certified radiologists and two image scientists. The board-certified radiologists included a general radiologist (PH), and specialists in chest (RMS) and musculoskeletal (DR).

2.5 Two Alternative Forced-Choice Protocol
Each of the test images (20-images × 7-bit rates × 2-algorithms) was presented to each observer as a paired comparison in the flicker mode on the ICW; one of the images was an original uncompressed image and the other was either another original or a compressed and reconstructed version. The test participants were instructed to select the "better" image for primary

diagnostic interpretation. The observers displayed the images and made their judgements from the 2X magnified view. The observers could vary the rate of flicker, including a mode for manual toggle between images. They could also vary the region of interest (ROI). Once they had made and recorded their judgement, the observers could select the next test image from the set through a menu provided on the GUI. The test image presentation sequence was randomized.

2.6 Original Revealed Forced-Choice Protocol

Each test image was again presented as a paired comparison to each observer in the flicker mode on the ICW. The same interactive controls and user interface instructions were provided. However, the difference in this experiment from the 2AFC experiment, is that the original, or control image was revealed to the observer. The observer was then asked to decide if the test image was another original, or a compressed and reconstructed version. As with the 2AFC experiment, the observers could record their answer via a button on the GUI, then select the next test image.

2.7 Spatial Resolution Rank-Order Protocol

The rank-order method was developed specifically for use with the new platform. The method required observers to compare in flicker mode on the ICW, the compressed and decompressed versions of an image against a set of reference images that had been parametrically degraded in spatial resolution. Upon initial display, the test image and the first reference image (the original) were presented in flicker mode on the ICW monitor. The observers were instructed to interactively adjust the reference image, via rolling the mouse wheel, until the best "overall diagnostic quality" match to the test image was found. The test image continued to flicker with the reference image as the control image was varied. The observers were provided additional controls for region of interest (ROI) selection and rate of flicker (continuously adjustable up to a maximum of 5 Hz in automatic mode or manual toggle). The observers were instructed to make their judgements at 2X magnification. A button was provided on the GUI for recording the number of the reference image that had the best overall diagnostic quality match to the test image. Once the observers had recorded their judgement, they could select the next test image for evaluation.

2.8 Side-By-Side versus Flicker Alternative Forced-Choice Assessment

A small pilot assessment was conducted to test the hypothesis that improved sensitivity could be realized over the traditional forced-choice methodology, i.e., side-by-side presentation on a light box of traditional screen film images or laser printed film examples, by using the flicker or sequential forced-choice methodology. This assessment was conducted entirely within the Health Imaging Research Laboratory at Kodak using four image scientists for observers. Three high-resolution (2K × 2.5K) digital radiographic images (1 Kodak Computed Radiograph - Chest, 1 Kodak Computed Radiograph - Bone, and 1 Thoravision - Upright Chest) were each JPEG compressed to 8 bit rates (2.0, 1.5, 1.0, 0.75, 0.5, 0.25, 0.125, and 0.0625 bits-per-pixel) and then decompressed. Twelve original images, four for each of the three unique images, were also included in the test set. Thus, a total of 36 test images were used (3 input images times 8 bit rates, plus the twelve originals). Hardcopy versions of each of the 36 test and 36 control (uncompressed originals) images were laser printed onto 14" × 17" film using a Kodak Ektascan laser printer 2180. The same images were also prepared for softcopy display for flicker evaluation on the ICW. The ORFC methodology was employed, and the experiment conducted twice. The first experiment was done using side-by-side presentation and comparison of the laser printed films. The second experiment was conducted on the ICW using the flicker methodology. The presentation sequence was randomized between the two experiments.

3. RESULTS

The results from all three compression experiments were consistent and indicate that the visually lossless threshold for images compressed with either the JPEG or wavelet algorithm occurs between 1.5 and 2.0 bits-per-pixel. This result is believed to be a conservative estimate because the experiments were conducted at 2X magnification, in ideal viewing conditions with unconstrained viewing distance. Moreover, the results from the pilot assessment show an increased sensitivity for observers to detect subtle differences between images when using the flicker presentation methodology versus traditional side-by-side forced-choice methods.

3.1 Two Alternative Forced-Choice

The results from the two-alternative forced-choice experiment are shown in Figures 5a and 5b. The figures show plots of the percent of the time (mean observer response) that the compressed image was selected as better than the original for JPEG and wavelet compression algorithms respectively; the observer responses are plotted as a function of bits-per-pixel. A distribution of responses near the 50 percent level is expected when images are indistinguishable to the observers. An estimate of the visually lossless threshold is indicated by the maximum bit rate at which images cannot be statistically distinguished from the original, i.e., a score that cannot be statistically separated from 50%. Note that 40 pairs of originals were also included in the experiment as a control, denoted in Figures 5a and 5b as 16 bits-per-pixel. By inspection, it is evident that at low compression, images are visually lossless with a significant change between 1.5 and 1.0 bits-per-pixel.

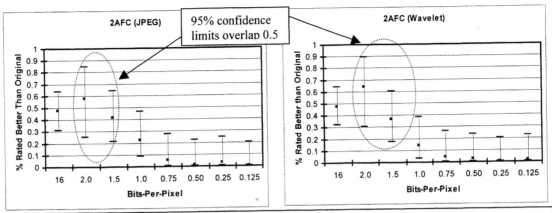

Figures 5a and 5b. Results of two alternative forced-choice experiment for JPEG (5a) and wavelet (5b) compression algorithms. Random scores centered on 50% are expected when the observers are guessing. Note the greatest change occurs between 1.5 and 1.0 bits-per-pixel.

3.2 Original Revealed Forced-Choice (ORFC)

The results of the ORFC experiment are shown in Figures 6a and 6b. The figures show plots of the percent of the time (mean observer response) that the test image was scored by the observer as another original; the scores are plotted as a function of the number of bits-per-pixel. The mean observer response for the case when the test image is another original is denoted as 16 bits-per-pixel. Note that the observers would sometimes mistakenly score an original as a compressed version. An estimate of the visually lossless threshold is indicated by the maximum bit rate at which the mean observer response cannot be statistically separated from the results of the original. By inspection of Figures 6a and 6b, the visually lossless threshold for images compressed with either JPEG or wavelet algorithms is above 1.5 bits-per-pixel, which is consistent with the results of the 2AFC experiment.

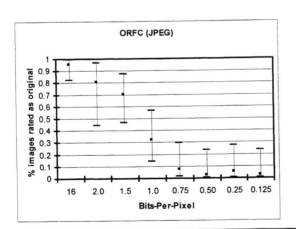
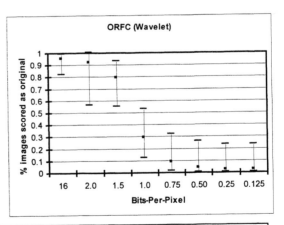

Figures 6a and 6b. Results of original revealed forced-choice experiment showing the % of images considered equivalent to the original at each bit rate. Notice that the observers did not always score images as equivalent when they were presented with another original. Note substantial change between 1.5 and 1.0 bits-per-pixel. Note that only the 95% confidence intervals for 2.0 overlap the mean values for the originals, unlike the 2AFC, suggesting that ORFC may be more sensitive.

3.3 Spatial Resolution-Based Rank-Order Method

The results from the spatial resolution-based rank-order experiment are shown in Figures 7a, 7b, 8, and 9. For convenience, the bit-rate values were converted to compression ratio, transformed onto a $\log_{10}$ scale, then plotted versus the $\log_{10}$ of one over the percent resolution of the corresponding reference image. Compression ratio was calculated as the ratio of the bit rate of the input image (16 bits-per-pixel) to the bit rate of the compressed image. Figures 7a and 7b show the results for one observer in the form of a bubble graph. The size of the bubble is proportional to the number of responses at a particular level. The x-axis intercept of the trend line represents an estimate of the visually lossless threshold because the x-axis corresponds to the reference image having 100% resolution of the original image. By comparing the degradation caused by compression for each algorithm against a common reference, the trend line offers additional insight about the relative image quality performance of the two algorithms at compression ratios beyond the visually lossless threshold. Figure 8 shows the calculated visually lossless thresholds and r^2 values from the linear fit for each observer and algorithm. The median visually lossless threshold calculated from the combined data from all observers was 12:1 for JPEG and 11:1 for wavelet, or roughly 1.5 bits-per-pixel. Starting at bit rates above 0.5 bits-per-pixel, i.e., below 32:1 compression ratio, the wavelet-compressed images are scored as more degraded than the JPEG compressed images. Figure 9 shows a comparison of the resolution versus bits-per-pixel relationships based on the curve fits established in Figures 7a and 7b. The results shown in Figure 9 again show that JPEG compression introduced less objectionable distortion than wavelet compression at bit rates above 0.5 bits-per-pixel. Below 0.25 bits-per-pixel, the wavelet-compressed images are preferred.

Figure 7a and 7b. Bubble plots and trend line showing relationship between rank-order scores correlated with spatial resolution plotted as a function of compression ratio. Relationships are shown in $\log_{10}$. The x-axis intercept represents an estimate of the visually lossless threshold.

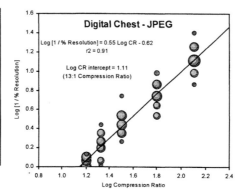

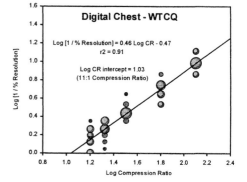

Figure 8 (below). *x-intercept (shown as bits-per-pixel) and r^2 from trend line for JPEG and wavelet compressed images for each observer.* **Figure 9 (right).** *Spatial resolution rank-order values corresponding to bit-rate.*

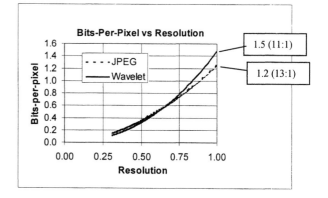

Observer	JPEG	r^2		Wavelet	r^2
A	1.2	0.91		1.5	0.91
B	1.5	0.86		2.6	0.9
C	1.5	0.86		1.3	0.9
D	1	0.93		1.1	0.92
E	1.3	0.9		1.6	0.93

3.4 Side-By-Side Versus Flicker Forced-Choice

The results of the side-by-side versus flicker ORFC experiment are shown in Figures 10a and 10b. The figures show plots of the percent of the time that the test image was scored by the observer as another original. The scores are plotted as a function of the number of bits-per-pixel.

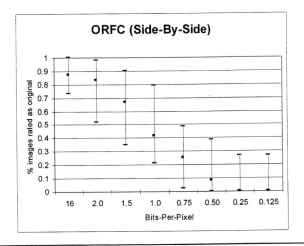
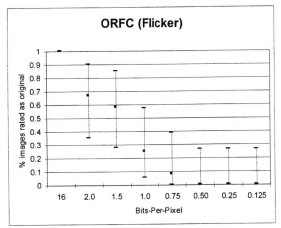

Figure 10a and 10b. Percent of compressed images rated as original shown as a function of bits-per-pixel. By inspection, it appears that compression distortion can be detected at a higher bit-rate using the flicker technique. Note that these results are based on a very limited set of data and should be treated as preliminary.

The results are consistent with the observation that subtle differences seem to be more readily detectable with the flicker methodology when images are viewed at 2X magnification than when using traditional side-by-side forced-choice-based experiment protocols. A sign test[35] was performed on the difference of the number of compressed images detected by each method for each of the five bit-rates of 0.5 or larger. If the probability of detection were the same for both methods, we would expect that each method would have a larger number detected than the other about half the time. Instead, the flicker method has detected more in all five categories. There is only a one in 16 chance that this would happen by chance if the detection probabilities were the same for the two methods. The results also suggest that the observers had greater confidence when rating test images that were in fact "originals" when using the flicker approach. Of the 48 ratings, (4 observers times 12 original images), 6 responses were scored as compressed from the side-by-side study. There were zero responses out of 48 that were scored as compressed when the flicker methodology was used. The time required to complete the evaluation was also recorded. It took (on average) 40 minutes for the observers to complete the side-by-side ORFC portion of the experiment, or just over 1 minute per image pair. The flicker portion of the study required on average 25 minutes, or roughly 40 seconds per image pair.

4. DISCUSSION

Three experiments based on dynamic viewing protocols were conducted for purposes of estimating the visually lossless threshold for images compressed using either 12 bit-per-pixel JPEG or a wavelet transform-based compression scheme. The viewing protocols were based on the sequential, or flicker, presentation of registered images on a softcopy workstation. All three experiments produced consistent estimates (between 1.5 and 2.0 bits-per-pixel) of the visually lossless threshold for both JPEG and wavelet-based compression methods. In addition, the spatial resolution-based rank-order technique provided information about the relative image quality performance of the wavelet and JPEG algorithms for bit rates below the visually lossless threshold by rating the test images using an image-based degradation scale. We believe the estimates of the visually lossless threshold for JPEG and wavelet compression are highly conservative, and thus robust across a range of viewing devices and conditions, because of the sensitive nature of the experimental protocol that was used.

Flicker-based comparison and evaluation methodologies intuitively provide increased sensitivity to detect subtle differences between image pairs. This intuition is supported, albeit not confirmed because of the extremely limited scope of experiment, by the side-by-side versus flicker sensitivity study. A more comprehensive experiment is currently in progress to further quantify the difference in sensitivity between the two approaches. We offer several plausible explanations for this based on our observations and experience with the ICW. First, the observers were not required to base their judgements about the differences between two images on memory, as is the case when images are presented for evaluation in a static side-by-side fashion. The complexity of image structures coupled with the time required to re-orient eye position to the same region on the image when looking side-to-side, causes the comparison process to be human memory taxing. The often-subtle visual effects being tested ostensibly makes the memory problem even more dominant, possibly confounding the interpretation of perception results obtained from forced-choice and subjective rank-order studies. Presenting image pairs sequentially, without any perceivable blanking time between test and control images, allows the observer to stare at select regions in the image while the test and control images toggle, hence mitigating the need to remember differences. One observer in the study commented that "flicker-based image comparison was similar to detecting motion". By mitigating the dependence on memory in the image comparison process, the visual effects in imagery that are caused just by differences in image processing can be isolated and, thus more specifically assessed. The flicker approach is particularly appropriate for evaluating the effects of irreversible compression on images because the compressed and reconstructed versions can be flickered with the originals and the distortion can be explicitly detected and assessed. The flicker approach provides the increased sensitivity to detect differences, but without the loss of image context.

The flicker comparison process can, however, be taken to an extreme. For example, it is common practice to construct the mathematical difference between an original and a compressed-reconstructed version, and then display the difference image after performing a gain and offset correction as a means of assessing the underlying structured noise introduced by the compression process. Using the aforementioned method, even single code value differences can be rendered at the minimum and maximum luminance settings. Although the assessment of difference images provides useful analytical information, to use the difference image to infer the visual impacts of compression distortion for an image when viewed under conditions suitable for diagnostic interpretation would be difficult, and could be misleading. Likewise, the flicker method, via tools provided on the ICW, allows for the image to be displayed in various ways such that virtually any difference between the compressed and reconstructed version and the original would be detectable. Thus, as part of the experimental protocol it was necessary to impose certain constraints on the observers' ability to adjust magnification, contrast, and brightness. Our goal was to establish a conservative estimate of the visually lossless threshold for high-resolution digital chest radiographs intended for primary diagnostic interpretation on a high addressable pixel monochrome softcopy display. As such, the viewing conditions for conducting the experiment were specified accordingly. Observers were allowed to view the images at either 1X or 2X magnification, but not at 4X. It was felt that a 4X magnified view of the image would represent an atypical practice. In addition, the observers were not allowed to vary the window width or window level settings, and consequently, were limited to viewing the images with predefined levels of contrast and brightness. This constraint was thought to be necessary at least for the first series of experiments because of the fear of confounding the experiment with an uncontrolled variable. We have discussed the need to understand the tolerances that need to be placed on window width and window level to ensure that a specified visually lossless threshold is maintained. This question will be addressed in future work.

Timing data was recorded during the three JPEG versus wavelet experiments that were conducted using the ICW. In addition, a direct comparison was made of the time required to complete the image comparisons using the side-by-side versus the flicker method, with the flicker method taking only 60% of the time that was required for the side-by-side study. Every observer that participated in the study had prior experience performing side-by side comparisons; each indicated that they preferred using the ICW for making forced-choice comparisons because they felt they could detect subtle differences both more easily and significantly faster. A more complete experiment is currently underway to quantify the evaluation speed differences between the side-by-side and flicker approaches. Should the flicker approach prove to be faster, it will offer the opportunity to increase statistical power by allowing more images to be evaluated in a specified time.

Sequential presentation offers one additional benefit over side-by-side presentation, in particular for softcopy experiments. Differences among display transfer functions can be an important factor in forced choice and preference experiments, and may, in fact, be the limiting effect if trying to "fine tune" processing parameters. By randomizing, errors caused by this effect can be distributed, but the consequence is decreased statistical power. Because images are presented on the same display with the flicker methodology, the display response variable can be "better-controlled" and random error mitigated. The variable display response effect also has the potential to confound softcopy-based ROC studies that make use of the rating method, especially if the experiment is conducted over the course of months as they often are. Even the most stable and carefully calibrated display systems are subject to a drift in sharpness and luminance response characteristics over time.[36]

The rank-order method employed a set of reference images that had been parametrically degraded in spatial resolution. The use of a reference image set for rank-ordering can provide advantages over rank-order methods that rely on word-based criteria because image-based scales are inherently less subjective. The ICW facilitated the use of a reference image set for rank-order experiments, perhaps providing a mechanism to obtain more widely acceptable rank-order results in the future. Because the distortion introduced by JPEG and wavelet compression is manifested in imagery in different ways, scoring the distortion against a standard reference as a means of comparing relative losses seemed appealing. The spatial resolution degraded images may be thought of in terms of larger pixels, and hence fewer pixels to cover the same image area (a simple, linear method of image compression). By relating the compressed-reconstructed images to a resolution series, we are comparing, or scoring, the loss in information content caused by a nonlinear process to a well-understood bandwidth reduction process. The results of our study demonstrate proof-of-concept for relating image quality losses caused by one type of degradation to losses caused by another. This may provide the foundation for rank-order rating quality losses in a standardized fashion and for laying the groundwork for building an image quality predictive model for an image ensemble in the future.

5. CONCLUSIONS

Dynamic viewing protocols that make use of the sequential display or flicker presentation of registered images on a high-resolution display device are powerful methods for evaluating image quality differences among image processing techniques. These methods are particularly useful for assessing information content loss caused by lossy image compression because the compressed and reconstructed versions can be directly compared against the original uncompressed image. The new viewing protocols increase observer sensitivity to detect the distortion introduced by irreversible compression over traditional side-by-side forced-choice and rank-order methods. Moreover, the use of new softcopy tools that are based on the flicker methodology can substantially reduce the time required to perform alternative forced-choice comparisons over traditional side-by-side forced-choice comparisons.

The visually lossless thresholds for high-resolution digital posteroanterior chest radiographs compressed with either 12-bit JPEG or wavelet/TCQ algorithms are equivalent and are estimated to be between 1.5 and 2.0 bits-per-pixel when the images are presented to radiologists at 2X magnification on a 2.0K X 2.5K diagnostic quality monitor.

Proof-of-concept has been demonstrated that image quality degradation caused by one type of irreversible compression can be related to another by comparing both types of degradation against a common spatial resolution-based reference standard.

ACKNOWLEDGMENTS

The authors gratefully acknowledge the time and expertise of Dr. David Rubin and Dr. Paul Ho from the Mallinckrodt Institute of Radiology, at the Washington University School of Medicine for participating in the three observer studies. In addition, the authors thank Dr. Thomas Pilgram from the Mallinckrodt Institute for statistically analyzing the observer response data. The authors thank Paul Jones and Rajan Joshi of the Image Science Technology Research Laboratory at Kodak for their assistance in developing the visually optimized quantization tables for the 12-bit JPEG and Wavelet/TCQ algorithms respectively. The authors thank Richard Van Metter, Xiaohui Wang, Kevin Kohm, and Lori Barski for participating as observers in the side-by-side versus flicker assessment. Finally the authors acknowledge Brian Terwilleger of the Commercial and Government Systems Division at Kodak for his time and expertise in writing the software for the Image Comparison Workstation. This work supported in part by Eastman Kodak Company and the Mallinckrodt Institute of Radiology.

REFERENCES

1. V. Savcenko, B. Erickson, P. Palisson, K. Persons, A. Manduca, T. Hartman, G. Harms, L. Brown, "Detection of Subtle Abnormalities on Chest Radiographs After Irreversible Compression." *Radiology* 1998; **206**, pp. 609-616.
2. D.R. Aberle, F. Gleeson, J.W. Sayre, et al., "The Effect of Irreversible Image Compression on Diagnostic Accuracy in Thoracic Imaging." *Invest. Radiol.*, **28**, pp. 398-403, 1993.
3. H. MacMahon, K. Doi, S. Sanada, et al., "Data Compression: Effect on Diagnostic Accuracy in Digital Chest Radiography." *Radiology*, **178**, pp. 175-179, 1991.
4. Pennebaker, W.B., Mitchell, J.L., *JPEG: Still Image Data Compression Standard*, Reinhold, New York. 1993.
5. M. Antonini, M. Barlaud, P. Mathieu, I. Daubechies, "Image Coding Using Wavelet Transform." *IEEE Trans. Image Proc.* Vol **1-2**, pp. 205-219, 1992.
6. http://www.crc.ricoh.com/CREW/
7. http://ipl.rpi.edu/SPIHT/spiht0.html
8. J.H. Kasner, M.W. Marcellin and B.R. Hunt, "Universal TCQ in Wavelet Image Coding." *Proceedings of the conference record of the Asilomer Conference on Signals, Systems and Computers*, **V2**, 1997, pp. 1279-1283.

9. Stein CS, Watson AB, Hitchner LE., "Psychophysical Rating of Image Compression Techniques." *Proc. SPIE* 1989; **077,** pp. 198-208.

10. Girod B. What's wrong with mean-squared error? [Chapter]. Watson AB, Editor. <u>Digital Images and Human Vision.</u> 1st ed. Cambridge, Massachusetts: MIT Press 1993; 207-220.

11. Daly S., "The Visual Difference Predictor." *Proc. SPIE* 1992; **1666,** pp. 2-15.

12. Barlow HB., "The Efficiency of Detecting Changes in Density in Random Dot Patterns." *Vision Res.* 1978; **18,** pp. 637-650.

13. Gardner K., Eastman Kodak Company - private communication 1997.

14. Good W., Lattner S., Maitz G., "Evaluation of Image Compression Using Plausible "Non Visually Weighted" Image Fidelity Measures." *Proc. SPIE* 1996; **2707,** pp. 301-309.

15. Metz CE., "Some Practical Issues of Experimental Design and Data Analysis in Radiological ROC Studies." *Invest. Radiol.* 1989; **24,** pp. 234-245.

16. Metz, Charles E., *Seminars in Nuclear Medicine, Vol VIII,* No. 4 (October), 1978.

17. Metz, Charles E., ROC Methodology in Radiologic Imaging. *Invest. Radiol.* 1986; **21,** pp. 720-733.

18. Hanley, J.A., and McNeil, B.J., "The Meaning and Use of the Area Under the Receiver Operating Characteristic Curve." *Radiology* **143,** pp. 29-36, April 1982.

19. Burgess, Arthur E., "Comparison of Receiver Operating Characteristic and Forced Choice Observer Performance Measurement Methods." *Med. Phys.* **22 (5),** May 1995.

20. S. Daley, "Applications of a Noise-Adaptive Contrast Sensitivity Function to Image Data Compression." *Opt. Eng.* vol. **29, no. 8,** pp. 977-987, 1990.

21. Cox, J.R., Muka, E., Wang, X., Blaine, G.J., "Factors Affecting the Selection of Compression Algorithms for Projection Radiography." *Proc. SPIE,* Vol. **3031,** pp. 256-264.

22. Slone, R.M., Hendrickson, D.D., Bhalla, S., Fisher, A.J., Kaltman, S.L., Woodard, P.K., et al, "Visually Lossless Compression of Digital Chest Radiographs." *Radiology* Vol. **209** (P), November 1998.

23. Slone, R.M., Foos, D.H., Young, S.S., Whiting, B.R., Muka, E., Kohm, K., "Demonstration of JPEG and JPEG 2000 Compression for Medical Images." *Radiology* Vol. **209** (P), November 1998.

24. Savcenko, V., Erickson, B.J., Palisson, P.M., Persons, K.R., Manduca, A., Hartman, T.E., Harms, G.F., Brown, L.R., "Detection of Subtle Abnormalities on Chest Radiographs After Irreversible Compression." *Radiology* 1998; **206,** pp. 609-616.

25. Bradley J. Erickson, et al, "Evaluation of Irreversible Compression of Digitized Postero-Anterior Chest Radiographs." *J. Digital Imag.,* Vol **10,** No 3 (August), 1997: pp 97-102.

26. Slone RM, et al, "Assessing Visually Lossless Irreversible Image Compression: A Comparison of Three Methods Using a Unique Image Comparison Workstation (ICW)." *Radiology,* in press.

27. J. M. Holbert, et al, "Selection of Processing Algorithms for Digital Image Compression: A Rank-Order Study." *Acad. Radiol.* 1995; **2,** pp. 273-276.

28. Gur D, et al, "Forced Choice and Ordinal Discrete Rating Assessment of Image Quality: A Comparison." *J. Digital Imag.* Vol **10,** No 3 (August), 1997: pp 103-107.

29. General Image Quality Equation User's Guide Version 3.0, HAE UAV Tier II+ Project Office, Arlington, VA (1994).

30. Driggers RG, Cox P, Kelly M, "National Imagery Interpretation Rating System and the Probabilities of Detection, Recognition, and Identification." *Opt. Eng.* **36**(7) 1952-1959 (July 1997).

31. Image Interpretability Rating Scale, Air Standard Agreement, AID STD 101/11A (Jan. 1980).

32. Marcellin MW, Fischer T., "Trellis Coded Quantization of Memoryless and Gauss-Markov Sources." *IEEE Trans. Communications,* January 1990.

33. Daley, S. , "Application of a Noise-Adaptive Contrast Sensitivity Function to Image Data Compression", *Opt. Eng.* vol **29,** no 8, pp. 977-987, 1990.

34. R. C. Gonzalez and P. Wintz, *Digital Image Processing,* Addison-Wesley Publishing Company, Inc., 1977.

35. R. E. Walpole and R. H. Myers, *Probability and Statistics for Engineers and Scientists,* Macmillan Publishing Company, 1985.

36. Reiman D, Flynn M, Ciarelli J, "A System to Maintain Perceptually Linear Networked Display Devices." *Proc. SPIE,* Vol **2431,** pp. 316-326.

SESSION 4

Perceptual Processes and Performance

An Eye-Position Study of the Effects of a Verbal Prompt and Pictorial Backgrounds on the Search for Lung Nodules in Chest Radiographs

Harold L. Kundel, Calvin F Nodine, Lawrence Toto

University of Pennsylvania School of Medicine, Philadelphia, PA 19104

ABSTRACT

Peripherally inconspicuous nodules on chest radiographs are frequently missed by competent readers. In order to find a peripherally inconspicuous nodule the reader must inspect the nodule site with the central vision and decide if the features at the site are sufficiently characteristic to report a nodule.

The experiment reported here was carried out to examine the effect of a nodule prompt and distraction by unrelated native abnormalities on the location and recognition of inconspicuous lung nodules on chest x-ray images.

On two occasions separated by 3 years, 4 radiologists had their eye-position recorded while viewing 24 chest radiographs, 12 with prominent native abnormalities and 12 with no abnormalities. An inconspicuous nodule was simulated in the lungs of half of the radiographs on the first viewing and in the other half on the second viewing. For the first viewing, the readers were instructed to report any abnormalities. For the second viewing the readers were told to report any abnormalities including nodules.

A nodule prompt triggers a scanning strategy that sends the central vision to high probability nodule sites early in search and at the same time relaxes the criteria used to evaluate nodule features resulting in more true positives and false positives without a change in absolute detectability. Prominent native abnormalities, unrelated to nodules, do not affect the search strategy but competitively inhibit the nodule feature recognition mechanism.

Keywords: Visual Perception, Visual Search, Decision Making, Eye Movements, Chest Radiography, Nodule Detection, Satisfaction of Search.

1. INTRODUCTION

Pulmonary nodules in chest radiographs are occasionally missed by competent image readers. On the basis of the analysis of eye-position recordings, three mechanisms: search, recognition and decision have been proposed as explanations for missing nodules that are truly visible when their location is known (1). In order to identify and report a nodule, the reader must find and inspect the nodule site with the central vision, recognize nodule features and decide if the features at the site are sufficiently characteristic to report a nodule (see Figure 1). Each of these mechanisms is influenced by characteristics of the image and of the mindset of the reader. The image characteristics that influence nodule detection include the features of the nodule (2), the interaction of the nodule with overlapping and surrounding structures (3, 4), effects of image cues such as lines, pointers and circles (5), and subtle aspects of the pictorial content of the entire image (4, 6). The influence of reader mindset is less well understood. Verbal prompts such as those provided by the clinical history improve the detection and interpretation of most abnormalities (7), however, their influence on lung nodules is controversial (8, 9). Anecdotal observations have been made that attribute the failure to find a subtle abnormality on an image to the prior recognition of a prominent abnormality. The phenomenon has been called "satisfaction of search" but it is not clear if incomplete visual search is really the mechanism for the effect (10, 11).

The experiment reported here was carried out to examine the combined effect of a nodule prompt and the presence of obvious lung parenchymal abnormalities on the process of finding and reporting inconspicuous lung nodules on plain chest x-ray images. The initial study was done with the assumption that the readers should not suspect that the images contained nodules in order to avoid having a nodule prompt wipe out the "satisfaction of search" effect (11). The prompt condition was added in order to test the assumption that prominent native abnormalities only interfered with the detection of unprompted nodules and at the same time shed some light on the mechanism of the effect.

122

Part of the SPIE Conference on Image Perception and Performance
San Diego, California • February 1999
SPIE Vol. 3663 • 0277-786X/99/$10.00

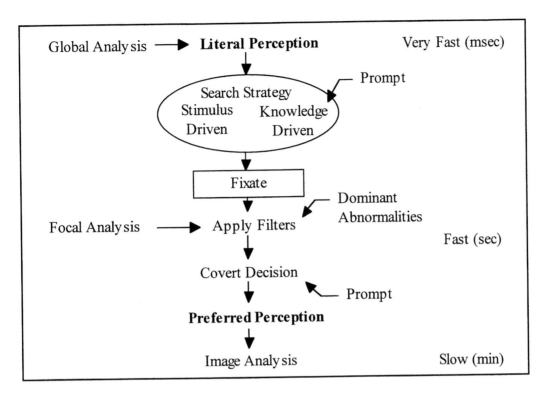

Figure 1. A flow diagram for nodule detection. During focal fixations the system analyzes (filters) the area within the useful field of view (UVF) for nodule features. Other dominant abnormalities compete for processing power with the nodule filters and render them less effective. A nodule prompt acts at two levels. First, it influences the search strategy determining where the foval fixations are directed and second, it influences the decision criteria when nodule features are identified generally making them less conservative.

2. MATERIALS AND METHODS

2.1 The Chest Images

The basic images in the test series were 12 PA chest images containing obvious native abnormalities and 12 PA chest images that were independently reported as disease-free by two chest radiologists. The 24 basic images were digitized to 100 micron resolution using a Lumisys Model 100 digitizer (Lumisys, Sunnyvale, CA). Once digitized, each image was duplicated and a pulmonary nodule that was 1 cm. in diameter with a Gaussian edge profile was digitally added to each of the 24 basic images to produce a final series consisting of 48 images where each image was represented with and without a nodule. The digitally synthesized nodules were placed by one of the investigators (LT) in the lung area of the disease-free images and in the non-diseased lung area of the images with native abnormalities. The available lung area included the region behind the heart.

The entire test series was divided into 4 sets of 12 images (A,B,C,D in Table 1). Each set contained 6 images with native abnormalities and 6 without native abnormalities. Two of the sets contained nodules and 2 sets were nodule free. The allocation of the sets to the 4 readers is shown in Table 1. The same allocation was used in the original (No Prompt) and follow-up (Nodule Prompt) study.

Table 1. The allocation of the 48 Images in the test series to the readers. The test sets are indicated by the uppercase letters (A,B,C,D) and the presence of a nodule by the lowercase (c and s). The number of images in each set is in parentheses.

Reader	Native Abnormality		Normal	
	Nodule	No Nodule	Nodule	No Nodule
1	Ac (6)	Bs (6)	Cc (6)	Ds (6)
2	Ac (6)	Bs (6)	Cc (6)	Ds (6)
3	Bc (6)	As (6)	Dc (6)	Cs (6)
4	Bc (6)	As (6)	Dc (6)	Cs (6)

2.2 Readers and Viewing the Images

Four readers who were attending radiologists participated in the study. All of them regularly read chest images on clinical rotations. Each reader viewed all of the images on two occasions separated by 2 years. On both occasions, eye-position was recorded using a Model 4000SU ASL eye tracker system (Applied Science Laboratories, Bedford, MA) . They were allowed a maximum viewing time of 30 seconds but were free to terminate viewing at any time prior to the limit. They were asked to report all abnormalities at the conclusion of viewing by dictating a brief diagnostic statement and a confidence rating for each abnormality. A "normal" or "negative" report also required a rating. A rating scale of 1 to 5 was used with 1 being most confident and 5 being least confident.

For the first phase of the study , designated as "the general task", they were read the following statement. "Each image may contain one, more than one, or no abnormalities. Report each abnormality using a short phrase and a confidence level from 1 to 5 where 1 is least confident and 5 is most confident. If an image is normal give your confidence rating as well". Two years later, in the second phase of the study, designated as "the nodule task", they were read the same statement with the phrase "*including pulmonary nodules*" added to the first sentence. This was the nodule prompt. The study was paired with regard to task, that is each reader saw the same set of images with and without being alerted for nodules (see Table 1).

2.3 Data Analysis

The eye position data were grouped into fixations and the time required for a fixation to hit a target site was calculated. A hit on a target site was scored when a visual fixation fell within a 4 degree diameter circle that was centered on the x,y coordinate of the nodule in both the nodule containing and the nodule-free image. This is equivalent to searching the image by moving a 4 degree visual field over the image. Our prior results show that the optimal visual field size for efficient search for low contrast nodules is between 4 and 6 degrees (12). Four degrees was used to keep the analysis on the conservative side. The target sites that did not contain a nodule are designated as control sites. The target hit times were grouped into those that occurred in the first 5 seconds, 10 seconds and 30 seconds. A target nodule that was reported was scored as a true positive independently of the confidence rating. The confidence ratings of the 4 readers were pooled and were used to compare the prompted and the unprompted readings using the computer program CORROC2. The statistical significance of the proportion of hits and nodule reports under various conditions was computed using the method described by Colton (13).

3. RESULTS

3.1 Visual Scanpaths

Visual scanpaths from 3 of the readers representing the three most common decision outcomes (true positive, false negative, and true negative) are shown in Figure 2. The scanpaths are superimposed on an outline of the chest x-ray image from a patient with a right pneumothorax and a synthesized nodule in the left mid lung. The scanpaths for the nodule prompt (lower row) were recorded in the same individuals 3 years after those for the unprompted task in the upper row.

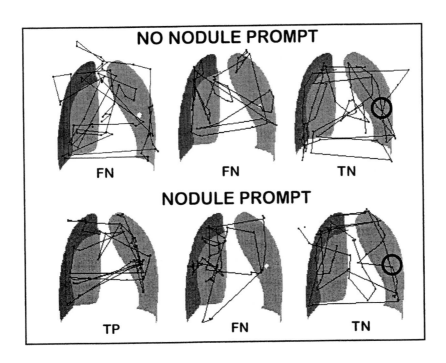

Figure 2. The scanpaths of 3 of the readers looking at the same chest image of a patient with a pneumothorax on the right side. The partially collapsed right lung is shown as a lighter gray. All of the readers look at the boundary between the collapsed lung and the air in the right hemithorax. Two of the images contain simulated nodules shown as a white blob and one does not. The zone where the nodule would have been, designated as the control region, is shown by a 4 degree diameter circle. The prompted and non-prompted viewings were separated by 3years.

3.2 The Effect of the Nodule Prompt on Visual Scanning for Nodules

The number of control and nodule sites hit by a 4 degree visual field during 5, 10 and 30 seconds of viewing is shown in Table 2. More nodule and control sites were hit in the first 5 seconds when there was a nodule prompt (18 v 26 nodule sites, p = .07 and 18 v 27 control sites, p = .05). By 30 seconds the number of hits on control sites was about equal for prompt and no prompt (40 v 41, p = .5) but the nodule sites received more hits when prompted (38 v 45, p = .03).

Table 2. The number of control and nodule sites that were inspected by a 4 degree diameter visual field with and without a nodule prompt and the probability of reporting a nodule when the site really contained a nodule.

	Nodule Prompt	Viewing time in seconds		
		5	10	30
Total hits on 48 control sites	No	18	25	40
	Yes	26	33	41
Total hits on 48 nodule containing test sites.	No	18	29	38
	Yes	27	38	45
Nodule test sites that were reported as positive	No	6	8	9
	Yes	12	19	20
True positive reports / Hit	No	.33	.28	.24
	Yes	.44	.50	.44

3.3 The Effect of the Nodule Prompt on Reporting Nodules

The number of nodules reported as positive is also shown in Table 2. When prompted, more nodules were reported (20 v 9 by 30 seconds) and the proportion of true positives per site that was hit was also greater (.44 v .24). Evaluation of the decision performance must consider the false positive as well as the true positive reports. This was done by computing the natural log of the odds ratio

$$LO = Ln \left[\frac{TPF \; x \; TNF}{FPF \; x \; FNF} \right] \tag{1}$$

The significance of the difference between two logodds values was tested using chi-square. The difference between the prompted and the non prompted condition is not significant (1.0 v .93, p = .88).

3.4 The Effect of the Presence of an Unrelated Native Abnormality on Reporting Nodules

Table 3 also shows the logodds values for images that either contained or did not contain a native abnormality. The logodds was smaller when the native abnormality was present no matter whether or not the readers were prompted about nodules. (no prompt; .45 v 1.30, p= .24 and prompt .52 v 1.47, p = .08). Taken together the difference is significant (.47 v 1.34, p = .04).

Table 3. Reader Performance expressed as true positives, false positives and the log of the odds ratio, broken down by whether the basic images was normal or abnormal and whether the reader s were prompted about the presence of nodules in the images.

Nodule Prompt	Contains Native Abnormality	Number of Nodule Images	True Positives	Total Number of Images	False Positives	Log Odds
No	Yes	24	3	48	4	.45
	No	24	6	48	4	1.30
	Total	48	9	96	8	.93
Yes	Yes	24	8	48	11	.52
	No	24	12	48	9	1.47
	Total	48	20	96	20	1.00

3.5 The Effect of the Presence of an Unrelated Native Abnormality on the Visual Scanning and Inspection of Nodule Sites.

The total number of control and nodule sites that were inspected by a 4 degree diameter visual field with and without a native abnormality on the image is shown in Table 4. There is no statistically significant difference between the normal and the native abnormality viewing conditions (39 v 42 and 44 v 39 at 30 seconds).

Table 4. The number of control and nodule sites that were inspected by a 4 degree diameter visual field with and without a native abnormality on the image.

	Native Abnormality	Viewing time in seconds		
		5	10	30
Total hits on 48 control sites	No	21	27	39
	Yes	23	31	42
Total hits on 48 nodule containing test sites.	No	24	35	44
	Yes	21	32	39

The median cumulative time spent looking at the nodule and control locations is shown in Table 5. for the true positive, true negative and false negative decisions on the nodule and the control sites. The presence of a native abnormality made no significant differences in the cumulative fixation time on nodule sites. There were no false positives on the control sites, so that category was not included in the analysis.

Table 5.   The median cumulative fixation dwell time on the 48 nodule sites (True Positive and False Negative) and the 48 control sites (True Negatives) during the 30 second viewing interval given as milliseconds.

Native Abnormality	Median Cumulative Dwell Time, (St.Dev.)		
	True Pos	False Neg	True Neg
No	4041 (18)	611 (26)	567 (39)
Yes	3200 (11)	581 (28)	681 (42)

4. DISCUSSION

Prompting for a nodule increases the concentration of visual attention on potential nodule sites in the image particularly early in the viewing process and increases the number of actual nodules that are inspected. This might occur because the peripheral vision is lowering its threshold for selecting nodule features and, therefore, finds more nodules or it could occur because of an alteration in the scanning strategy that allocates more attention to the apparently normal appearing lung zones earlier in the scanning process. The control sites were not rich in nodule features since they did not elicit a single false positive response, yet they were hit as often as the corresponding nodule sites and with comparable cumulative fixation time. This suggests that the prompt affects the scanning strategy and does not affect the peripheral feature recognition mechanism.

The nodule prompt also increases both true positives and false positives. This suggests that when image areas are fixated, the central nodule recognition mechanism is either more sensitive to nodule features or has a lower threshold. However, the overall detectability as measured by the logodds is not changed indicating that the affect of the prompt is to lower the decision threshold without changing the sensitivity of the nodule feature filters.

The presence of an unrelated native abnormality does not affect the number of nodule sites that are hit during visual scanning but it does result in a decrease in the total number of nodules reported. The proportion of true positives to false positives changes resulting in an absolute decrease in detection performance as shown by the logodds. This is the so called "satisfaction of search" effect, but the results indicate that it is not due to a failure of the scanning mechanism to fixate potential nodule sites. Furthermore, the average time spent gazing at the nodule and control sites is unchanged as was also found by Berbaum et al. (14). This suggests that the presence of native abnormalities affects the sensitivity of the central feature recognition mechanism perhaps by shifting attention to other channels. So, "satisfaction of search" or SOS although a catchy phrase is misleading as far as mechanism is concerned and perhaps should be called something like "recognition inhibition".

5. ACKNOWLEDGMENTS

We would like to thank Bruce Kneeland Curtis Langlotz, Wallace Miller, Jr., Harvey Nisenbaum for their help with this study.

6. REFERENCES

1. Kundel HL, Nodine CF, Carmody DP. Visual scanning, pattern recognition, and decision making in pulmonary nodule detection. Invest Radiol 1978;13:175-181.
2. Brogdon BG, Kelsey CA, Mosely RD. Factors affecting perception of pulmonary lesions. Radiologic Clinics of North American 1983;21(4):633-654.
3. Revesz G, Kundel HL, Graber MA. The influence of structured noise on the detection of radiologic abnormalities. Invest Radiol 1974;9:479-486.
4. Kundel HL. Predictive value and threshold detectibility of lung tumors. Radiology 1981;139:25-29.

5. Krupinski EA, Nodine CF, Kundel HL. Perceptual enhancement of tumor targets in chest x-ray images. Percep & Psychophys 1993;53:519-526.
6. Kundel HL, Nodine CF, Thickman DI, Carmody DP, Toto LC. Nodule detection with and without a chest image. Invest Radiol 1985;20:94-99.
7. Aideyan UO, Berbaum K, Smith WL. Influence of prior radiologic information on the interpretation of radiographic examinations. Academic Radiology 1995;2:205-208.
8. Berbaum KS, Franken JEA, Dorfman DD, Barloon TJ. Influence of clinical history upon detection of nodules and other lesions. Invest Radiol 1988;23:48-55.
9. Swensson RG. The effects of clinical information in film interpretation: Another perspective. Invest Radiol 1988;23:56-61.
10. Berbaum KS, Franken JEA, Dorfman DD, Rooholamini SA, Kathol MH, et.al. Satisfaction of search in diagnostic radiology. Invest Radiol 1990;25:133-140.
11. Samuel S, Kundel HL, Nodine CF, Toto LC. Mechanism of satisfaction of search: Eye position recordings in the reading of chest radiographs. Radiology 1995;194:895-902.
12. Kundel HL, Nodine CF, Thickman DI, Toto LC. Searching for lung nodules a comparison of human performance with random and systematic scanning models. Invest Radiol 1987;22:417-422.
13. Colton T. Statistics in Medicine.Little, Brown and Co. Boston, 1974.
14. Berbaum KS, Franken JEA, Dorfman DD, et al. Role of faulty visual search in the satisfaction of search effect in chest radiography. Academic Radiology 1998;5:9-19.

Medical image compression using attention modelling

Anthony J. Maeder

School of Electrical and Electronic Systems Engineering
Queensland University of Technology, PO Box 2434 Brisbane 4001, Australia

ABSTRACT

This paper describes the use of a simple model of visual importance in digital images, based on the use of contrast statistics for prediction of areas of detail which influence observer attention, to allow image compression to be undertaken at varying quality within an individual image. The effects of this strategy on expert observer perception of the reconstructed images, based on subjective image quality judgement and analysis of eye-position patterns, are considered by applying the model to sample mammograms, cervical and thoracic X-rays. The results indicate that consistent observer performance can be attained with images compressed in this way, at compression rates in excess of those reported for uniformly compressed images.

Keywords: image compression, perceptual image quality, observer performance, eye-position recording, visual attention, visual importance.

1. INTRODUCTION

The effects of various forms of image manipulation on human observer performance caused by their influence on assimilation and appraisal via the human visual system (HVS) raise important issues in medical image analysis[1]. Many studies have been undertaken to investigate observer response to particular manipulations applied to particular classes of medical images[2]. Image compression is one such class of image manipulations which is of special interest, as it is often applied in constructing the stored image at the time of the raw image capture, and may thus be outside the control of subsequent observers. In selecting the compression technique and extent of compression to be applied, it is thus desirable to know whether observer performance would be impaired, and if so to what extent.

Compression techniques for medical images are often subjected to stringent numerical error analysis to quantify the effects on the reconstructed image. The numerical measures commonly used are based on approximating fundamental human visual system characteristics (e.g. mean square error (MSE)) or on signal processing theory (e.g. peak signal-to-noise ratio (PSNR)). Alternatively, the effects on observer performance of specific tasks undertaken using the reconstructed image can be studied. These studies can be subjective (e.g. diagnostic decisions leading to receiver operating characteristic (ROC) analysis) or objective (e.g. eye-position recording for visual search and attention monitoring).

Often the above approaches cannot adequately take into account the complex characteristics of the HVS of observers. That is, they generally treat the image as a single, indivisible entity to which operations are applied globally and about which facts are established globally. They tend to ignore the capacity of the HVS to process visual information distributed spatially within the visual field differently depending on the level of relevance to the task, or in undirected observations, depending on the intrinsic significance of the visual information to the observer. If it were possible to identify the places in the image where the most significant information was located, these could be preserved more rigorously than others, and so be more readily interpreted. Correspondingly, less significant or irrelevant visual information could be degraded and stored less fully, without affecting the accuracy of interpretation.

2. VISUAL ATTENTION AND IMPORTANCE

It is difficult to define where the most significant visual information in an image is located. Any model proposed needs to be widely applicable and incorporate only a few variables, if it is to be easily applied and not overly sensitive to variations in

Part of the SPIE Conference on Image Perception and Performance
San Diego, California • February 1999
SPIE Vol. 3663 • 0277-786X/99/$10.00

image types. Studies of human observers suggest that a strong indicator of visual significance is obtained by considering eye-position and eye-movement patterns, which are determined by elements of the image contents which attract observer visual attention sufficiently to cause fixation to occur[3]. Some effort has been expended in devising models which will predict these patterns in an overall sense. A basic model that has been proposed by psychophysics researchers is visual "salience" and methods have been developed to compute the local salience values for an image[4]. This model assumes unskilled and undirected observers, that is, those who have little or no prior conception or expectation of the image contents or the task to be performed using the image.

An approach for compression of ordinary natural scenes has been developed based on this model, by combining early vision factors such as color, contrast, direction, edges and texture, to produce a map of image "importance"[5]. This map indicates the relative importance of a local area of the image (typically a regular neighbourhood or block of pixels) to the observer, relative to the scene as a whole. Only a few levels of importance need to be distinguished (typically up to 4), as it is acknowledged that other aspects of HVS processing (e.g. template recognition) take effect once salience is established. The importance map approach has been used amongst other things to allow compression improvements in ordinary natural scenes and image sequences[6]. Areas deemed to be of lesser importance were compressed with lower quality, with little if any effects on overall image perception.

In extending this model to apply to compression of medical images, two major differences need to be considered. First, expert medical image observers (such as radiologists) are not "unskilled", in the sense that they are accustomed to looking at images of the given type and tend to have predisposed viewing habits for them. Second, they are also not "undirected", as they have an overall task expectation (whether explicit or implicit), that is the conducting of a diagnosis based on the conditions visible in the image.

Thus the importance model would be more useful for medical images if it could be derived and applied in harmony with expert observer bias, that is without producing changes which degrade the performance of these skilled and directed observers. This means that the factors and weightings chosen when constructing the importance map for an image must be appropriate for emphasizing the type of visual details expected by an observer and used in the diagnostic process, or equivalently, de-emphasizing other details. A range of such factors could be considered, such as edges, texture, shape features etc. The choice of which are most significant for the expert observer warrants further study, but there is substantial evidence in the literature that contrast and the corresponding sensitivity response affected by contrast (CSF) is a dominant influence in HVS response, especially in early vision and thus in stimulating primary attention shifts and fixations, but also more specifically in radiological viewing. The investigation reported here concentrates on contrast as the basis for generating importance maps.

3. IMAGE COMPRESSION AND QUALITY

Current trends in PACS and teleradiology commonly make use of lossy image compression. For instance, lossy compression is often necessary to achieve acceptable storage or transmission efficiencies for delivering images to radiologists at remote locations. Compression rates quoted in the literature for diagnoses involving a wide range of medical image types are typically in the range of 10:1 to 15:1, and some authors claim rates of 20:1 to 25:1 are acceptable for certain applications[2]. The effects of compression losses in degrading the image information content are reflected in expressions of image "quality". A distinction is often drawn between physical quality of the image, as determined by acquisition and storage properties, and diagnostic quality, which affects the accuracy with which human observers can perform analysis of the image.

The image compression standard JPEG[7] is widely used for medical images, as it discards information to which the HVS optical and early vision components are least sensitive, via selective preservation of spatial frequencies extracted by the discrete cosine transform (DCT). Subband, wavelet and fractal compression techniques have also been proposed as candidates for medical image applications as they offer some theoretical advantages and can be matched well to individual images. However, they are less popular than JPEG as they lack universal implementations, which in turn limits their portability and interoperability.

The JPEG standard requires a fixed choice of image compression parameters to be made for each image. Often this is achieved by specifying an image quality factor, which is used to drive the level of quantization applied to reduce the values computed in the DCT (e.g. in the well-known CJPEG implementation). The quality factor must be set at a level high enough to ensure that the most detailed information to be retained in the image is not degraded, and consequently less detailed information will be preserved with similar quality, perhaps unnecessarily. Quality factors of 90 to 95 are often selected, to yield compression ratios of around 10:1. Although the JPEG standard does not permit quantization variations within the image, it has been shown that theoretical modelling of HVS response can be used to adjust quantization dynamically to achieve a given level of visual quality[8].

The errors introduced by JPEG compression at high quality factors are typically minor variations in individual pixel intensity values, with contrast, edges and texture well preserved. At intermediate quality factors, some blurring of edges and "ringing" or ghosting may occur, while at low quality factors contrast is reduced and visible "block" artifacts occur. Such errors are typically quantified by numerical measures, which although indicative of perceived quality, are far from accurate. Some models have been suggested which allow aspects of HVS response to be incorporated[9]. As a simpler alternative, subjective quality assessments can be obtained using mean opinion score (MOS) observer ratings.

Combining these observations with those of section 2, it is proposed that a map of image importance be constructed based on the type of image detail regarded as significant by expert medical image observers, and this map be used to select the local level of image quality required by the compression technique. Previous work[10] has considered the construction of such maps using several conventional image statistics to provide importance factors for medical images, with only modest benefits. Here it is demonstrated that by confining the choice of such factors to a single (and arguably the most influential) visual stimulus, viz. contrast, greater compression gains can be obtained without degradation of observer performance.

4. EXPERIMENTAL RESULTS

Three types of medical images were considered in the experiments reported here. Each type was represented by 5 sample images drawn from a large collection of such images. Minimal image processing had been applied automatically to the images at the time of digitization with no subsequent manual enhancements. The three image types comprised mammograms of 1024 x 1024 x 8b, cervical x-rays of 1708 x 1414 x 12b, and thoracic x-rays of 2048 x 2048 x 12b. When presented under the standard experimental viewing conditions, the effective resolution of these images on the display monitor was approximately halved, by a combination of cropping and interpolation, and intensity dynamic range was reduced where necessary to 8 bits. Examples of the three image types are shown in Figure 1.

A program was developed for constructing a bi-level importance map for a given image, based on contrast statistics derived for 8x8 pixel blocks in the image. Two such importance factors were adopted: contrast at pixel scale was computed using the sum of adjacent pixel absolute intensity differences across the block, while contrast at JPEG block scale was computed from the absolute difference of the average intensities for the uppermost and lowermost 10-percentiles of the intensity distribution for the block. Thresholds for these two importance factors were obtained by ranking the values obtained and selecting a cutoff higher than the values obtained for background areas in the image at around the 20-percentile point of non-background values, i.e. preserving the higher contrast useful image data. The resulting bi-level importance maps for the images of Figure 1 are shown in Figure 2. High importance areas are expected to offer greatest potential for attracting observer visual attention.

Two sets of experiments were conducted to investigate the effects on observer performance of using the importance map to vary the compression quality. Both experiments were undertaken using a CCIR Rec.500 standard subjective viewing room. First, compressed images were prepared using the conventional JPEG uniform compression strategy (CJPEG implementation) to form uniform quality images from highest quality factor 95 down to lowest quality factor 20, and also using the bi-level importance maps to construct images of varying quality. Two numerical measures, MSE and PSNR, were used to assess image quality, and four expert observers (practicing radiologists) were asked to rate the image quality using a 5-point MOS scale. Sample images at the highest and lowest quality available were presented first, and thereafter observers viewed a set of reconstructed compressed images of different qualities, each of which was based on a different raw image. The results from this experiment are summarised in Table 1.

Second, the same expert observers were subjected to eye-position monitoring, using an ASL-210 eye tracker. The observers were presented with a set of images, each displayed for 10 seconds duration, with the instruction to perform an unguided diagnostic examination of the image. Again, each reconstructed compressed image presented was based on a different raw image. The observer eye-positions were recorded at 125Hz (8ms) intervals and classified as fixation or saccade positions according to the distance between successive positions. The fixation points were then grouped by dividing the image into a rectangular grid, with each grid element constituting about 4% of the total image area. Grid elements were identified as areas of high or low fixation rates by simple thresholding. Details of the aggregated eye-position patterns for the images are summarised in Table 2, and the areas of high and low fixation rates for the sample images are shown in Figure 3. Note that high fixation rate here indicates experimentally observed high importance in terms of visual attention.

From the results shown in Table 1, it can be seen that image quality for the uniformly compressed images as indicated by numerical measures falls off rapidly at quality factors below 80. The aggregated MOS results for each image quality level indicate consistent overall ranking of the uniform quality images, with greater uncertainty for images in the middle of the quality range. In Table 2, it can be seen that the percentage of the image area subject to high fixation values is less for the images of uniform low quality, and comparable for the uniform high quality and varying quality images. Similarly, the percentage of image area subject only to saccadic eye-position presence is much higher for the uniform low quality images. Table 3 shows the fraction of overlap of high fixation areas in pairs of the images used for the Table 2 results. It can be seen that the fixation patterns differ very little between the uniform high quality and the varying quality images, as compared with the smaller overlap between high and low quality images, as the high attention locations are more widespread or shifted. This suggests that the uniform low quality in images has a distracting effect on observer visual attention (i.e. the important attention attracting details have been lost), but selective low quality in unimportant locations in the image does not.

5. CONCLUSION

Although the results reported here are derived from relatively simple experiments, they nevertheless provide a strong indication that the proposed approach of allowing varying compression quality, with higher quality where image detail is of greater importance to the expert observer, provides improved compression ratios without discernible degrading of observer performance. The further investigation of this approach requires more detailed analysis of observer viewing patterns and ultimately ROC studies should be undertaken to provide definitive performance results.

It is conceivable that other more sophisticated factors could subsequently be incorporated in the importance map computation, for example to allow the inclusion of known areas of interest for the structure of the given image type, or to allow for known typical viewing patterns of the particular expert observer. However, the benefits of such improvements are likely to be comparatively small and less universal than the use of fundamental importance factors, owing to the variable nature of individual viewing strategies and the potential distracting effects of many small areas of low image quality in close proximity to areas of higher quality.

ACKNOWLEDGEMENTS

This work was supported by the Australian Research Council under the Collaborative Grants program. Dr Ken Thomson of Western Hospital Footscray provided valued advice and images, and Mr Derek Carter of University of Ballarat undertook the necessary programming, experimentation and processing of results.

REFERENCES

1. W.R. Hendee and P.N.T. Wells (eds), "The perception of visual information," *Springer, New York,* 1997 (2nd ed).

2. Society for Computer Applications in Radiology (SCAR), "Understanding compression," *Reston VA,* 1997.

3. C. Koch and S. Ullman, "Shifts in selective visual attention: towards the underlying neural circuitry," *Human Neurobiology* **4**, pp 219-227, 1985.

4. E. Niebur and C Koch, "A model for the neuronal implementation of selective visual attention based on temporal correlation among neurons," *Journal of Computational Neuroscience* **1**, pp 141-158, 1994.

5. A.J. Maeder, "Importance maps for adaptive information reduction in visual scenes," *Conference Proceedings of ANZIIS 1995*, pp 24-29, Perth (Australia), 1995.

6. A. Maeder, J. Diederich and E. Niebur, "Limiting human perception for image sequences," *Electronic Imaging 1996, SPIE Proceedings* **2657**, pp 330-337, 1996.

7. G. Wallace, "The JPEG still picture compression standard," *Communications of the ACM* **34(4)**, pp 30-44, April 1991.

8. A.B. Watson, "DCTune: a technique for visual optimization of DCT quantization matrices for individual images," *SID Digest of Technical Papers* **24**, pp 946-949, 1993.

9. S. Daly, "The visible differences predictor: an algorithm for the assessment of image fidelity, in A.B. Watson (ed), Digital images and human vision," *MIT Press, Cambridge MA,* pp179-206, 1993.

10. A.J. Maeder, "Tuning of JPEG quantization matrices for x-ray images," *Medical Imaging 1997, SPIE Proceedings* **3034/2**, pp 653-658, 1997.

Table 1: Summary of compression ratios and quality indicators for the test images

Images	QF	CR	MSE	PSNR	MOS μ	MOS σ
Mammo	20	57:1	4.3	41.8	1.4	0.5
	40	44:1	2.8	43.7	3.1	0.6
	60	36:1	1.6	46.2	3.7	0.7
	80	26:1	1.0	48.0	3.8	0.8
	90	17:1	0.7	49.6	4.1	0.4
	95	11:1	0.5	51.3	4.1	0.6
	90/20	21:1	0.5/3.1	50.9/43.2		
Cervical	20	41:1	7.8	39.2	1.7	0.5
	40	30:1	3.7	42.4	3.2	0.6
	60	24:1	2.3	44.5	3.6	0.5
	80	16:1	1.3	47.1	3.9	0.9
	90	10:1	0.7	49.5	3.9	0.9
	95	7:1	0.5	51.5	3.9	0.8
	90/20	15:1	1.0/4.0	47.7/42.1		
Thoracic	20	45:1	9.0	38.6	1.1	0.3
	40	34:1	4.6	41.5	2.0	0.5
	60	26:1	3.5	42.7	3.0	0.7
	80	17:1	2.4	44.4	3.3	0.5
	90	10:1	1.8	45.7	4.2	0.7
	95	6:1	1.2	47.1	4.2	0.6
	90/20	14:1	1.3/3.0	46.9/43.3		

Table 2: Summary of eye-position details for the test images

Images	QF	Fixation Area %	Saccade Area %
Mammo	20	23	50
	90	38	38
	90/20	33	33
Cervical	20	30	46
	90	42	42
	90/20	42	38
Thoracic	20	22	46
	90	25	38
	90/20	23	38

Table 3: Overlap fraction for high fixation area locations for the test images

Images	QF Pairs	Fixation Area Overlap
Mammo	90 - 20	0.83
	90 - 90/20	0.92
Cervical	90 -20	0.58
	90 - 90/20	0.83
Thoracic	90 - 20	0.83
	90 - 90/20	0.92

Figure 1: Three sample images from the test sets used to obtain the experimental results

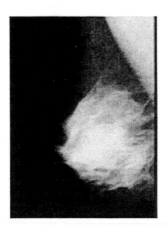
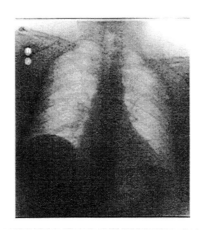
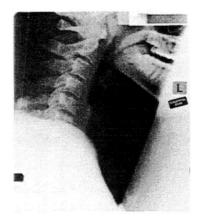

Figure 2: Importance maps for the three sample images above, based on contrast factors

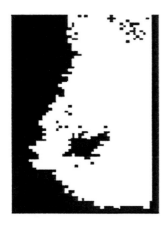
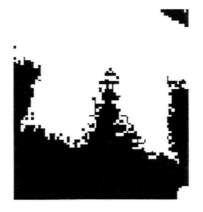
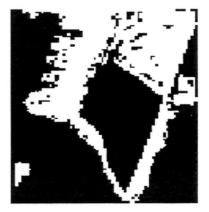

Figure 3: Areas of high and low fixation rates for the three sample images above

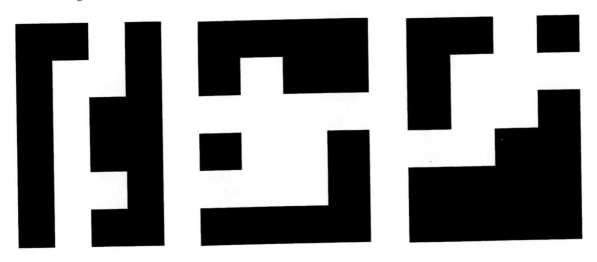

The Development of the Eye-movement Response in the Trainee Radiologist

David S. Wooding[a], Geraint M. Roberts[b], and Jane Phillips-Hughes[b]

[a]Applied Vision Research Unit, University of Derby, Derby, UK, DE3 5GX
[b]Diagnostic Radiology, University of Wales College of Medicine, Cardiff, Wales, CF4 4XN

ABSTRACT

In order to explore the initial response of the visual system to radiological images in groups of individuals with increasing degrees of radiological training and experience, the locations of fixations made during visual inspection of digitised chest radiographs were examined for 4 groups of observers: 10 experienced radiologists, 9 first-year "novice" radiologists, 11 "trainee" radiologists in the second and third years of their training, and 7 naive controls. Each observer viewed 12 digitised chest radiographs (6 normal and 6 showing some abnormality) on a VDU for 8s each. Eye movements were recorded throughout and observers indicated via a button box whether they thought the radiograph to be normal or abnormal. A least squares index[27] was utilised in order to quantify the similarity in fixation location between pairs of eye movement traces over the first 1.5 and 3 seconds of an inspection. The similarities thus produced were then averaged to give intra- and inter-group similarities in fixation location.

The fixation locations of experienced radiologists were found to be highly similar as a group, as were those of the novices. While the fixation locations of controls showed less similarity, it was the fixations of trainees which were the least similar (i.e. showed the most variability) within their group. The fixation locations of novices showed a greater similarity to those of radiologists than those of controls, and a decreased similarity to those of controls than those of the controls themselves. However, rather than showing that the fixation locations of individuals become increasing similar to those of radiologists as training progresses, the data show that the more variable fixation locations of trainees are the least similar to those of radiologists than those of any of the groups, even the controls.

Control observers examine every day images in a similar way[27] and this is also true of radiological images. Experienced radiologists view radiological images in a similar way to each other, but their training has resulted in differences between them and controls. In becoming experienced radiologists, it appears that trainees may move through a developmental phase characterised by more idiosyncratic eye movements; their eye movements becoming less similar to controls or experienced radiologists than they were. With experience the eye movements of trainee radiologists may become more similar to both groups, but the transition of the trainee from novice to experienced radiologist is not a simple one: the change involves a period of some disorder.

Keywords: Eye movements, radiologists, training, visual perception

1. INTRODUCTION

1.1 The Guidance of Eye Movements over Images

The pattern of eye fixations made by an observer in viewing an image provides a measure of the visual processing involved in this complex task. Although the locations of such fixations are not in general randomly distributed[7,14,37], there is no consensus regarding the relationship between the eye movement pattern and the properties of the image under examination. Further, the relative contributions of low level visual processing and higher level cognitive mechanisms to the control of search eye movements are also unclear. It has been argued that informative areas of an image are identified with the first few seconds during a sequence of eye movements[24,26] and that knowledge about the setting of a scene and of the main objects contained within it is obtained during the first fixation[6,31]. The visual system appears to take a snapshot of a scene by utilising its low spatial frequency content to achieve coarse, global recognition[30] as was suggested by Gould[11].

It has been suggested that a number of different image features may be responsible for attracting fixations during brief visual inspection, e.g. irregular contours[1,2], edges[34], symmetry[23] and low spatial frequency regions[10]. Mackworth and Morandi[26] noted that in their experiments fixation locations corresponded to regions of the image rated subjectively as "informative" and Loftus and Mackworth[25] reported that frequency of fixation during picture viewing related to the novelty, or unexpectedness, of objects. Such objects were, however, also distinguished by their unusual spatial structure[33]. Both peripheral visual mechanisms responsive to specific image features and higher level cognitive mechanisms have been implicated by different investigators.

Intra-observer comparisons between eye movements made by the same observer to repeated presentations of the same image indicate, however, that the locations of fixations are preserved, but their sequence is not[23,36]. Mannan et al.[27] revealed a high degree of similarity between the locations of fixations made by different observers viewing unfamiliar images, especially during the initial 1.5s period of presentation. The ability of observers to recognise the images did not influence the fixation patterns, and it was concluded that for a given image, the fixation pattern was determined by its spatial properties. Mannan et al.[28], however, reported only weak similarities between the locations of fixations and those of spatial features examined.

1.2 The Guidance of Eye Movements in Radiology

The radiological image presents the observer with a range of complex and novel features, and the nature of the radiologist's examination of this image remains largely a mystery, both to scientists attempting to describe it, and to the radiologists themselves.

Radiologists do not look where they think they are looking, and large areas of the image can remain unsearched[18,21,22], often with the belief they had been[8].

There is debate as to how much the radiologist is in conscious control of his/her examination of the image. Lesions are more likely to be examined and to be examined for longer, even if they are not reported[20], suggesting they are picked up by a relatively low level, unconscious system. This suggests that the unconscious visual system might be better able to guide the eyes than the conscious Radiologist. Tuddenham and Calvert[35] suggest that systematic search actually *impedes* detection, and Kundel et al.[19] find that radiological search patterns are best modelled by a random scanning model, suggesting no conscious pre-determined strategy, but a more unconscious driving of the eyes. For an information-rich radiological image, Nodine and Kundel[29] suggest that the higher level, more cognitive, functions only begin to operate only as long as 10 seconds into a presentation.

Whatever the radiologist is doing, he/she is doing it very quickly. Kundel and Nodine[17] show remarkable detection rates for very brief (0.2 second) presentation times, the observers detecting a variety of abnormalities of varying sizes in a single glimpse of the image, without the need for scanning eye movements. This suggests the operation of a highly trained or expert system.

1.3 The Development of Expertise in Radiology

Whatever the arguments about the performance of radiologists, it remains true that the competent radiologist can meaningfully describe the features inherent in a radiological image while the control observer cannot. This expertise is presumed to develop as a result of the specific training and experience to which the trainee radiologist is exposed, but it is not known how skills of perception, detection, cognition, visual memory, interpretation, deduction and communication interact to produce the radiologist, nor which of them can be influenced by this training.

In a study of chess expertise, Chase and Simon[9] argue that the main difference between novice and expert is that the experts have immediate access to relevant knowledge and superior pattern recognition. Even the latter, more fundamental ability can be receptive to training. Karni and Sagi[15] described the time course of learning for a simple line orientation detection task, suggesting that the new perceptual task triggered neural changes in the early processing stages of the adult visual system, and that the changes were permanent.

As a number of studies claim no difference between the detection performance of experienced and junior Radiologists of only a year's training[4,5,12,32], it would appear that learning in some areas takes place within an initial short period only.

Kundel and La Follette[16] show similarities between the initial fixations of experienced observers (from the second year of medical school onwards) when confronted with a radiographic image, in contrast with the eye movements of inexperienced observers. The radiologist broadly scanned the image, following the lines made by the anatomical features of the image, while laymen used a less structured pattern of eye movements and novices scanned localised regions in the centre. The search patterns of the residents and the experienced radiologists were similar, which suggests that the development of the search strategy depends on the knowledge of anatomy and pathology which are learnt at medical school. They also found that the experienced radiologists moved to the abnormality faster and interpreted the abnormality more accurately than the students. Nodine and Kundel[29] claim that the experienced radiologist covers more of the relevant target area. Whether this is as a result of the conscious direction of the eyes to key areas on the basis of clinical knowledge (as the authors suggest), or of an improvement in basic search function as a result of experience is unclear.

This study aims to provide quantifiable evidence for the development of the acquisition of expertise in terms of a measurable change in an unconscious low-level system: the eye movement response to a radiological image. It is also hoped that it will offer some insight into the curious change which is taking place in the visual and perceptive systems of trainee radiologists.

2. METHODS

In order to explore the initial response of the visual system to radiological images in groups of individuals with increasing degrees of radiological training and experience, the locations of fixations made during visual inspection of digitised chest radiographs were examined.

2.1 Experimental Measurements

4 groups of observers took part in the experiment: 7 naive control observers ("controls"), 9 first-year radiologists ("novices"), 11 radiologists in the second and third years of their training ("trainees") and 10 experienced radiologists ("radiologists"). The mean experience of each group (with standard deviations in parenthesis) was 0.0 (0.0), 2.3 (0.7), 16.5 (4.3) and 90.0 (85.4) months respectively. The mean ages (with standard deviations in parenthesis) of observers in each of the groups were 27.0 (2.0), 28.8 (1.9), 29.8 (1.8) and 34.7 (7.6) years respectively. Snellen acuity (after refractive correction if required) was 6/6 or better. All observers were taken from the Department of Diagnostic Radiology, University of Wales College of Medicine, Cardiff.

Each observer viewed a total of 12 digitised chest radiographs (6 normal and 6 showing some abnormality) on a VDU, with each image being presented for 8s. The images were divided into two sessions of six images, and the presentation order of the different images within a given session was randomised. Eye movements were recorded throughout and observers indicated via a button box after each presentation whether they thought the radiograph to be normal or abnormal. The elicitation of responses was included solely to give observers a task, rather than to have them aimlessly look at the image.

Images were presented on a 256 grey level, high resolution (1280 pixel x 1024 pixel) 20 inch Hewlett Packard VDU (D1187A). Each image subtended 27 x 21 degrees, i.e. approximately the size of a conventional radiograph on a viewing light box. All the digitised images were inspected by JPH, an experienced radiologist, who subjectively evaluated the overall appearance of the image and the appearance of the general features and abnormalities (if present) and judged them to be within the limits of that which might be expected if the image was a conventional radiograph.

Eye-movements were tracked with the P-scan system[3], a binocular, video-based, eye-movement tracker with 20 ms temporal resolution and ±0.5 degrees spatial resolution. The observer's head was held firmly in place by clamping at the temples and with the support of a chin-rest. Observers were instructed to avoid blinking during the presentation period and traces were eliminated from the analysis if blinks occurred during the analysis period. A full screen calibration of eye-movement position was performed at the start of each group of 6 images. Drift of calibration between images was minimised by the presentation of a small centrally positioned cross which the observer was requested to fixate before each image and which was removed 60ms before the image appeared.

2.2 Identification of Fixations

Spatial locations of the eye's position were recorded for each 20ms frame and the data were analysed in terms of fixations and saccades by the method described by Jacobs[13]. The results of the analysis were examined together with the raw data in order to check on the analytical method employed. A fixation was defined by a minimum of three successive 20 ms frames in which eye position was maintained within 0.5 degrees, and successive fixations were distinguished by a separation of at least 0.5 degrees between eye positions in successive frames.

2.3 Comparing the Similarity of Eye-Movements

The study was concerned with the initial response of the visual system to the radiological image, and as a result, analysis was performed over the first 1.5s and 3s of each eye movement trace only.

A least squares index, I_s, was utilised in order to quantify the similarity in fixation location between pairs of eye movement traces[27]. This was defined as:

$$I_s = \left[1 - \frac{D}{D_r} \right] 100$$

where D is a measure of dissimilarity, given by:

$$D^2 = \frac{n_1 \sum\limits_{j=1}^{n_2} d_{2j}^2 + n_2 \sum\limits_{i=1}^{n_1} d_{1i}^2}{2 n_1 n_2 \left(a^2 + b^2 \right)}.$$

n_1 and n_2 are the number of fixations in the two eye-movement traces under comparison, d_{1i} is the distance between the location of the ith fixation in the first trace and its nearest neighbour in the second trace, and d_{2j} the distance between jth fixation in the second trace and that of its nearest neighbour in the first. The quantities a^2 and b^2 are the squares of the side length of the image, the term $(a^2 + b^2)$ ensuring that D is dimensionless. D_r is defined in the same way as D, but refers to two sets of random locations, the numbers of which equal n_1 and n_2 in the two traces under comparison. The behaviour of the distribution as a function of n_1 and n_2 has been examined by Mannan *et al*[27]. The index of similarity compares the locations of two sets of fixations without regard to the order in which they were made. It should be noted that at the start of each image presentation, the observer was fixating the centre of the screen and this initial fixation was been omitted from the computations.

The similarities between trace pairs were then averaged to give intra- and inter- group similarities in fixation location.

3. RESULTS

In order to investigate any change in eye movement response to the radiological image with training, the analysis was focused on comparisons between each of the groups and the groups representing the two "end-points" of development, namely the controls and the experienced radiologists. In addition, the similarity of eye fixations *within* each of the groups was also examined.

There were essentially no differences in the trends observed when the analysis was performed over 1.5s or over 3s. The average similarity values over 3s are lower across the board, a feature of increasing numbers of fixations already described in previous work[27]. For this reason, only the results of analysis performed over the first 1.5s will be examined here (though figure 4 offers the 3s data for comparison).

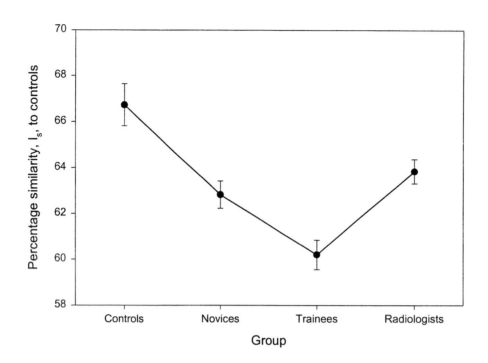

Figure 1
Mean percentage similarity, I_s, in fixation location over 1.5s for each of the four groups (controls, novices, trainees and radiologists) when compared with fixation location in controls. The error bars show the standard error of the mean.

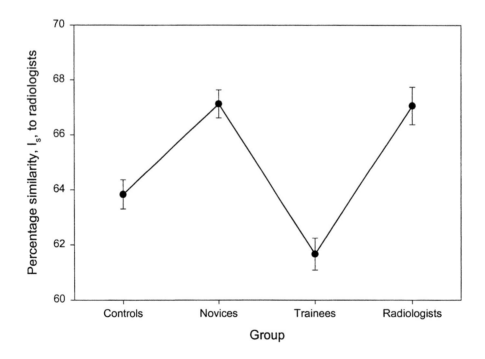

Figure 2
Mean percentage similarity, I_s, in fixation location over 1.5s for each of the four groups (controls, novices, trainees and radiologists) when compared with fixation location in radiologists. The error bars show the standard error of the mean.

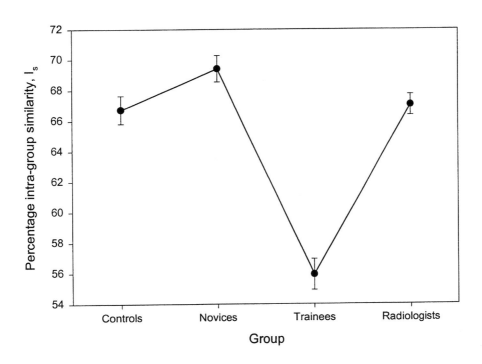

Figure 3
Mean intra-group percentage similarity, I_s, in fixation location over 1.5s for each of the four groups (controls, novices, trainees and radiologists). The error bars show the standard error of the mean.

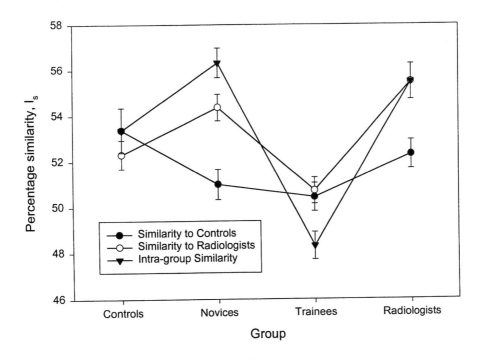

Figure 4
Mean percentage similarity, I_s, in fixation location over 3s for each of the four groups (controls, novices, trainees and radiologists) when compared with fixation location in controls (closed circles), radiologists (open circles) and within the groups themselves (closed triangles). The error bars show the standard error of the mean.

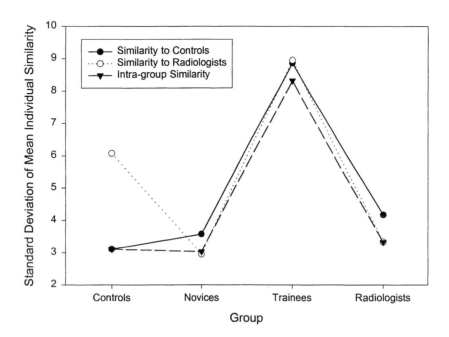

Figure 5
Standard deviation of the mean individual similarity in fixation location over 1.5s for observers in each of the four groups (controls, novices, trainees and radiologists) when compared with fixation location in controls (closed circles), radiologists (open circles) and within the groups themselves (closed triangles).

For each image the similarity of an individual's eye-movement trace to that of each other individual was calculated. These similarities were then averaged to give mean inter- and intra-group similarities.

Figure 1 shows the mean percentage similarity, I_s, when fixation locations for each of the four groups in turn (controls, novices, trainees and radiologists) were compared with fixation locations of controls. Controls have the highest similarity at around 67% when compared with controls, novices and radiologists show around the same degree of similarity to controls at around 63%, and trainees show the least similarity to controls, around 60%. The error bars show the standard error on the means.

As the order of the groups on the horizontal axis has been organised with increasing radiological experience to the right, figure 1 can also be thought of as illustrating the change in similarity with controls as radiological experience increases. The "mean" individual starts with no radiological experience and with eye-movements very similar to his/her fellow controls. As the individual acquires experience, his/her similarity with controls drops through the first year on into the second and third years of training. On qualifying as a radiologist, the individual regains some similarity with controls, though never reaching the initial similarity he/she shared with controls.

The mean percentage similarity, I_s, when fixation locations for each of the four groups in turn (controls, novices, trainees and radiologists) were compared with fixation locations of radiologists is shown in Figure 2. Novices and radiologists show around the same degree of similarity to radiologists at around 67%, with controls showing less similarity at around 64%. At around 62%, trainees show the least similarity to radiologists. The error bars show the standard error on the means.

As with figure 1, the horizontal axis of figure 2 has been organised with increasing radiological experience to the right, so that the graph can be read as illustrating the change of the "mean" individual's similarity with radiologists as the individual gains radiological experience. The graph shows that as the individual becomes a novice, his/her eye movements become more similar to radiologists. As the individual moves through the second and third years of training, his/her eye movements become less similar to radiologists than they were when the individual had no radiological experience, finally regaining similarity with radiologists.

Finally, the mean percentage similarity, I_s, when the similarity of fixation locations between members of each of the four groups in turn (controls, novices, trainees and radiologists) was examined. Figure 3 shows the novices having the highest intra-group similarity at around 69%, with controls and radiologists at a lesser level of around 67%. The lowest intra-group similarity by far was recorded for trainees at around 56%. Again, the error bars show the standard error on the means.

Viewing figure 3 as illustrating the change in intra-group similarity with increasing radiological expertise (moving right along the horizontal axis), we see the "mean" control exhibiting a reasonably high degree of similarity to his/her fellow controls. Novices show slightly higher intra-group similarity, but with increasing radiological experience, the "mean" individual becomes much less similar to his/her peers, regaining similarity as he/she becomes an experienced radiologist.

As stated earlier, only the initial 1.5s of the eye movement traces have been considered here, but figure 4 shows a similar analysis to that in figures 1 to 3 for analysis over 3s. It is included to illustrate that the trends observed over 1.5s are maintained over 3s.

The accuracy of the values in figures 1 to 4 is denoted by error bars representing the standard error on the means. It is also useful to consider the *spread* of values for each of the groups. Mean similarities were calculated for each of the individuals in the study when compared with all controls, all radiologists, and all others within the individual's group. These individual measures were then averaged for each group to give a mean similarity for members of that group. Figure 5 shows the standard deviation on those means, in order to illustrate the spread of individual means within a group. In comparisons with controls, radiologists, and within their own group, the trainees show markedly higher standard deviation and hence spread of individual means than any of the other groups. There was therefore much variation in the response of individuals in the trainee group.

4. DISCUSSION

Figures 3 and 5 demonstrate a high degree of similarity in the locations of fixations for individuals within the same group, for controls, novices and for radiologists. However, the trainees show considerably more variability in response within their group. There is clearly less of a standard "trainee" response in terms of the locations of fixations, unless the group is characterised by this idiosyncratic quality.

Differences between the trainee response and that of the other groups are also visible in figures 1 and 2, which show how the eye movement response of an individual develops with experience relative to that of a control and radiologist respectively. The response of novices appears to be less similar to controls and more similar to radiologists than that of the inexperienced controls. However, a gradual progression, in terms of the eye movement response becoming more like a radiologist and less like a control as experience increases, is not observed in the data. The novices are as similar to the radiologists as the radiologists are to themselves, and as similar to the controls as are the radiologists. The trainees, on the other hand, are less like the controls and less like the radiologists than are any of the groups.

The responses of the two extremes of radiological experience, namely the controls and the radiologists, are what one might expect. The radiologists tend to look at the image in a similar way as a group, using the same cues in the image, and lacking similarity with the controls. This is significant in that it shows that in terms of this low level response to the radiological image, radiologists are not the same as controls. The controls also tend to look at the image in a similar way as a group, lacking similarity with the radiologists, and presumably using a set of non-radiologically derived cues. Experienced radiologists share some similarity with controls, so perhaps the experienced radiologist learns to use the basic visual information available to controls in tandem with the radiological visual information unavailable to controls. After all, the visual system of an experienced radiologist developed from that of a control, and trained radiologists still have to deal with the everyday images of the world.

Moving on to the novice group, since these are individuals who have had only a few months of experience it might seem surprising that at this early stage their eye movements are as similar to radiologists and controls as are the radiologists themselves. However, "similar" does not mean "the same"; we cannot tell from the data the nature of the similarity, i.e.

whether the way in which novices are similar to radiologists is the way that radiologists are similar to each other. It would appear that what little experience the novices have gained has had an effect on their response to the radiological image since they are more similar to radiologists than controls, though it may be that their years of medical (rather than radiological) training have had an input. This similarity to radiologists occurs so early in the presentation of the image (i.e. within the first 1.5s), that it must be largely unconscious, and driven by the appearance of the stimulus rather than by a slow reasoned radiological or medical appraisal of the image.

Finally, the trainees present the most interesting data of all the groups and merit further study. Their members are more idiosyncratic in their responses, in that there is a less well-defined "typical" way that trainee radiologists examine chest radiographs, compared with controls, novices or experienced radiologists. Trainees show less similarity to both controls and radiologists than any of the groups. The gain in similarity to radiologists with training observed in the novices is gone, and to become more like the radiologists they will also have to become more similar to the controls!

Trainees are less like controls than experienced radiologists and less like radiologists than controls. It could be argued that this results from the trainee consciously trying to drive the visual system rather than sitting back and trusting it like the other groups. In chasing for what it thinks might be there, the trainee shuns cues available to the controls resulting from the basic features of the image and misses the radiological cues available to the radiologist. This is unlikely as this study was performed on the first 1.5s of eye-movement data, limiting the conscious driving of eye-movements and the planning of a search strategy. Another possibility is that in the development from control to experienced radiologist the visual system does not undergo a smooth transition - it becomes eccentric, disordered, as it reorders itself to handle both radiological and everyday images. The trainee state is therefore neither one thing nor the other. In order to become more similar to the radiologist, it maybe that the trainee must first become less similar as a drastic "rewiring" is taking place at a neural level.

5. CONCLUSION

Control observers examine every day images in a similar way and this is also true of radiological images. Experienced radiologists view radiological images in a similar way to each other, but their training has resulted in differences between them and controls. In becoming experienced radiologists, it appears that trainees may move through a developmental phase characterised by more idiosyncratic eye movements; their eye movements becoming less similar to controls or experienced radiologists than they were. With experience the eye movements of trainee radiologists may become more similar to both groups, but the transition of the trainee from novice to experienced radiologist is not a simple one: the change involves a period of some disorder.

ACKNOWLEDGEMENTS

The authors would like to thank the staff and students of the Department of Diagnostic Radiology, University of Wales College of Medicine, Cardiff for volunteering as patient observers. David Wooding was supported by a grant from the Welsh Scheme for the Development of Health and Social Research (under the aegis of the Welsh Office).

REFERENCES

1. J. R. Antes, "The time course of picture viewing." *J. of Exp. Psychol.* **103**(1), pp. 62-70, 1974.
2. F. Attneave, "Informational aspects of visual perception." *Psychol. Rev.* **61**, pp. 183-193, 1954.
3. J. L. Barbur, W. D. Thomson, and P. M. Forsyth, "A New System for the Simultaneous Measurement of Pupil Size and Two-Dimensional Eye Movements." *Clinical Vision Sciences* **2**(2), pp. 131-142, 1987.
4. J. C. Bass, C. Chiles, "Visual Skill. Correlation with Detection of Solitary Pulmonary Nodules." *Invest. Radiol.* **25**(9), pp. 994-998, 1990.
5. K. S. Berbaum, W. R. Smoker, and W. L. Smith, "Measurement and prediction of diagnostic performance during radiology training." *Am. J. Roentg.* **145**(6), pp. 1305-11, 1985.
6. I. Biedermann, R. J. Mezzanotte, and J. C. Rabinowitz, "Scene perception: Detecting and judging objects undergoing violation." *Cog. Psychol.* **14**, pp. 143-177, 1982.
7. T. Buswell, *How people look at pictures.* University of Chicago Press, Chicago, 1935.

8. D. P. Carmody, H. L. Kundel, and L. C. Toto, "Comparison scans while reading chest images. Taught, but not practiced." *Invest. Radiol.* **19**(5), pp. 462-466, 1984.

9. W. G. Chase, and H. A. Simon, "The mind's eye in chess." In: *Visual information processing,* W.G. Chase (Ed.), Academic Press, New York, 1973.

10. P. Ginsburg, *Visual information processing based on spatial filters constrained by biological data.* Ph.D. Thesis. University of Cambridge, 1978.

11. D. Gould, "Looking at pictures" In: *Eye movements and psychological processes.* R. A. Monty, and J. W. Senders (Eds.), pp. 323-345, Erlbaum Associates, Inc., New Jersey, 1978.

12. P. G. Herman, and S. J. Hessel, "Accuracy and Its Relationship to Experience in the Interpretation of Chest Radiographs." *Invest. Radiol.* **10**(1), pp. 62-67, 1975.

13. A. M. Jacobs, "Eye-movement control in visual search: How direct is visual span control?" *Perception and Psychophysics*, **39**(1), pp. 47-58, 1986.

14. M. Jeannerod, P. Gerin, and J.Pernier, "Déplacements et fixations du regard dans l'exploration d'une scene visuelle." *Vision Res.* **8**, pp. 81-97, 1968.

15. A. Karni, and D. Sagi, "The time course of learning a visual skill." *Nature* **365**, pp. 250, 1993.

16. H. L. Kundel, and P. S. La Follette Jr., "Visual search patterns and experience with radiological images." *Radiology* **103**(3), pp. 523-528, 1972.

17. H. L. Kundel, C. F. Nodine, "Interpreting Chest Radiographs Without Visual Search." *Radiology* **116**, pp. 527-532, 1975.

18. H. L. Kundel, and D. J. Wright, "The Influence of Prior Knowledge on Visual Search Strategies During the Viewing of Chest Radiographs." *Radiology* **93**, pp. 315-320, 1969.

19. H. L. Kundel., C. F. Nodine, D. Thickman, and L. Toto, "Searching for Lung Nodules. A Comparison of Human Performance with Random and Systematic Scanning Models." *Invest. Radiol.* **22**(5), pp. 417-422, 1987.

20. H. L. Kundel, C. F. Nodine, and E. A. Krupinski, "Searching for lung nodules. Visual dwell indicates locations of false-positive and false-negative decisions." *Invest. Radiol.* **24**(6), pp. 472-478, 1989.

21. E. Llewellyn Thomas, "Search Behavior." *Rad. Clin. North Am.* **7**(3), pp. 403-17, 1969.

22. E. Llewellyn Thomas, and E. L. Lansdown, "Visual search patterns of radiologists in training." *Radiology* **31**, pp. 288-92, 1963.

23. P. J. Locher, and C. F. Nodine, "Symmetry catches the Eye." In: *Eye movements: From Physiology to Cognition.* J. K. O'Regan and A. Lévy-Schoen (Eds.), pp. 353-361, Elsevier Science Publishers B.V. (North-Holland), 1987.

24. G. R. Loftus, "Eye fixations and recognition memory for pictures." *Cog. Psychol.* **3**, pp. 525-551, 1972.

25. G. R. Loftus, and N. H. Mackworth, "Cognitive determinants of fixation location during picture viewing." *J. Exp. Psychol.: Hum. Perc. Perf.* **4**, pp. 565-572, 1978.

26. N. H. Mackworth, and A. J. Morandi, "The gaze selects informative detail within pictures." *Perc. Psychol.* **2**(11), pp. 547-551, 1967.

27. S. K. Mannan, K. H. Ruddock, and D. S. Wooding, "Automatic Control of Saccadic Eye Movements made in Visual Inspection of briefly presented 2-D images" *Spatial Vision* **9**(3), pp. 363-386, 1995.

28. S. K. Mannan, K. H. Ruddock, and D. S. Wooding, "The relationship between the locations of spatial features and those of fixations made during visual examination of briefly presented images." *Spatial Vision* **10**(3), pp. 165-188, 1996.

29. C. F. Nodine, and H. L. Kundel, "The Cognitive Side of Visual Search in Radiology." In: *Eye Movements: From Physiology to Cognition.* J. K. O'Regan and A. Lévy-Schoen. (Eds.), pp. 573-581, Elsevier Science Publishers B.V., North-Holland, 1987.

30. A. Oliva, P. G. Schyns, and G. Tiberghien, "Regularity of Spatial Organisation in Scene Categories and Coarse-to-Fine Identification." *Perception* **22**, Supplement: 16th European Conference on Visual Perception Abstracts, pp. 102, 1993.

31. M. C. Potter, "Short-term conceptual memory of pictures." *J. Exp. Psychol.: Human Learning and Memory* **2**, pp. 509-522. 1976.

32. P. L. Rackow, V. M. Spitzer, W. R. Hendee, "Detection of low-contrast signals. A comparison of observers with and without radiology training." *Invest. Radiol.* **22**(4): pp. 311-314. 1987.

33. K. Rayner, and A. Pollatsek, "Eye movements and Scene Perception." *Can. J. Psychol.* **46**, pp. 342-376, 1992.

34. W. Richards, and L. Kaufman, "'Centre-of-gravity' tendencies for fixations and flow patterns." *Perc. and Psychol.* **5**, pp. 81-84, 1969.

35. W. J. Tuddenham, and W. P. Calvert "Visual Search Patterns in Roentgen Diagnosis." *Radiology* **76**, pp. 255-256, 1961.

36. G. J. Walker-Smith, A. G. Gale, and J. M. Findlay, "Eye movement strategies in face perception." *Perc.* **6**, pp. 313-326, 1977.

37. A. Yarbus, *Eye movements and Vision.* Plenum press, New York, 1967.

A Chronometric Analysis of Mammography Expertise

Claudia Mello-Thoms[1], Calvin F. Nodine and Harold L. Kundel

University of Pennsylvania School of Medicine, Philadelphia PA 19104

ABSTRACT

This paper studies the effects of training and experience on decision time and performance in mammography. We compared the performance of three groups of observers representing different levels of expertise: dedicated breast imagers (mammographers), radiology residents undergoing a mammography rotation, and mammography technologists, when reading a test set that contains benign and malignant lesions, as well as lesion free images. We show that the number of cases read significantly impacts performance, as measured by the area under the AFROC curve. We also show that different levels of expertise have different decision structures during the time course of image viewing. In fact we show that the mammographers should stop reading an image after 60-80 seconds, because at this point they have found all of the true targets present, and they are much more likely to make a mistake. On the other hand residents and technologists mistakes plague their performance throughout the time course of image viewing.

Keywords: expertise, mammography, AFROC analysis, time course of image viewing.

1. INTRODUCTION

Breast cancer is one of the leading causes of death among American women. It is estimated that one woman is diagnosed with this disease every three minutes, and from these, 46,000 will die each year (3). Many techniques are available for diagnosing breast cancer; the most widely used is Mammography, due to its cost/effectiveness ratio, which allows for the screening of large parcels of the population. It has been shown (4) that mammography screening leads to a reduction of breast cancer mortality of 29-45% in women in their forties, and 34% for older women.

In this paper the roles of experience and training in mammography expertise are studied. We compared the performance of experienced radiologists dedicated to breast imaging (mammographers), radiology residents undergoing a mammography rotation and mammography technologists, when reading a test set composed of 78 two-view mammograms containing benign and malignant lesions, as well as lesion free cases. These three groups differ in their levels of formal learning (training) and total number of cases read (experience). As a consequence, the speed and accuracy relationship, which is a hallmark of expertise, is clearly observed in the decision structures of these three groups.

Although it is almost impossible to find one measure that defines an expert in mammography, one can consider that each case read, with or without feedback, corresponds to a learning trial. In this sense it has been estimated (1) that expertise in mammography translates roughly to an average of 12,000 cases a year over a period of 3 years. If one considers that the average radiology resident sees, over a period of 4 years, around 900 cases, of which perhaps a dozen are actual cancers, then it becomes clear that many more years of dedicated work will be necessary to elevate that radiologist to the level of his or her expert peers. This paper will explore the relationship between the number of cases read and performance, as measured by the area under the AFROC curve.

Also, the features that signal breast cancer may be very small and difficult to find. This is translated in a False Negative rate of 10 to 30%, of which 2/3 are seen in retrospect (2). Because these False Negatives (FNs) may have potentially deadly consequences, experts learn to over-read the cases, which generates high rates of False Positives (FPs). When these FPs occur in the time course of decision making will also be examined in this paper.

2. MATERIALS AND METHODS

The test set used consisted of 78 image pairs representing the cranial-caudal (CC) and the medial-lateral oblique (MLO) views of the breast. It was digitized using a Lumiscan Model 100 digitizer (Lumisys Inc., Sunnyvale, CA) using a 100 micron spot size. This test set was assembled from cases considered normal for two years by mammographic assessment and cases with benign and malignant lesions that were biopsied and thus confirmed as being either benign or malignant.

---

[1] Correspondence: Email: cthoms@mipgsun.mipg.upenn.edu

146

Part of the SPIE Conference on Image Perception and Performance
San Diego, California • February 1999
SPIE Vol. 3663 • 0277-786X/99/$10.00

The test set was displayed on a single 19-inch 2048 x 2048 gray scale monitor (GMA 201, Tektronix, Beaverton, OR) interfaced to a Sun Sparc 10 workstation (Sun Microsystems, Sunnyvale, CA). Each display consisted of two views of the same breast: on the left hand side was the CC view, and on the right hand side was the MLO view.

The observers were instructed to indicate malignant lesions only. They were free to search the image for as long as they wished. Upon encountering a malignant lesion, they were supposed to move a mouse controlled cursor to the center of that malignant lesion, and click. This action would cause a window to open, in which they had to indicate the type of the lesion (mass, calcification, architectural distortion), and their level of confidence that that lesion was indeed malignant (definitely malignant, highly suspicious for malignancy, moderately suspicious for malignancy and low suspicious of malignancy). Note that the observers were instructed to indicate the same lesion in the other view of the breast, if they could see it. If only benign lesions were found, the observers were instructed to go to the next image, by clicking a button entitled "Return to Screening". Similarly, if no lesions were found the observers were instructed to go to the next image. Also, in order to get information about the different experience levels, we obtained data on the number of mammographic reports generated by the residents and mammographers.

3. RESULTS

Detection and Localization of Malignant Lesions: We assessed the observers abilities to detect and localize malignant breast lesions as a function of the observers' expertise. The area under the AFROC, A1, was used to compare the three groups. The average area per observer derived from analysis of variance of A1 values was .840(.039) for mammographers, .653(.058) for residents and .592(.062) for technologists. Analysis of variance indicated that the mammographers were significantly better (p<.01, Scheffe test) than either residents or technologists. Furthermore, these last two groups did not differ significantly from one another.

Performance vs. Experience: The 19 radiology residents who were part of our study were primarily third- and forth-year residents, and three of them were fellows at the time of these tests. They had a mammography reading experience that varied from 10 to 2465 cases over a 3-year interval. Over the same period the mammographers read between 9459 and 12145 cases. The relationship between A1 and the log (base 10) number of cases (we used the log because of the power law of learning (5)) shows a significant linear regression fit (R2=.667), having a positive slope, which indicates that case reading experience indeed influences A1 performance over a wide range of experience (F(1,22)=44.15,p<.0001). This is shown in Figure 1.

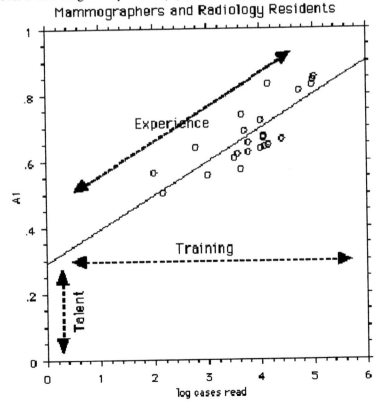

Figure 1. The roles of experience and training in observer performance, as measured by the area under AFROC, A1.

Note that the regression line intercepts the y axis at A1=.293. This implies that, with zero reading case experience, the observers performed close to the chance line, which is A1=.00 for AFROC. The fact that the performance is still above the chance line in the beginning of a mammography rotation can be explained by taking into account that these residents were already exposed to general radiology residence training.

Decision Times vs. Decision Outcomes: We also looked at the decision times as a function of decision outcome. Note that because the observers were instructed to indicate the lesion pair (that is, the same lesion on both views of the breast), when possible, they made on average two or more decisions per case (a case being a set with two images, one CC and one MLO view of the same breast, displayed simultaneously). For these paired decisions, decision times to the first decision were inversely proportional to the level of expertise. The mammographers were significantly faster than the residents (p<.01, Scheffe test), and residents significantly faster than technologists (p<.0001, Scheffe test). When comparing the mammographers with the residents we found that 32% more of these first decisions were True Positives, and they were reported faster than residents'. Mean decision time for the correct decision per pair was 15.66 sec v. 21.56 sec, t(376)=3.91, p<.001. On the other hand the technologists detected even fewer True Positives, and did so at a much slower pace (28.08 sec).

Time Course of Image Viewing: Finally we looked at the question of when the True (TPs) and False Positive (FPs) decisions occurred in the time course of image viewing. We have divided the FPs into two types, namely, the ones that correspond to a benign lesion (that is, they are due to the actual presence of a lesion in the image, except that the lesion was benign), which we called FPBs, and the ones that were due not to the presence of lesions themselves, but rather to a misinterpretation of the image features, which we called FPNs. This is shown in Figure 2.

Figure 2. Time Course of Image Viewing. The first curve shows the mean number of decisions for the mammographers as a function of time. Note that the FP curves do not overtake the TP curve for the initial 140 seconds of image viewing. The second curve shows how the residents perform under the same conditions. Note that there is much more competition among the FPs and the TPs. The final curve shows the results for the technologists. In this case the FPs overtake the TPs very early on, and this leads to fewer true lesions found and many more mistakes.

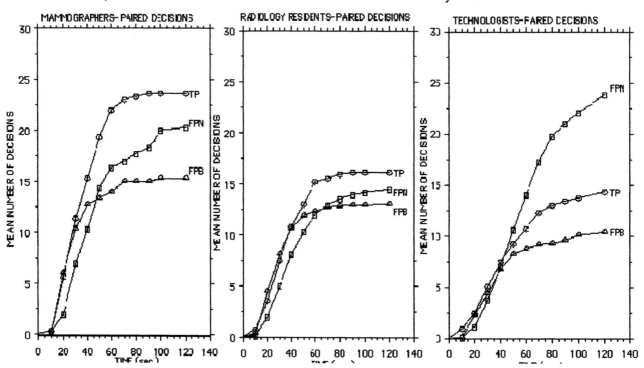

For the mammographers, although there is competition between the FPNs and the TPs during the time course of image viewing, the former never overcomes the latter, which provides further evidence that mammographers are in fact well trained target detectors. Furthermore, the FPBs are the first ones to die off, probably because, being the most common type of lesion seen on their daily practices, they are easier to discriminate from malignant lesions. For the residents the behavior is different. Although the FPNs never overtake the TPs, the competition is much more fierce. Moreover, there is also competition from the FPBs, which reflects the fact that the residents have been exposed to a smaller number of cases, and so to them it is harder to differentiate between benign and malignant lesions, as well as artifacts (that is, object-like structures that they may see in the image but that do not correspond to an actual lesion).

The technologists behavior is quite different than the other two groups. Due to a combination of lack of formal training in reading mammograms and lack of experience in doing so, they use what we chose to call 'the shot-gun strategy'. This means that anything that looks even slightly suspicious gets called as being malignant. This low threshold forces them to make many False Positive calls, and these calls overtake, very early on, the decision course of the TPs. As a consequence the technologists not only make many more calls per image but also commit many more errors, and have the lowest rate of true malignant lesions found.

4. DISCUSSION

The analysis of our data from three perspectives, namely, performance, experience and decision time, has shown that the mammographers performed significantly better than either residents or technologists when reading a test set composed of 78 two-view mammograms. We hypothesized that this better performance is directly related to the number of cases seen, because by seeing more cases they become more attuned to the features that signal a malignant lesion. They also become better at differentiating benign from malignant lesions, as well as they are less responsive to features in the image that potentially mimic a lesion, such as superposition of structures, etc. We believed that the number of cases seen has a reflection in the perceptual process, making the mammographers better target detectors and better target classifiers, in the sense that the memory schema for separating malignant from benign lesions is larger than that of either of the other two groups.

We showed the importance of experience by the significant correlation between the logarithm of the number of cases read and the performance, as measured by the area under the AFROC curve.

Furthermore, we have showed that the mammographers are significantly faster decision makers than either residents or technologists, and they are better at classifying lesions as being benign or malignant. They make many more first calls that are True Positives. Note that this reflects a speed-accuracy relationship, which is a hallmark of expertise.

In order to understand when the True and False Positive calls are made during the time course of image viewing we have studied the decision behavior of the three groups. The mammographers, being better target detectors, find most of the TPs within the first minute of image viewing. Moreover, because of their familiarity with the benign lesions, they are able to find most of these within 30 seconds of viewing the image. The interesting information in this curve is that after 60 seconds their FPNs start to rise, and eventually they overtake the TPs. This seems to indicate that the mammographers would make less errors if they stopped reading the image after 60-80 seconds, while their TPs are still dominating the FPB and FPN curves.

In the case of the residents this behavior is somewhat different, although the same pattern set by their mentors is present in that the TP curve still dominates the FP curves. In this case, however, competition is more fierce, as indicated by the longer decision times, and thus attention is very divided. The differentiation between the benign lesions (FPBs) and ones that are due to misinterpretation of image features (FPNs) becomes less pronounced, possibly as a result of having seen fewer benign lesions. Furthermore, the TPs have to constantly compete with these erroneous calls, which depresses the TP decisions.

For the technologists the situation is even worse. Their perceptual decision making process appears to have a very low threshold, causing them to call anything that seems slightly suspicious in the image as being malignant. This behavior obtains that very early on the FPs overcome the TPs, which leads the technologists to make many more errors and to find many fewer true lesions.

5. CONCLUSIONS

We have studied the roles of experience and training in mammography expertise. We have shown that not only is there a significant difference in performance as a function of level of expertise but also a difference in decision making strategies that impacts on decision time.

Our results showed that the experts are faster and better at localizing malignant lesions in a mammogram test set. This is a reflection of the speed-accuracy relationship. Furthermore, our results have shown when the experts should stop reading the films, because at a certain point in the time course of decision making False Positives overtake the True Positives. Note that this results provide support for how the experts are better, but the problem of why they are better is still a very open one.

ACKNOWLEDGEMENTS

This work has been partially supported by Grant DAMD17-97-1-7103 between the USAMRMC and CF Nodine.

REFERENCES

(1) CF Nodine, HL Kundel, SC Lauver, LC Toto. "Nature of Expertise in Searching Mammograms for Breast Masses". *Academic Radiology* 3, pp. 1000-1006, 1996.
(2) M Giger, H MacMahon. "A Perspective on False Positive Screening Mammograms". *The American College of Radiology Bulletin* 34:3, pp. 565-596, 1996.
(3) CM Kocur, SK Rogers, LR Myers, T Burns, M Kabrinsky, JW Hoffmeister, KW Bauer, JM Steppe. "Using Neural Networks to Select Wavelet Features for Breast Cancer Diagnosis". *IEEE Engineering in Medicine and Biology Magazine*, pp. 95-102, 1996.
(4) SA Feig. "A Perspective on False Positive Screening Mammograms". *The American College of Radiology Bulletin* 54:6, pp. 8-9, 1998.
(5) JR Anderson. *Cognitive Psychology and its Implications.* WH Freeman, 1995.

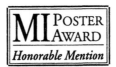

Influence of monitor luminance and tone scale on observers' search and dwell patterns

Elizabeth A. Krupinski*, Hans Roehrig

Dept. Radiology University of Arizona, Tucson, AZ 85724

ABSTRACT

The goal of this study was to measure the influence of monitor display luminance and tone scale on diagnostic performance and visual search behavior. Radiologists viewed 50 pairs of mammograms in two experiments. The first experiment changed the monitor's tone scale from its default (non-linearized) scale to the DICOM Barten scale (perceptually linearized). The second study compared an 80 ftL with a 140 ftL monitor. Eye-position was recorded. Performance with the Barten was higher than with the default curve. Performance with the 140 ftL was higher than with the 80 ftL monitor. Viewing time did not differ for tone scale, but was significantly shorter for 140 ftL vs 80 ftL. The number of fixation clusters generated was higher for the 80 ftL and the default tone scale. The difference was significant for lesion-free images. Median decision dwell times were longer in the default and 80 ftL conditions. Display luminance and tone scale affect diagnostic and search performance when using monitors. Lower luminance levels and a non-linearized display prolong search and recognition of normal, lesion-free areas compared to lesion-containing areas - radiologists are having more trouble deciding that areas are truly normal. It is recommended that such factors as monitor luminance and choice of tone scale be taken into account when deciding to use CRT monitors for viewing radiographic images in the clinical environment.

Keywords: monitors, luminance, tone scale, visual search

1. INTRODUCTION

In mammography full-field digital mammography systems may soon replace traditional film acquisition and display systems.[1-3] However, one potential impediment to regular use of digital display systems is that optimal display design and performance factors are not yet completely understood for reading radiographs from CRT monitors. There are numerous perceptual, learning and ergonomic factors that must be considered when transitioning from film to filmless radiographic reading.[4] The question of how to best display digitally acquired mammograms on a computer workstation is being addressed by a number of groups.[5-8] In fact, a recent workshop of the Working Group on Digital Mammography[9] dedicated an entire meeting to discussing "Digital Displays and Workstation Design". In addition to such issues as how to design a navigation system for viewing digitally displayed mammograms, two very important and basic factors that were recommended to consider were display luminance and tone scale. Radiographic view boxes for reading film are quite bright compared to CRT monitors. A luminance of over 1000 ftL (3500 nits) is recommended for mammography.[10] Monitors at about 200 ftL are available today, but cost and useful lifetime are important considerations when considering use of these monitors. Tone scale (the characteristic curve, comparable to gamma with film) is also very important. There is fairly good evidence[11] that a perceptually linearized display, which optimizes the display by taking into account what the capabilities of the human visual system are, is better than a non-perceptually linearized display. Basically perceptual linearization produces a tone scale in which equal changes in driving levels yield changes in luminance that are perceptually equivalent for the whole luminance range.[12-14]

The goal of the present study was to determine if changes in luminance and tone scale affect diagnostic accuracy of radiologists viewing mammograms on high-resolution CRT monitors. In addition to evaluating diagnostic performance, we were also interested in determining if changes in luminance and tone scale affect the visual search patterns of the radiologists as evaluated by recording eye position.

Part of the SPIE Conference on Image Perception and Performance
San Diego, California • February 1999
SPIE Vol. 3663 • 0277-786X/99/$10.00

151

2. METHODS & MATERIALS

2.1. Displays & Images

The same general paradigm was used for both studies. A series of 50 pairs of mammograms (craniocaudal and mediolateral views, right or left breast) was collected from the Tucson Breast Center. Eighteen of the cases had a single subtle mass, eighteen had a single subtle cluster of microcalcifications, and fourteen were lesion free. Cases with masses or microcalcifications were all biopsy proven, and the lesion-free cases had confirmed lesion-free status for at least three years. The films were digitized using a Lumisys digitizer (Lumisys, Sunnyvale, CA) with a spot size of 80 microns and a contrast resolution of 12 bits. The images were displayed on two DataRay DR110 monitors (DataRay Corp., Westminster, CO). One of the monitors had a maximum luminance of 140 ftL, and the other had a maximum luminance of 80 ftL. The monitors were the same in every other respect except for the front panel, which accounted for the 60% difference in luminance. See Table I for basic specifications of the monitors. A Dome MD4 display controller board (Dome Imaging Systems, Inc. Waltham, MA) was used in both monitors. For the luminance study the default tone scale (non-perceptually linearized) was used for image presentation. In the tone scale study only the 140 ftL monitor was used. The images were seen once using the default scale and once using the Barten (perceptually linearized) scale. In both studies, ambient room lights were turned off in order to make viewing conditions as similar as possible in both studies.

Table 1. Basic specifications for the DR110 DataRay monitors.

Display Type	Portrait Mode
CRT Size	21" FS
Deflection Angle	90 deg
Active Display Area	11.5" x 15.5"
Phosphor	P-45
Bulb Transmission	52%
Panel	92% and 62%
Resolution	1728 x 2304
Refresh Rate	70 Hz

2.2. Viewing Procedure

Six radiologists participated in each study. The same six radiologists did not participate in both studies because in each study they had to view each image in each of two conditions. A counterbalanced randomized experimental design was used for each study. For the luminance study, three of the radiologists saw half of the images on the 140 ftL monitor in the first session and the other half on 80 ftL monitor in the second session. After a period of at least six months (to promote forgetting of the images), the observers came back and viewed the images in the opposite conditions. The other three observers viewed the images in the reverse order. The protocol was the same for the six observers in the tone scale study. Each session lasted about one hour. The pairs of images appeared side-by-side (CC on the left, MLO on the right). No image functions were available during the monitor reading sessions. Observers could view images for as long as desired. Viewing time per case was recorded. For each case, the observers had to report their decision in two parts. For the first decision observers had to decide if the case was lesion-free or if it contained a mass or microcalcification cluster. They then had to report their confidence in that decision using a six-level rating scale, where 1 = no lesion, definite and 6 = lesion present, definite. If a mass or microcalcification cluster was reported, observers had to indicate its position on an outline of the breast provided for that purpose. Observers could indicate more than one finding per case.

2.3. Eye-Position Recording & Analysis

Eye position was recorded using an Eye-Tracker 4000SU system with head tracker (Applied Science

Laboratories, Waltham, MA). Complete details of the procedures used to record eye position and calibrate the position of the observers can be found in a report by Nodine et al.[15] For initial calibration purposes in the present study, the observers were seated 45 cm from the display. After calibration observers were free to move in closer to the display and move their head. A detailed account of the methods used to analyze the x,y fixation data can be found in Nodine et al.[15] For this study, if 50% of the area of a fixation cluster overlapped a mass or microcalcification cluster, it was considered a "hit". The same criterion was used for a false-positive decision, except the cluster overlapped the erroneously reported image location. True-negative decisions constituted those areas with fixation clusters that were lesion free.

3. RESULTS

3.1. Diagnostic Accuracy

The diagnostic accuracy results have been presented in detail previously.[16] Briefly, however, performance was measured using Alternative Free Response Receiver Operating Characteristic Analysis. The average area under the curve (A1) in the luminance study was 0.9594 for the 80 ftL monitor and 0.9695 for the 140 ftL monitor. The difference was not statistically significant (t = 1.685, df = 5, p = 0.1528). The true-positive rate was slightly higher (85% vs 83%) for the 140 ftL monitor and the true-negative rate was slightly higher (88% vs 86%). In the tone scale study, A1 was 0.9720 for the Barten scale and 0.9511 for the default. The difference was statistically significant (t = 5.423, df = 5, p = 0.0029). The true-positive rate was higher (88% vs 84%) for the Barten curve, as was the true-negative rate (87% vs 82%).

3.2. Visual Search

The eye-position data were analyzed along a number of parameters. The first parameter analyzed was total viewing time per case. In the luminance study, average viewing time with the 80ftL monitor was 52.71 sec (sd = 24.08, min = 6 sec, max = 99 sec). The average viewing time with the 140 ftL monitor was 48.99 sec (sd = 22.15, min = 10 sec, max = 99 sec). The difference was statistically significant (t = 1.99, df = 299, p = 0.047). Total viewing time with the Barten curve was 49.53 sec (sd = 20.55, min = 11 sec, max = 98 sec).

The eye-position dwell time data were analyzed with respect to median dwell times for true and false, positive and negative decisions. The results of these analyses are presented in Table 2.

Table 2. Median decision dwell times (msec) for the tone scale and luminance studies. TP = true positive, FN = false negative, FP = false positive, TN = true negative.

	TP	FN	FP	TN
Barten Curve	1636	1299	1853	586
Default Curve	1748	1411	1945	613
140 ftL	1684	1329	1527	604
80 ftL	1737	1647	1741	627

As Table 2 illustrates, all decision dwell times were greater for the default vs Barten tone scale and for the 80 ftL vs 140 ftL monitors. In the luminance study, the difference for the true negative dwells was statistically significant ($X^2 = 4.08$, df = 1, p < 0.05). Another eye-position parameter related to dwell times is number of clusters generated during search. For this analysis, the number of clusters generated during search was examined for the lesion-free images, those with microcalcifications and those with masses. The results of this analysis are presented in Table 3.

Table 3. Average number of clusters generated during search in the luminance and tone scale studies for lesion-free, microcalcification containing and mass containing cases.

	Lesion-Free	**Microcalcification**	**Mass**
Barten Curve	11.04	9.17	8.64
Default Curve	11.49	9.19	8.68
140 ftL	10.55	9.18	8.52
80 ftL	12.05	9.30	8.89

As Table 3 illustrates, the number of clusters generated was consistently higher for all types of images for the default vs Barten scales and for the 80 ftL vs 140 ftL monitors. In the luminance study the difference for the lesion-free images was statistically significant ($t = 2.83$, $df = 166$, $p < 0.01$).

4. DISCUSSION

When using CRT monitors to view radiographic images, diagnostic accuracy and visual search are influenced to some degree by both luminance levels and the type of characteristic curve or tone scale that is used. The higher luminance monitor yielded slightly higher diagnostic performance than the lower luminance monitor; and the perceptually linearized (Barten curve) monitor yielded slightly higher diagnostic performance than the non-linearized default curve. For the tone scale study, the difference in diagnostic performance was statistically significant and the greater true-positive and true-negative rates for the Barten curve show why this difference exists. The difference in the luminance study was not statistically significant, but the same trend for higher true positives and true negatives was evident in this study for the higher luminance monitor. In both studies, AFROC A1 values were quite high. This probably has to do with the fact that the radiologists were merely asked to perform a detection task – determine if a lesion is present and identify it as either a mass or microcalcification. They were not asked to follow this up with a classification of benign or malignant. If they had been asked to perform a classification task, diagnostic performance assessed in this manner may not have been so high. It is still interesting to note, however, that even the basic detection task was affected by the luminance and tone scale of the monitor.

The eye-position data were quite interesting as well. The data from both studies indicate that monitor conditions can significantly affect visual search behavior. Overall viewing times were longer with the lower luminance and non-linearized displays than with the higher luminance and linearized displays. The time differences may seem small when looking at the raw numbers, but if you add the differences up over a day's worth of cases that need to be read, these relatively small differences can add up. This could result in greater fatigue associated with reading images or fewer images being read in a given period of time. The dwell and number of clusters data suggest one possible reason for the overall prolonged viewing times. For the lower luminance and non-linearized displays, dwell times were longer for every type of decision and more clusters were generated on every type of image (lesion-free or lesion-containing) than for the higher luminance and linearized displays. Since it is generally assumed that dwell time is a reflection of information processing [15,17-18], one possible conclusion is that more information processing is needed in the lower luminance and non-linearized viewing conditions. Specifically, it seems that the true negative decisions and searches of lesion-free image areas is most affected by changes in luminance and tone scale. Radiologists seem to be having a more difficult time deciding that normal image areas are indeed normal. Radiologists must alter their regular search strategies and patterns to compensate difficulties in interpreting certain image areas due to shortcomings in the display parameters.

The results of these two studies suggest that if radiologists are to regularly review radiographic images from CRT monitors, care must be taken in choosing which monitors should be used and how they should be set up. Higher luminance monitors with a perceptually linearized tone scale seem to result in improved diagnostic and visual search performance. To what degree this holds true with even brighter monitors those we tested remains to be seen. There may come a point where the luminance is too high and a significant amount of eye strain and fatigue results. Further testing and experience in the clinical environment will help clarify this issue. Whether there are better tone scales available other than the Barten curve also needs to be investigated further. It is clear however hat perceptual linearization does provide a significant benefit both in terms of diagnostic performance and search behaviors.

ACKNOWLEDGMENTS

This work was supported in part by Toshiba Medical Systems, Tokyo, Japan and DataRay Corporationm, Westminster, CO.

REFERENCES

1. R.B. Schilling, J.D. Cox, S.R.D. Sharma, "Advanced digital mammography", *J Digital Imaging* **11**, pp. 163-165, 1998.

2. R.H. Moore, D.B. Kopans, L.T. Niklason, P.J. Slanetz, K.A. McCarthy, D.A. Hall, et al. "Initial clinical experience with full-field digital mammography", *Radiology* **205(P),** pp. 274, 1997.

3. L.L. Fajardo, M.B. Williams MB. The clinical potential of digital mammography. In: Doi K, Giger ML, Nishikawa RM, Schmidt RA, eds. Digital Mammography '96. New York, NY: Elsevier, 1996;43-52.

4. Wang J, Langer S. A brief review of human perception factors digital displays for Picture Archiving and Communications Systems. J Digital Imaging 1997;10:158-168.

5. Williams MB, Mangiafico PA, Simoni PU, Stanton MJ, Phillips W, Rosen D. Workstation display of images from a prototype detector for digital mammography. Radiology 1997;205(P):742.

6. Zeffiro T, Sterling VA, VanMeter J. Digital mammography review station. Radiology 1997;205(P):742.

7. Hemminger BM, Dillon A, Pisano ED, Johnston RE. Demonstration of a softcopy display system for digital mammography. Radiology 1997;205(P):743.

8. Jahangiri MI, Lou SL, Hoogstrate DR, Huang HK. Full-field direct digital mammogram (FFDM) display workstation (DWS). Radiology 1997;205(P):745.

9. Working Group on Digital Mammography: Digital Displays and Workstation Design. Meeting held March 9-10, 1998; Washington, DC.

10. American College of Radiology. Recommended specifications for new mammography equipment: screen-film systems, image receptors, and film processors. Reston, VA: ACR, 1995;43-45.

11. S.M. Pizer, "Intensity mappings: linearization, image-based, user-controlled", *Proc SPIE* **271**, pp. 21-27, 1981.

12. R.E. Johnston, J.B. Zimmerman, D.C. Rogers, S.M. Pizer, "Perceptual standardization", *Proc SPIE* **536**, pp. 44-49, 1985.

13. B.M. Hemminger, R.E. Johnston, J.P. Rolland, K.E. Muller, "Perceptual linearization of video display monitors for medical image presentation", *Proc SPIE* **2164**, pp. 222-241, 1994.

14. M.I. Sezan, K.L. Yip, S.J. Daly, "Uniform perceptual quantization: applications to digital radiography", *IEEE Trans Syst Man Cybern* **SMC-17**, pp. 622-634, 1987.

15. Nodine CF, Kundel HL, Toto LC, Krupinski EA. Recording and analyzing eye-position data using microcomputer workstation. Behav Res Methods Instrum Comput 1992;24:475-485.

16. E.A. Krupinski, H. Roehrig, T. Furukawa, C. Tang, "Influence of monitor luminance and tone scale on observer detection performance", *Proc SPIE* **3340**, pp. 99-104, 1998.

17. M.A. Just, P.A. carpenter, "Eye fixations and cognitive processes", *Cognitive Psychology* **8**, pp. 441-480, 1976.

18. M.A. Just, P.A. Carpenter, "Reading and spatial cognition: reflections from eye fixations", In: G. Luer, U. Lass, J. Shallo-Hoffman, Eds. *Eye movement research: physiological and psychological aspects*, pp. 193-213, Hogrefe Publishers, Lewiston, NY, 1988

*Correspondence: Elizabeth Krupinski, PhD Department of Radiology, University of Arizona 1609 N. Warren Bldg 211 Rm 112 Tucson, AZ 85724 520-626-4498 (ph) 520-626-4376 (f) krupinski@radiology.arizona.edu

Breast cancer screening: Comparison of radiologists' performance in a self-assessment scheme and in actual breast screening

Helen C. Cowley[*] and Alastair G. Gale

Institute of Behavioural Sciences, University of Derby, Derby. UK

ABSTRACT

The PERFORMS self-assessment scheme[1,2,3] is used by the UK Breast Screening Programme as an educational tool. From this scheme a radiologist can gain insight into their own sensitivity, specificity, feature and cancer detection performance. Such data may, however, be questionable if they are not well related to the radiologist's performance in actual breast screening. Consequently, data from the scheme were compared with those from actual breast screening performance. Some correlations were found in performance, this indicates that continued use of the scheme is important to identify any areas of individual difficulty.

Keywords: PERFORMS, breast screening, performance, radiologist, sensitivity, specificity

1. INTRODUCTION

The PERFORMS (PERsonal perFORMance in Mammographic Screening) self-assessment scheme has been used by breast screening radiologists in the UK since 1991. It currently consists of five film sets of mammographic cases with known pathology (abnormal cases) or a normal three-year follow up (normal cases). Each case has also been inspected independently by 20 experienced breast screening radiologists and a 'radiological standard' diagnosis subsequently determined. Over 90% of UK radiologists have participated in the original PERFORMS film set and three rounds have been completed. Subsequent to this, a new film set, PERFORMS 2, has been developed and this has been in use for over a year. Various advanced training film sets are also available. The scheme is used by the National Health Service Breast Screening Programme in the UK (NHSBSP) as an educational tool. Results include information concerning an individual's:

- Sensitivity
- Specificity
- Cancer detection performance and
- Feature detection and interpretation performance.

Such information is useful to the radiologist in providing insight into their individual skill, but it is important that such performance measures also describe an individual's actual breast screening performance. Consequently, three different measures of performance in actual breast screening were compared with performance on the film set. These measures were: interval cancer data, detailed breast screening and symptomatic data and annual performance data.

2. METHOD

2.1. Interval cancer data

In the UK an interval cancer database has been established by the NHSBSP. An interval cancer is a cancer in a woman who has had a previous negative mammogram ('Screening' in Table 1) and who then presents with a symptomatic cancer ('Diagnostic' in Table 1) before the next screening mammogram. The four different types of interval cancers are shown in Table 1.

---

[*] Correspondence: Email: H.C.Cowley@derby.ac.uk   Telephone/Fax: (0)1332 622287

Part of the SPIE Conference on Image Perception and Performance
San Diego, California ● February 1999
SPIE Vol. 3663 ● 0277-786X/99/$10.00

Table 1. Types of interval cancers

Type of interval cancer	Mammography	
	Screening	Diagnostic
True interval	Normal	Abnormal
False negative	Abnormal	Abnormal
Occult	Normal	Normal
Unclassifiable	No mammography at diagnosis	

At screening all interval cancers are reported as normal by the radiologist: either due to there being no abnormality visible (i.e., true interval, occult and possibly unclassifiable) or because the abnormality was not detected or misinterpreted by the radiologist (i.e., false negative and possibly unclassifiable). The types of interval cancers that are relevant for the current research are the false negatives as it is these that have been missed by a radiologist. False negative interval cancers are ones where the radiologist missed a suspicious feature on the screening mammogram and this eventually becomes symptomatic. False negative cancers can have either **minimal** signs on the screening mammogram, e.g. subtle architectural distortion, or they can have **malignant** signs, e.g. spiculate mass. Radiologists should miss very few screening cases which have malignant signs, but those with minimal signs are more problematic and can be more easily overlooked. Increased training of radiologists can reduce the number of false negative interval cancers.

The interval cancer database contains details of 2655 interval cancers. Of these, 24% were classed as false negatives, the majority (45.5%) being false positive cases. The features missed in the false negative interval cancers were compared with those not detected or misinterpreted in rounds two and three of the original version of PERFORMS to determine whether similar features were missed.

2.2. Detailed breast screening and symptomatic performance

Anonymous 'real-life' breast screening and symptomatic data for three radiologists from one breast screening unit were compared with their performance in the self-assessment scheme. The real-life data used were provided by the radiologists from accumulated audit data from their symptomatic and breast screening practices. The breast screening data were collected from cytologically proven cases between February 1990 and December 1994 and the symptomatic data between January 1993 and December 1994.

The diagnostic accuracy for the symptomatic mammograms was determined by the use of ROC analysis on the routine audit data collected in the department. These data comprised single reader opinions of 'benign' or 'malignant', based on the symptomatic mammogram. The data were obtained from pathology and radiology departments and the mammography decisions were linked to outcome data, i.e. biopsy or fine needle aspiration cytology results. In total, 1220 cases were included in the analysis, the number of these cases read by an individual radiologist ranged from 288 to 548. The outcome data were classified as either benign or malignant. Each mammogram was scored by the radiologist using a five point scale (from -2 = benign to 2 = malignant). From these data, ROC curves were constructed for each radiologist using ROCFIT[4].

Breast screening data were collected in a similar way, the information used was based on the cases recalled for review and the mammograms taken at this stage were single read. In total, 1090 cases were included and the number of cases read by a single radiologist ranged from 267 to 413 cases. A five point rating scale was again used to score each mammogram and ROC analysis performed.

2.3. Annual breast screening performance

All radiologists in the NHSBSP keep a record of the number of women screened, recalled, cancers detected, size of these cancers, missed cancers etc. These data are fed into a computer system at each breast screening unit and are collated to provide national performance values. Thirty-six radiologists were able and willing to release their individual data on a strictly confidential basis. They provided values concerning the number of cases read and recalled; and the number of malignant cases detected and missed each year. The data ranged from 1993 to 1997 inclusive, the number of radiologists that provided data for each of these years are detailed in the following table.

Table 2. Number of radiologists providing data per year

	1993-1994	1994-1995	1995-1996	1996-1997
Number of radiologists	5	16	20	28

3. RESULTS

3.1. Interval cancer data

The percentage of the occurrence of each feature in the false negative interval cancers was compared with the percentage of each feature missed in rounds two and three in the recall cases (abnormal cases requiring recall for further assessment) and the malignant cases in the original PERFORMS film set. These percentages are shown in Table 3, with each column in the table summing to 100%. This table shows a difference in the proportion of features in the interval cancers showing malignant and minimal signs. Those showing minimal signs contain more well defined masses, architectural distortions and asymmetries, abnormalities that have a positive predictive value (PPV)[5] for malignancy of 2%, 40% and less than 1% respectively and are therefore only slightly suspicious of malignancy. Whereas those with malignant signs show more ill defined and spiculate masses, these abnormalities have a PPV of 50% and 90% respectively and are therefore highly indicative of malignancy.

Table 3. Percentage of each feature missed

| | Interval Cancer Database | | | PERFORMS | | | | |
	Malignant signs	Minimal Signs	Mean	Round 2 recall cases	Round 2 malignant cases	Round 3 recall cases	Round 3 malignant cases	Mean
Wdm	1.7	5.0	4.5	3.5	3.8	5.1	5.2	4.3
Idm	27.6	18.7	20.2	16.4	15.5	14.5	11.3	15.1
Sm	22.4	8.63	11.0	9.6	6.3	10.0	7.1	9.1
Pd	13.8	21.6	20.2	18.6	17.9	18.3	17.0	18.2
Asym	20.7	26.3	25.3	28.4	18.0	27.7	22.9	26.2
Calc	13.8	19.8	18.8	23.5	38.5	24.3	36.5	27.2

Key:
Wdm	Well defined mass	Pd	Architectural distortion
Idm	Ill defined mass	Asym	Asymmetry
Sm	Spiculate mass	Calc	Calcification

A Pearson correlation was carried out to determine whether there was any similarity between these groups of data. The significant correlations are shown in Table 4.

Table 4. Significant correlations

	Pearson correlation	Significance	N
Minimal signs x Round 2 recall	0.957	0.003	6
Minimal signs x Round 3 recall	0.925	0.008	6
Minimal signs x Mean PERFORMS	0.899	0.015	6
Mean Interval x Round 2 recall	0.940	0.005	6
Mean Interval x Round 3 recall	0.892	0.017	6
Mean Interval x Mean PERFORMS	0.864	0.027	6

This table indicates a correlation between the features found in the false negative cases with minimal signs and the features found in the recall cases in the self-assessment scheme. There is also a correlation between the features found in the false negative cases (regardless of minimal or malignant signs) and the recall cases in PERFORMS.

The similarity in the proportions of the features missed in PERFORMS and the interval cancer database (ICD) is shown in Figure 1, this compares the mean percentage of each feature missed in the two sets of data, mean values are from Table 3.

Figure 1. Mean percentage of each feature missed

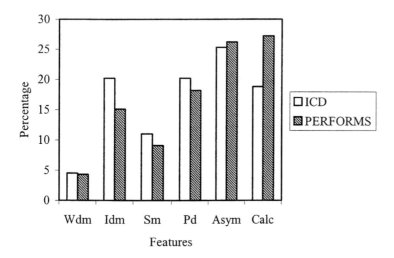

3.2. Detailed breast screening and symptomatic performance

To ascertain that the performance on the PERFORMS scheme of the three radiologists was similar to the performance of the other radiologists in their health region on the scheme, the classification A_z values (area under the ROC curve) for the three radiologists were compared with those of their colleagues. Analysis of variance found no significant differences for either round one or round two. This suggests that the classification performance of the three radiologists on the film set was similar to the other radiologists. Data for the first two rounds of PERFORMS were used because the majority of radiologists in the region had already completed these rounds. Pooled ROC curves for the two groups of subjects (Regional radiologists and the three radiologists) are shown in Figure 2. The markers on the lines are for purposes of identification only.

Figure 2. ROC curves for the three radiologists and the region

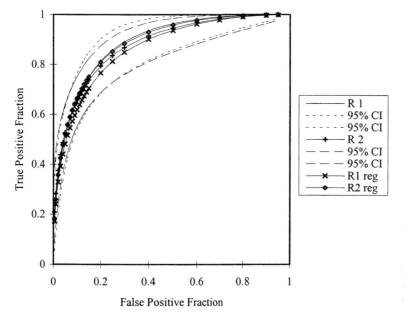

Key:
R 1   Round one data (three radiologists)
R 2   Round two data (three radiologists)
R1 reg Round one data (region)
R2 reg Round two data (region)
95%   95% confidence intervals for the
CI   R 1 and R 2 data

Ideally, the ROC curves for three radiologists for their symptomatic and breast screening data should be the same as those for the PERFORMS scheme, i.e. their PERFORMS ROC curves need to lie within the 95% confidence intervals for their real-life data and vice versa. ROC curves for the scheme were constructed for rounds one and two and for PERFORMS 2 (data were included for <u>all</u> the film sets that the radiologists had participated in). These ROC curves are shown in Figures 3 to 5. The three radiologists involved have been labelled A, B and C in order to maintain anonymity.

Figure 3. ROC curves for radiologist A

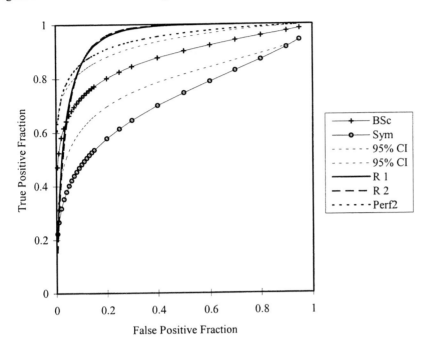

Key:
BSc   Breast screening data
Sym   Symptomatic data
95% CI   Lower and upper boundaries of the asymmetric 95% confidence intervals for breast screening
R 1   PERFORMS data, round one
R 2   PERFORMS data, round two
Perf2   PERFORMS 2 data

Figure 3 indicates that, for Radiologist A, performance on the PERFORMS scheme was better than in breast screening and symptomatic performance was the worst. The PERFORMS ROC curves do not lie within the 95% confidence intervals for breast screening or symptomatic performance. Real-life and PERFORMS performance are therefore not the same for this radiologist and performance in the self-assessment scheme was better than performance in breast screening. The symptomatic 95% confidence intervals have not been included to aid clarity.

Figure 4. ROC curves for radiologist B

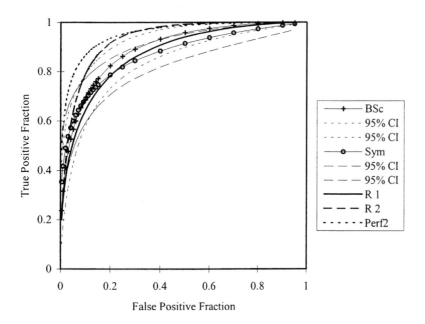

Figure 4 shows that, for Radiologist B: breast screening; symptomatic and round one data were the same (they lie within the 95% confidence intervals for the breast screening and symptomatic curves). The ROC curves for PERFORMS 2 and round two of PERFORMS lie just outside the upper boundary of the breast screening curve. This figure therefore indicates that performance in round one of PERFORMS was the same as the breast screening and symptomatic performance for this radiologist.

Figure 5. ROC curves for radiologist C

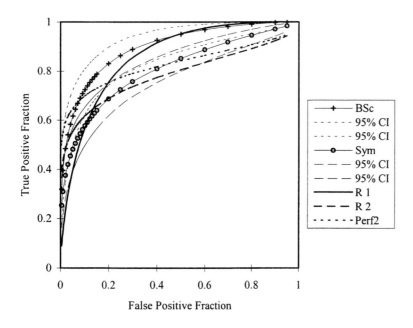

This figure shows that, for Radiologist C, round one PERFORMS data lie within the 95% confidence intervals for breast screening. The other ROC curves for PERFORMS and the symptomatic ROC curve lie just below the lower boundary of breast screening, the PERFORMS curves lying within the 95% confidence intervals for the symptomatic data. Performance in PERFORMS is therefore the same as breast screening and symptomatic performance for this radiologist.

The results for the three radiologists show that performance on PERFORMS is sometimes the same as breast screening or symptomatic performance, but other times is not. To clarify whether results from this scheme are the same as those from actual screening, the data for the three radiologists were pooled, these ROC curves are shown in Figure 6. This figure shows that for the three radiologists, performance in the self-assessment scheme lies within the 95% confidence intervals for breast screening, apart from for PERFORMS 2 which lies just above the upper boundary. Symptomatic performance lies just below the lower boundary for breast screening. Performance in PERFORMS 2 may be expected to be better than in the original version of PERFORMS as the radiologists completed this film set in 1997, rounds one and two were completed in 1992 and 1994 respectively, the breast screening data were from 1990 to 1994 and symptomatic data from 1993 to 1994. The radiologists' performance should therefore be better in PERFORMS 2 as they have increased breast screening experience at this time.

Figure 6. Pooled ROC curves for the three radiologists

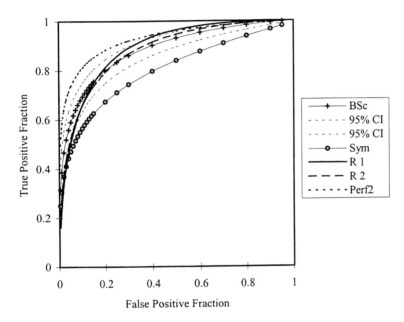

In addition to examining the ROC curves themselves, it is important to compare the A_z values for each ROC curve. These are shown in Table 5 with their standard deviation. The A_z values correspond to the curves in Figure 3 to Figure 6.

Table 5. A_z values for individual radiologists (A-C) and pooled data

A_z Values (St. Dev.)	A (Fig. 3)	B (Fig. 4)	C (Fig. 5)	Pooled (Fig. 6)
Round 1	0.95 (0.03)	0.87 (0.05)	0.86 (0.04)	0.89 (0.03)
Round 2	0.95 (0.03)	0.94 (0.03)	0.79 (0.06)	0.88 (0.03)
PERFORMS 2	0.94 (0.05)	0.95 (0.02)	0.83 (0.10)	0.93 (0.03)
Symptomatic	0.72 (0.03)	0.87 (0.02)	0.81 (0.02)	0.80 (0.01)
Breast Screening	0.87 (0.03)	0.90 (0.02)	0.90 (0.02)	0.88 (0.01)

These data were analysed using the INDROC program[6] to determine whether there were any significant differences between any of the ROC curves. This program uses a univariate z-score test of the difference between the areas under the two ROC curves. The results are shown in Table 6 and significant differences are highlighted.

Table 6. Significant differences between ROC curves

PERFORMS		Radiologists					
		A		B		C	
		BSc	Sym	BSc	Sym	BSc	Sym
R 1	P (2 tailed)	0.0870	*0.0001*	0.7198	0.9572	0.4187	0.2503
	z value	1.7117	5.0070	-0.3587	0.0537	-0.8087	1.1495
R 2	P (2 tailed)	0.0672	*0.0001*	0.2917	0.1017	0.0776	0.7227
	z value	1.8302	5.3901	1.0543	1.6366	-1.7648	-0.3548
Perf 2	P (2 tailed)	0.2411	*0.0002*	0.0630	*0.0125*	0.4968	0.8600
	z value	1.1723	3.7148	1.8594	2.4970	-0.6795	0.1764

Key:
R 1   Round one (PERFORMS)
R 2   Round two (PERFORMS)
Perf 2   PERFORMS 2
BSc   Breast Screening
Sym   Symptomatic

Table 6 shows that there were significant differences between the symptomatic ROC curve and the PERFORMS curves for radiologist A. There was also a significant difference for radiologist B between PERFORMS 2 and the symptomatic ROC curve. There were no other significant differences in performance. This indicates that although some of the ROC curves for PERFORMS and actual breast screening were not the same (i.e. did not lie within each others 95% confidence intervals), the differences in performance were never significant. Some significant differences were found between symptomatic and performance in PERFORMS, but these were mainly for radiologist A.

3.3. Annual breast screening performance

A Pearson correlation was used to compare recall rate and sensitivity for each of the years with performance in the self-assessment scheme, where:

$$\text{Recall rate} = \frac{\text{number of women recalled}}{\text{number of women screened}} \times 100$$

and

$$\text{Sensitivity} = 1 - \frac{\text{number of malignant cases missed}}{\text{number of malignant cases detected} + \text{number missed}}$$

Performance in round one of PERFORMS was compared with 1994 screening data. Second round PERFORMS data were obtained between September 1993 and December 1994, this was therefore compared with screening data from 1994 to 1995 inclusive. Finally, third round data were collected from February 1996 onwards, these were therefore compared with screening data from 1995 and 1996. Few of the 36 radiologists that supplied breast screening data had participated in PERFORMS 2 at the time of this report and so data for this film set were therefore excluded.

Table 7 shows the correlations between the performance variables in the self-assessment scheme and breast screening performance. Significant positive correlations were found between the recall rates and correct recall performance (sensitivity) in PERFORMS and significant negative correlations were found with the correct return to normal screen (specificity) percentages and the number of malignant cases missed. In addition to the recall rate of individual radiologists, breast screening data concerning sensitivity were obtained. Significant correlations for sensitivity were only found for the number of malignant cases missed in round three and sensitivity for one particular year - 1996, ($r = -0.658$, $p = 0.004$, $N = 17$).

Table 7. Correlations between PERFORMS and the recall rate

PERFORMS Round	Year of Recall Rate	CR			CS			Miss		
		r	sig	N	r	sig	N	r	sig	N
1	1994	0.734	**	15	-0.662	**	15	-0.535	*	15
2	1994	0.654	**	15	-0.681	**	15	-0.399		15
	1995	0.545	**	19	-0.576	**	19	-0.464	*	19
3	1995	0.386		17	-0.555	*	17	-0.536	*	17
	1996	0.287		24	-0.460	*	24	-0.384	*	24

Key:

*   Correlation significant at the 0.05 level (1 tailed)

**   Correlation significant at the 0.01 level (1 tailed)

The following figures show the significant results for the three rounds of PERFORMS.

Figure 7. Comparison of performance in round one and recall rate in 1994

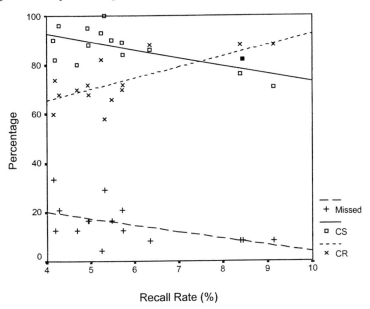

This figure indicates that as the recall rate in breast screening increased, so the correct recall (CR) rate in PERFORMS significantly increased and the correct return to normal screen (CS) rate significantly decreased. Correspondingly, the percentage of malignant cases missed (Missed) also decreased significantly.

Figure 8. Comparison of performance in round two and recall rate

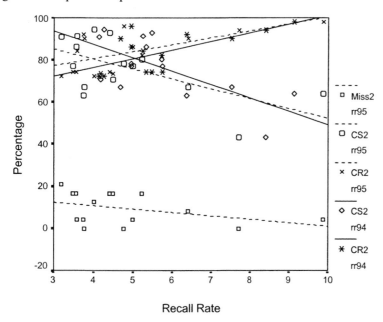

This figure indicates that in the second round of PERFORMS, a decrease in the correct return to screen (CS2) rate in PERFORMS correlated significantly with an increase in the recall rate in 1994 (rr94) and 1995 (rr95). Also, an increase in the correct recall (CR2) rate corresponded with an increase in the recall rate in 1994 (rr94) and 1995 (rr95). Finally, a decrease in the number of malignant cases missed (Miss2) correlated with the recall rate in 1995 (rr95).

Figure 9. Comparison of performance in round three and recall rate

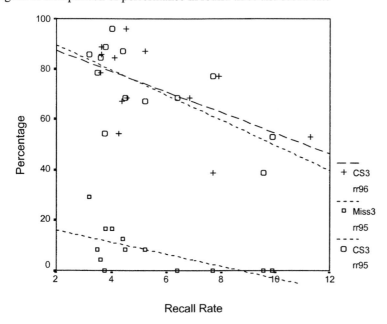

This figure indicates that for round three of PERFORMS, a decrease in correct return to screen (CS3) correlated significantly with an increase in the recall rate in the screening programme in 1995 (rr95) and 1996 (rr96). Also, a decrease in the percentage of missed malignant cases (Miss3) corresponded with an increase in recall rate in 1995 (rr95).

166

4. DISCUSSION

The PERFORMS self-assessment scheme has been in use for some time in the UK and is used as part of the quality assurance of the NHSBSP. However, results from this scheme have greater impact if performance is comparable with actual breast screening performance. The purpose of this research was therefore to assess whether there was any similarity between screening performance and PERFORMS. Although the various PERFORMS film sets comprise cases from the NHSBSP, these film sets are weighted with difficult malignant and abnormal cases. Additionally, the mammograms in the original version of the scheme may be of lower quality than later screening cases as the density of the image and the technique for taking the mammograms has changed [7]. The mammograms in PERFORMS 2 were taken between 1992 and 1994 and were therefore higher quality than those in the original version.

4.1. Interval cancer data

Comparison of the features missed in the false negative interval cancers and those not detected and misinterpreted in PERFORMS found that radiologists miss similar proportions of features. In other words, feature detection performance in the self-assessment scheme is directly comparable with that of actual breast screening.

4.2. Detailed breast screening and symptomatic performance

The purpose of this study was to ascertain whether an individual radiologist's data from the PERFORMS self-assessment scheme compared with their performance in actual breast screening. The results indicate that for radiologist C, round two PERFORMS and PERFORMS 2 data were the same as symptomatic performance and round one data was the same as breast screening performance. No significant differences in performance were found for any of these values. Radiologist B showed similarity between breast screening, symptomatic and round one data. Data for PERFORMS 2 and round two were better, the data for PERFORMS 2 being significantly different from the symptomatic performance. Radiologist A showed no similarity between PERFORMS, breast screening or symptomatic performance. Performance in the self-assessment scheme was best, then breast screening and finally symptomatic. Significant differences were found for the areas under the symptomatic and PERFORMS curves for this radiologist. When pooled ROC curves were constructed for the three radiologists, breast screening performance correlated with round one and round two performance. Symptomatic performance was lower and performance in PERFORMS 2 was higher. Overall these results indicate that some correlations were found between performance in PERFORMS and actual breast screening and there were few significant differences in performance, especially when compared with breast screening. Given the well known variability in a radiologist's performance, then these results are very positive.

4.3. Annual breast screening performance

These results found that classification performance (correct recall and correct return to normal screen percentages) and the number of malignant cases missed in the self-assessment scheme did correlate with the recall rate in breast screening. In addition, sensitivity values for 1996 to 1997 correlated significantly with the number of malignant cases missed in the self-assessment scheme in round three. These results therefore indicate that performance in the self-assessment scheme does correlate with some performance measures in actual breast screening, this therefore further validates this schemes use as a quality assurance mechanism.

5. CONCLUSIONS

Data from the interval cancer database, detailed performance values for three radiologists and annual performance values from 36 radiologists were compared with performance in PERFORMS. Results indicated that performance in the self-assessment scheme does correlate with **some** performance values from actual breast screening. The main findings were:
- The features missed in the self-assessment scheme were in the same proportions as those missed in actual breast screening.
- There were some correlations between an individual's performance in the various PERFORMS film sets and their symptomatic or breast screening performance.
- Performance for the original version of the film set correlated with breast screening performance when the data for the three radiologists were pooled, symptomatic performance was worst (lowest A_z value) and performance in the new film set was best (highest A_z value).

- There were some correlations between the annual recall rate and the CR and CS percentages in the self-assessment scheme and sensitivity in one year correlated with the number of malignant cases missed.

As the cases in the original version of PERFORMS were of somewhat lower quality and it was weighted with difficult cases, it may be expected that performance would be poorer on this film set than in actual breast screening, but this did not prove to be the case. The similarity therefore in performance for the film set and breast screening may be due to the cases being screening cases. This therefore suggests that continued participation in the original version of the scheme is important as results do indicate performance in the NHSBSP.

The cases in PERFORMS 2 were newer than those in the original version, and dated from a similar time as the breast screening cases, particularly the cases used in the study with the three radiologists. It may be expected therefore that performance on this film set be similar to breast screening performance, because of the similarity of the cases. Performance, however, on PERFORMS 2 proved to be better than performance in breast screening. There are several explanations for this, for instance: the radiologists had previous experience with the PERFORMS film sets. The cases in PERFORMS 2 have the same benign to recall and benign to malignant ratios and also contain similar proportions of features as the original version of this film set, suggesting that results from this scheme are indicative of actual performance.

ACKNOWLEDGEMENTS

We gratefully acknowledge the continued support of the National Health Service Breast Screening Programme and all the radiologists that participate in the PERFORMS scheme.

REFERENCES

1. H.C. Cowley and A.G. Gale. "Minimising human error in the detection of breast cancer." *Contemporary Ergonomics*. S.A. Robertson, (Ed.). London: Taylor and Francis, 1996.
2. A.G. Gale, A.R.M. Wilson and E.J. Roebuck. "Mammographic screening: radiological performance as a precursor to image processing." *Biomedical Image Processing and Biomedical Visualisation*. R.S. Acharya and D.B. Goldof, (Eds.). SPIE 1905: 458-464, 1993.
3. A.G. Gale, C.J. Savage, E.F. Pawley, A.R.M. Wilson and E.J. Roebuck. "Breast Screening: visual search and observer performance." *Image Perception*. H.L. Kundel, (Ed.), Proceedings SPIE Vol. 2166: 66-75, 1994.
4. C.E. Metz. "Some practical issues of experimental design and data analysis in radiological ROC studies." *Investigative Radiology;* 24: 234-245, 1989.
5. H.C. Burrell, D.M. Sibbering, A.R.M. Wilson, S.E. Pinder, A.J. Evans, L.J. Yeoman, C.W. Elston, I.O. Ellis, R.W. Blamey and J.F. Robertson. (1996). "Screening Interval Breast Cancers: Mammographic Features and Prognostic Factors." *Radiology;* 199: 811-817.
6. C.E. Metz and H.B. Kronman. 'INDROC' program: June 1989 (IBM-PC version), 1989.
7. K.C. Young, M.G. Wallis, R.G. Blanks and S.M. Moss. "Influence of number of views and mammographic film density on the detection of invasive cancers: results from the NHS Breast Screening Programme." *British Journal of Radiology;* 70: 482-488, 1997.

SESSION 5

Technology Assessment and Observer Performance I

Psychophysical Evaluation of the Image Quality of a Dynamic Flat-panel Digital X-ray Image Detector using the Threshold Contrast Detail Detectability (TCDD) Technique

Andrew G Davies, Arnold R Cowen & Tom J Bruijns[a]

Medical Physics, University of Leeds, The General Infirmary, Leeds LS1 3EX, UK.

[a]Philips Medical Systems, 5680 DA Best, NL.

ABSTRACT

We are currently in an era of active development of the digital X-ray imaging detectors that will serve the radiological communities in the new millennium. The rigorous comparative physical evaluations of such devices are therefore becoming increasingly important from both the technical and clinical perspectives. The authors have been actively involved in the evaluation of a clinical demonstration version of a flat-panel dynamic digital X-ray image detector (or FDXD).

Results of objective physical evaluation of this device have been presented elsewhere at this conference. The imaging performance of FDXD under radiographic exposure conditions have been previously reported, and in this paper a psychophysical evaluation of the FDXD detector operating under continuous fluoroscopic conditions is presented. The evaluation technique employed was the threshold contrast detail detectability (TCDD) technique, which enables image quality to be measured on devices operating in the clinical environment. This approach addresses image quality in the context of both the image acquisition and display processes, and uses human observers to measure performance. The Leeds test objects TO[10] and TO[10+] were used to obtain comparative measurements of performance on the FDXD and two digital spot fluorography (DSF) systems, one utilising a Plumbicon camera and the other a state of the art CCD camera. Measurements were taken at a range of detector entrance exposure rates, namely 6, 12, 25 and 50 µR/s. In order to facilitate comparisons between the systems, all fluoroscopic image processing such as noise reduction algorithms, were disabled during the experiments. At the highest dose rate FDXD significantly outperformed the DSF comparison systems in the TCDD comparisons. At 25 and 12 µR/s all three systems performed in an equivalent manner and at the lowest exposure rate FDXD was inferior to the two DSF systems.

At standard fluoroscopic exposures, FDXD performed in an equivalent manner to the DSF systems for the TCDD comparisons. This would suggest that FDXD would therefore perform adequately in a clinical fluoroscopic environment and our initial clinical experiences support this. Noise reduction processing of the fluoroscopic data acquired on FDXD was also found to further improve TCDD performance for FDXD. FDXD therefore combines acceptable fluoroscopic performance with excellent radiographic (snap shot) imaging fidelity, allowing the possibility of a universal x-ray detector to be developed, based on FDXD's technology. It is also envisaged that fluoroscopic performance will be improved by the development of digital image enhancement techniques specifically tailored to the characteristics of the FDXD detector.

1. INTRODUCTION

The development of solid state x-ray detectors is currently being undertaken by a number of x-ray manufacturers. It seems likely that these devices will form the basis for much of the digital image acquisition devices in the next millennium. A clinical demonstrator version of one such device, called "flat dynamic x-ray detector", or FDXD, has been installed within the Clarendon Wing x-ray department of the General Infirmary at Leeds. The assessment of the imaging and clinical performance of the system has been undertaken as a joint project between the University of Leeds, The General Infirmary, and Philips Medical Systems.

FDXD has been developed by the research laboratories of Philips Medical Systems in Germany and the Netherlands. FDXD is capable of continuous fluoroscopy, pulsed fluoroscopy, single shot and serial exposures. The detector comprises a 550 μm thick thallium activated cesium iodide layer deposited upon an amorphous silicon photo-diode sensor thin film transistor read-out array. The device has a 20 x 20 cm field size, and a 1,024 x 1,024 pixel matrix. The detector is mounted below a floating top patient table. The other elements of the system have been described previously[1].

Figure 1: Snapshot of a sialogram acquired on FDXD.

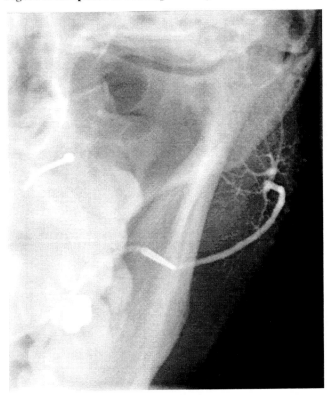

The experimental FDXD system has been installed within the General Infirmary for over one year, and early experimental studies have concentrated on single shot radiographic imaging performance. Physical measures of performance and early clinical experiences have been encouraging[1,2]. Detective Quantum Efficiency of the detector is superior to current generation photostimulable phosphor computed radiography (CR) devices at radiographic doses, and a range of clinical examinations, or parts of these examinations, have been undertaken, including:

- double contrast barium studies (Ba swallows, small bowel meals, Ba enemas)
- arthrography of the wrist
- sialography (an example snapshot image is presented in Figure 1)
- macrodacro examination
- Intravenous Pyelography
- snapshot radiography of the extremities (hand, knee, shoulder, and elbow).

The factors limiting the range of examinations performed have been related to the form factor of the experimental installation, such as the field coverage, and detector and tube mounting. In this paper the fluoroscopic performance is examined in relation to existing DSF systems. The assessment of performance was performed in three ways: physical measures of performance, early clinical experiences, and a psychophysical assessment of image quality. The physical measures of performance are presented elsewhere[3], and this paper concentrates upon the psychophysical investigation.

The low x-ray doses used in modern x-ray image intensifier television (IITV) fluoroscopy pose a challenge for any competing dynamic x-ray acquisition technology. The low fluence of incident x-ray photons per pixel require the detector to have very low noise levels. IITV systems are the current mainstay of fluoroscopic systems. These systems used an analogue TV camera to record the image formed on the output screen of the image intensifier. Digital Spot Fluorography (DSF) systems digitise the signal from the TV camera, thus allowing computer based image enhancement and noise reduction to be applied to the image data. The latest generation of DSF systems use a CCD camera to record the digital data, offering many imaging and operational benefits.

Within this paper we compare FDXD to a Plumbicon IITV system and a state-of-the-art CCD based fluoroscopy system. Both the Plumbicon and CCD based system used the same design of 35 cm x-ray image intensifier tube. The comparisons are performed at a range of dose levels, which cover the range of doses found in clinical examinations. In addition to the basic fluoroscopy performance, the impact of noise reduction processing algorithms on the data is also investigated.

1.1. Evaluation of System Performance

Threshold contrast detail detectability (TCDD) measurements are an established method of assessing image quality[4,5]. TCDD experiments rely upon human observers reading a set of radiographs (or live fluoroscopy) of a test object. The test objects contain discs, referred to as *details*, arranged in rows. Each consecutive row in the test object contains details of decreasing diameter. Details within the test object are made from metals of varying thickness, giving a range of detail contrasts. Within a row, the contrast of the details decreases. An example radiograph of such a test object is shown in Figure 2. In this example the radiographic conditions for the exposure were set to illustrate the layout of the details, whereas under normal operating conditions not all of the details within a row are visible. When scoring a test object the observer is required to specify the last detail in each row that is visible. These results are then averaged over a number of observations of the test object, and a number of observers (four observations by four experienced observers is common).

Figure 2: Radiograph of the Leeds TO[10] test object.

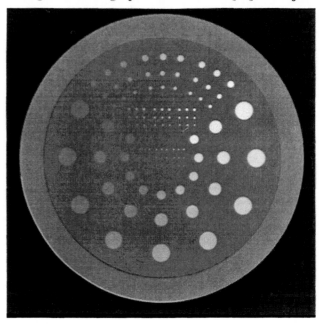

The average contrast threshold for each row is referred to as $C_t(A)$, where A is the area of the details within the row. TCDD results can then be represented on a plot of the threshold index, $H_t(A)$, where

$$H_t(A) = \frac{1}{C_t(A) \times \sqrt{A}}$$

Under ideal conditions the threshold index diagram would produce a horizontal straight line, with uniform values of $H_t(A)$, for all detail sizes. Higher values of $H_t(A)$ indicate better performance. However, unsharpness of the imaging system reduce performance smaller detail sizes. Inhibition in the human visual system and noise within the imaging system, reduce performance for larger detail sizes.

TCDD offers a method of assessing imaging performance which takes into account the physical performance of the acquisition system, manipulations on the digital image data such as image processing, the image display sub-system, and the human visual system. TCDD therefore allows analysis of the complete imaging chain unlike physical measures of performance, such as DQE, which to date have addressed the performance of the detector alone.

Criticisms of the TCDD technique include bias from the subjective nature of the human observers and the fact that the process of detecting disks in a uniform background does not necessarily mimic the same processes as a human reading a clinical radiograph[6]. Whatever, when implemented in a rigorous and controlled manner, TCDD experiments produce reproducible results, for example Launders et al.[7] describe a procedure for using the TCDD methodology that achieved a relative standard error of approximately 5%. The preferred alternative method of assessment to TCDD is a study of clinical observer's diagnostic accuracy. However, studies of observers' diagnostic performance reporting clinical images, such as the Receiver Operating Characteristic (ROC) technique, also suffer from a number of serious drawbacks. Often no non-radiological confirmation as to the presence of an abnormality can be obtained thus leaving the study with a questionable "gold-standard" and can provide potential bias. Additionally clinical data is difficult and time consuming to collect, and large demands are placed on observer's time.

TCDD therefore allows the rapid assessment of imaging performance of the whole imaging chain, with a conveniently acquired data set, and relatively low demands on observer's time and system usage. Achievable accuracies are sufficient to provide a useful tool for first line assessment, allowing the assessment of a reasonably large set of variables or systems prior to a full clinical study.

1.2. Noise reduction processing in digital fluoroscopy

The processing of fluoroscopic images, by a recursive filtering algorithm can have a large impact on image quality. The basic concept of the recursive filter is to impose temporal averaging into the fluoroscopy sequence. If P_n is the processed fluoroscopy frame n, and I the input (most recent) fluoroscopy frame, then:

$$P_{n+1} = \alpha(I) + (1-\alpha)(P_n)$$

where α controls the degree of averaging and takes values between 0 and 1. As α decreases the temporal averaging effect increases, and the effective SNR is increased thus one would expect better performance in the TCDD experiments, and eight-fold increases in DQE have been claimed by using very low values of α on a solid state fluoroscopy system[9]. However, as α is decreased temporal unsharpness is introduced into the image where movement occurs. This motion blur can make the image clinically unacceptable, and therefore sets an upper bound on the improvement which can be expected over the unprocessed fluoroscopic performance of the detector in a clinical environment.

2. MATERIALS AND METHODS

2.1. Fluoroscopy systems

2.1.1. FDXD

The FDXD clinical demonstrator is capable of acquiring continuous fluoroscopy at 25 frames per second. The images are read into a real time video processor, which was configured to hold the last 180 fluoroscopy frames acquired. Each frame is acquired at a spatial resolution of 1,024 x 1,008 pixels, with a 14 bit greyscale depth. The FDXD demonstrator has a detector size of 200 x 200 mm, therefore making the pixel size approximately 200 µm.

FDXD, and indeed any solid state x-ray detector, requires calibration of the detector system in order to correct for the non uniform response of the pixels within the array. The calibration scheme for FDXD applies gain and offset correction for each pixel in the array, and this is performed by the real time video system. In addition to the calibration, the real time video system also applies defect pixel corrections, i.e. values for the defective pixels in the array are interpolated from neighbouring pixels.

Image display on the FDXD was on a 1,024 x 1,024 pixel interlaced monitor. It is possible to store the 180 fluoroscopy frames in the real time video system to disk, allowing the impact of post processing of the data on threshold contrast to be investigated.

2.1.2. Comparison systems

FDXD was compared to two other fluoroscopy systems:
- Philips XTV16 installed within Philips' research laboratories, Best, NL
- Philips C2000 DSI system installed within the radiology department of the General Infirmary.

Both of these systems incorporate 35 cm diameter x-ray image intensifiers of the same design, and both were evaluated in the 25 cm (10") field selection.

XTV16 is a state of the art digital fluoroscopy system which utilises a CCD camera for image acquisition. It is capable of continuous fluoroscopy at both 30 and 25 frames per second, the latter of which was selected for these experiments. Image acquisition for the XTV16 is at a spatial resolution of 1,024 x 1,024 pixels, with a ten bit greyscale depth. Display of the data is via a 1,024 x 1,024 non-interlaced monitor.

The C2000 uses a Plumbicon camera for image acquisition and is a established widely used IITV system. The fluoroscopy mode that was selected on the C2000 for this experiment was "*Bypass Fluo HLR*". In the bypass mode, the analogue output from the camera is displayed on a 1,024 x 1,024 interlaced monitor.

2.2. Exposure rates

Within a fluoroscopy run on a patient, a single frame will cover a wide range of exposure rates to the detector, depending upon the radio-opacity of the subject. Average entrance exposure rates to the detector for a modern fluoroscopy system are approximately 25 μR/s. In order to cover the clinically relevant range of exposure rates, the systems were compared at 50, 25, 12 and 6 μR/s.

2.3. Test Procedure

2.3.1. Standard fluoroscopic performance

The Leeds TO[10] threshold contrast test object was used at the 6, 12, and 25 μR/s exposure rates on all three systems. The test object consists of twelve rows of nine details. The diameter of details decreases with row order, and the contrast of the details within a row decreases. Observers are required to allocate a score for each row of the test object, indicating the last detail visible within the row. Contrasts values for each detail were calculated using published spectral and filter models[8], and are shown in Figure 3. At the 50 μR/s exposure rate all nine details were visible on some rows of the TO[10] test object on the XTV16 and FDXD systems thus making this test object unusable under these conditions. The TO[10+] test object was therefore used instead at this dose on the XTV16 and FDXD. TO[10+] is of similar design to TO[10], although the details extend to lower contrast.

Figure 3: Contrasts values for TO[10] at 70 kVp, 1.5 mm Cu added filtration.

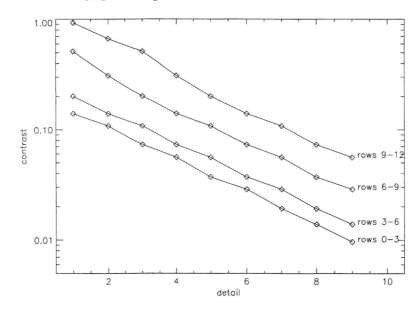

Three observers each read four fluoroscopy runs of the test object at each exposure rate. Due to time limitations all four observations of the test object were performed in the same session. Ideally readings of the test object would have been performed individually with enough time between readings to prevent observers remembering their previous scores.

In all cases the x-ray generator was operated in fixed kVp and mA mode. All acquisitions were performed at 70 kVp with 1.5 mm of added copper filtration. Where present, the anti-scatter grid, amplimat and table were removed from field of view, and the test object placed as close as possible to the detector surface. In order to achieve the required dose rates, the mA and SID were adjusted accordingly.

On the C2000 and XTV16 systems test object observations were performed in live fluoroscopy, whereas for FDXD 180 fluoroscopy frames were read into the real time video system, and played back for viewing in a loop of approximately seven seconds. On the FDXD gain, offset and defect pixel correction were performed by the real time video system. "Bypass Fluo HLR" and unprocessed (i.e. non noise reduced fluoroscopy) were selected on the C2000 and XTV16 respectively.

Ambient lighting within the viewing rooms was dimmed in all cases. Viewing monitors were positioned at head height, and observers were encouraged to vary their viewing distance during the experiment in order to optimise the visibility of each of the detail sizes within the test object. No time limit was imposed on the observers.

2.3.2. Impact of post processing

In order to assess the impact of noise reduction processing on the fluoroscopic performance of FDXD, an eight second run of the TO[10] test object was post processed by a noise reduction algorithm utilising recursive filtering. A recorded run from the 25 µR/s detector entrance exposure rate was selected. This runs was reread four times each by the observers and compared to original unprocessed run.

3. RESULTS

3.1. Standard Fluoroscopic Performance

Figure 4: TCDD performance at 50 µR/s.

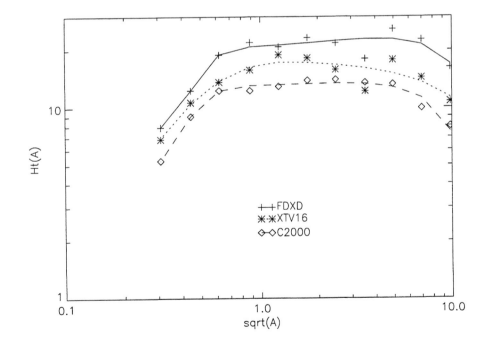

Figure 5: TCDD results at 25 µR/s.

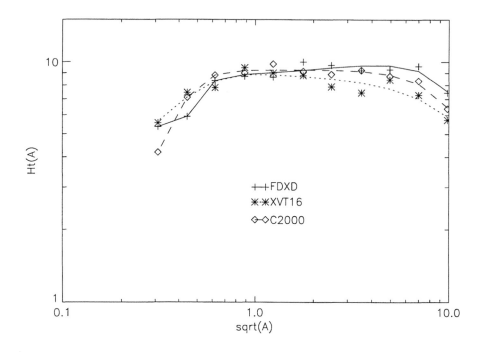

Figure 6: TCDD results at 12 µR/s.

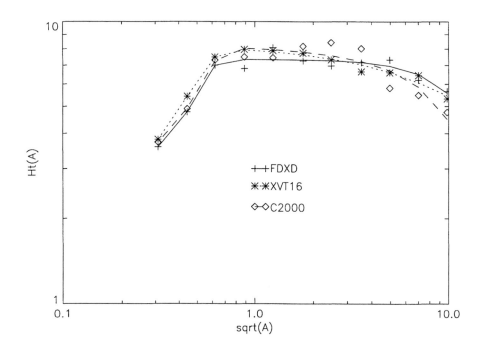

Figure 7: TCDD results at 6 µR/s (superior C2000 performance is due to increased camera lag).

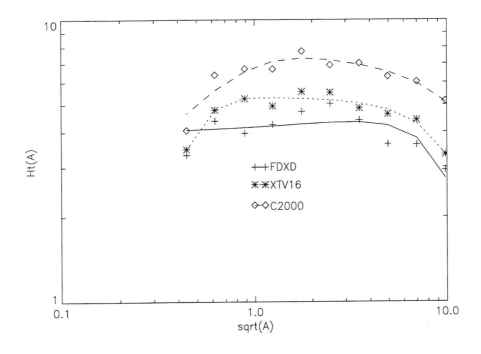

3.2. Noise reduced fluoroscopy

Figure 8: FDXD Noise reduction.

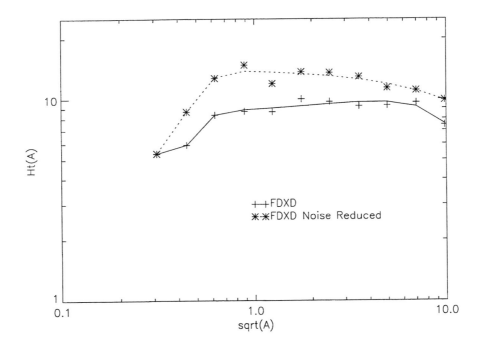

4. CONCLUSIONS

The performance of an experimental solid state fluoroscopic x-ray detector, FDXD, has been compared to that of two existing DSF technologies (Philips XTV16 CCD-based DSF system and a Philips C2000 Plumbicon-based DSF system) using the TCDD technique. The comparisons were undertaken over a range of detector entrance exposure rates, namely 50, 25, 12 and 6 μR/s. The impact of computer based noise reduction via recursive filtering was also investigated.

At the highest exposure rate of 50 μR/s, FDXD significantly outperformed both reference DSF systems. Under standard fluoroscopic exposure rates, namely 25 and 12 μR/s, FDXD performed in an equivalent manner to the reference systems. At the lowest exposure rate of 6 μR/s, FDXD was significantly worse than the other two systems. At this exposure rate the C2000 Plumbicon based IITV system was superior to the CCD-based XTV16.

The high performance of the C2000 at the lowest exposure rate can be attributed to the inherent lag in the plumbicon camera, and not due to superior efficiency of the detector system. At low dose levels, illumination of the camera target layer is reduced, the lag in the Plumbicon camera increases leading to the improved TCDD performance. By contrast the XTV16's CCD camera has no inherent lag, as the entire pixel charge is read out of the array at each frame interval (40 ms). At these low dose rates, electronic noise within the FDXD system is the dominant noise source, and limits performance at these dose rates.

At the highest fluoroscopy exposure rates, and at radiographic exposure doses electronic noise within the FDXD is much less significant, and performance improves accordingly. In IITV systems, structure noise is prevalent at higher doses and limits performance, whereas this structure noise is largely removed by the calibration process of FDXD.

It is therefore concluded that at comparable exposure rates within the ranges used in clinical routine in modern fluoroscopy, FDXD performs at an equivalent level to IITV fluoroscopy systems with regard to TCDD performance. This would suggest that FDXD should provide similar fluoroscopic performance to IITV systems for the broad range of clinical examination types, and our initial clinical experiences support this. The processing of the fluoroscopy runs by a moderate noise reduction algorithm produced a significant improvement in FDXD's TCDD performance at 25 μR/s. With the use of a noise reduction processing of fluoroscopy, it may therefore be possible to reduce the mean detector exposure rate and still maintain acceptable fluoroscopic performance.

In order to investigate this, two eight second fluoroscopy runs were obtained from the same patient (double contrast small bowel meal) on FDXD, one at a mean detector entrance exposure rate of 25 μR/s, and the second at 12 μR/s. A noise reduction algorithm was applied to both fluoroscopy runs, and presented to panel of clinical staff at the General Infirmary. Initial opinions were that the processed half exposure rate fluoroscopy run would be acceptable for the majority of clinical procedures. Obviously a more thorough investigation is required and this is being planned by the authors.

In summary, the fluoroscopic performance of the FDXD was found to be equivalent to modern IITV reference systems using the TCDD technique. This combined with our clinical experiences with the experimental system, and also physical measures of FDXD detector performance, indicate that FDXD is capable of adequate fluoroscopic performance in a clinical environment.

ACKNOWLEDGEMENTS

The authors would like to thank the scientific staff at the University of Leeds and PMS, Best, who acted as observers, and also the clinical staff involved with the project in Leeds.

REFERENCES

1. T.J.C. Bruijns, P. L. Alving, E.L. Baker, R. Bury, A.R. Cowen, N. Jung, H.A. Luijendijk, H.J. Meulenbrugge & H.J. Stouten "Technical and clinical results of an experimental flat dynamic digital x-ray image detector (FDXD) system with real-time corrections" Proc. SPIE Medical Imaging 98: Physics of Medical Imaging, **3336**, 1998.

2. R.F. Bury, A.R. Cowen, A.G. Davies, E.L. Baker, P. Hawkridge & T.J.C. Bruijns, "Initial experiences with an experimental solid state universal x-ray image detector" Clinical Radiology, **53**, pp923-928, 1998.

3. T.J.C. Bruijns, R. Bury, F. Busse, A.G. Davies, A.R. Cowen, W. Rutten & H. Reitsma, "Technical and clinical assessments of an experimental flat dynamic x-ray image detector system". Proc. SPIE Medical Imaging 99: Physics of Medical Imaging **3659**, 1999.

4. G.A. Hay, O.F. Clarke & A.R. Cowen, "A set of x-ray test objects for quality control in TV fluoroscopy", British Journal of Radiology, **58**, pp335-344, 1985.

5. A.R. Cowen, "The physical evaluation of physical performance of TV fluoroscopy and digital fluorography systems using the Leeds x-ray test objects: A UK approach to QA in the diagnostic radiology department" In: Specification, acceptance testing and QC of diagnostic x-ray imaging systems, Eds.: JA Seibert, GT Barnes & RG Gould, American Association of Physicists in Medicine Monograph No. 20, Pub AIP Press, Woodbury NY, pp499-568, 1994.

6. ICRU Report 54: Medical Imaging: the assessment of image quality, Pub: International Commission on Radiological Units and Measurements, Bethesda, MA, 1996.

7. J. Launders S. McArdle, A. Workman & A.R. Cowen "Update on the recommended viewing protocol for FAXiL threshold contrast detail detectability test objects used in TV fluoroscopy" British Journal of Radiology, **68**, pp70-77, 1995.

8. IPEM Report No. 78, "Catalogue of diagnostic x-ray spectra and other data" Pub: Institute of Physics and Engineering in Medicine, York. ISBN 0 904181 88X, 1996.

9. R.E. Colbeth, M.J. Allen, D.J. Day, D.L. Gilblom, R. Harris, I.D. Job, M.E. Klausmeir-Brown, J. Pavkovich, E.J.Seppi, E.G. Shapiro, M.D.Wright, J.M. Yu, "Flat panel imaging system for fluoroscopy applications", Proc. SPIE Medical Imaging 98, **3336**, pp376-387, 1998.

Evaluation of angiograms obtained from a laser-based x-ray source in DESA regime

Ernest M. Scalzetti[a], Andrzej Krol[*a], George M. Gagne[a], Ted T. Renvyle[a], Charles C. Chamberlain[a], Jean-Claude Kieffer[b], Zhiming Jiang[b], and Jianfan Yu[b]

[a]SUNY Health Science Center at Syracuse, NY 13210

[b]INRS, University of Québec, Varennes, Canada J3X 1S2

ABSTRACT

Contrast resolution of angiograms created using a laser-based x-ray source in Dual Energy Subtraction Angiography (DESA) regime has been investigated. It has been compared to contrast in angiograms obatined using an x-ray tube-based clinical angiography unit in DSA mode. Contrast detail phantoms and rats with opacified vascular structures were imaged. A table top terawatt laser was used (10^{19} Wcm^{-2}, 150 fs or 450 fs per pulse). For Iodine contrast agent, an Iodine filter was used with the BaF$_2$ target to obtain images with mean x-rays energy below the Iodine K-edge. La target and La filter was used to obtain images with mean x-rays energy above the Iodine K-edge. For Ba contrast agent, a Nd filter was used with the Nd target to obtain images with mean x-rays energy below the Ba K-edge. Gd target and Nd filter was used to obtain images with mean x-rays energy above the Barium K-edge. It has been determined that the laser-based DESA with properly selected targets demonstrates better contrast than a standard x-ray tube-based DSA angiography. We conclude that laser-based x-ray source has promise for angiography in DESA regime providing that sufficient x-ray flux can be delivered by the laser.

Keywords: dual energy subtraction angiography, contrast resolution, laser-produced x-ray spectra

1. INTRODUCTION

Through application of synchrotron x-ray sources it has been recently demonstrated that Dual Energy Subtraction Angiography (DESA) offers an attractive alternative to Digital Subtraction Angiography (DSA).[1] Dichromatic[2] contrast enhancement involves subtraction of two images obtained at two different x-ray energies at the same phase of the cardiac cycle. Two x-ray beams are used: one with mean energy below (E^-) and the other with mean energy above (E^+) the Iodine K-edge (33.2 keV). The contrast enhancement is achieved due to discontinuity of the photoabsorption coefficient of Iodine at the Iodine K-edge. While absorption, due to various type of tissue, decreases relatively slowly and continuously with increasing energy, the absorption due to Iodine effectively "jumps" by a factor of six at 33.2 keV. As a result, the overall sensitivity of angiography performed in DESA mode, as compared to DSA, is enhanced. It is possible that, in some cases, angiography could be even performed via simple intravenous administration of the contrast agent thus eliminating selective catheterization and offering a non-invasive diagnostic tool. It is well known that DSA is susceptible to motion artifacts due to possible missregistration of the mask images obtained pre-Iodine administration and the images acquired post-Iodine administration. In DESA approach, however, the motion artifacts could be avoided, if the low- and high-energy images were acquired in a sufficiently short time interval, i.e. below 250 ms.

---

* Correspondence: Email: krola@vax.cs.hscsyr.edu; Telephone: (315) 464-7054; fax: (315) 464-7068

Part of the SPIE Conference on Image Perception and Performance
San Diego, California • February 1999
SPIE Vol. 3663 • 0277-786X/99/$10.00

X-rays produced by a standard x-ray tube cannot be used in DESA system due to their broad polychromatic structure. Modern ultra-fast high power lasers[3] are able to generate high-power, ultra-short laser light pulses that form foundation of new type of x-ray source, called laser-produced plasma (LPP) x-ray source. We have initiated investigations on feasibility of utilization of this new source of x-rays in DESA applications. A laser-based DESA system was constructed, see Fig. 1. It utilizes filtered LPP x-ray radiation obtained using rare-metal metal target (such as La) with a rare-metal filter for the high-energy beam (E^+ =33.4 keV) and BaF_2 target with I filter for the low energy beam (E^- = 32.2 keV) for Iodine contrast imaging. For Ba contrast agent, a Nd filter was used with the Nd target (E^- = 37.2 keV) to obtain images with mean x-rays energy below the Ba K-edge (37.4 keV). A Gd target (E^+ =42.6 keV) and a Nd filter was used to obtain images with mean x-rays energy above the Barium K-edge.

2. MATERIALS AND METHODS

2.1. Phantoms and contrast media

Four phantoms were constructed of acrylic plastic with dimensions of approximately 13 cm x 5 cm x 2 cm. A series of 14 cylindrical wells was drilled in each phantom to a depth of approximately 2.5 cm. The channel diameter was the same in individual phantoms, but varied from phantom to phantom. The well diameters used were 0.6 mm, 1.0 mm, 2.0 mm and 4.0 mm. The subtraction phantom was constructed similarly but without channels.

The wells in each contrast-detail phantom were filled with a commercially available iodine-based contrast medium[4] and sealed with waterproof plastic tape. The concentration gradient used is given in Table 1:

Table 1

Well No.:	Concentration (mg I/ml)
1	50
2	45
3	40
4	35
5	30
6	25
7	20
8	15
9	10
10	5
11	2.5
12	1.25

2.2. Animal model used

The rats were euthanized with an intraperitoneal injection of barbiturate. The thoracic cavity was opened. The ascending aorta was identified and cannulated using a butterfly needle. The vascular system was flushed with saline after renting the right atrium. The insoluble copper iodide solution was suspended in water and maintained in suspension by forceful to-and-from injection between two syringes connected by a three-way stopcock. The tubing from the butterfly needle was attached to this stopcock, and 5-ml aligots of the aqueous suspension are administered into the ascending aorta, alternating with re-suspension of the salt.

The thoracic cavity is then washed and closed. The specimen was radiographed to demonstrate the distribution of the contract agent. It was then stored in a freezer.

2.3. Angiographic images with x-ray tube

The individual contrast-detail phantoms were attached directly to the II housing and digital images obtained in the radiographic mode at a tube potential of about 50 kilovolts-peak,[5] giving an effective photon energy of 25 to 30 keV. Magnification at the II input phosphor was estimated to be approximately 1.02. Image subtraction was accomplished by imaging the acrylic blank, or a rat before contrast agent administration, storing this image as the subtraction mask, and subtracting the mask from the stored contrast-detail images. Digital images were transferred to a Fuji Model FI-LM laser printer and printed on Fuji CR-780-H film. Processing was done at 90 seconds at $34°$ C.

2.4. Angiographic images with laser-based x-ray source

Using a horizontal geometry, the phantoms or rats were placed at a distance of ~40 cm from the laser target and ~2 cm from the film plane.[6] This gave a magnification factor of ~1.02. The objects were centered to the film-screen cassettes (Fuji). Film processing was done at $35°C$ with 90 second processing.

3. RESULTS

X-ray spectra were obtained[6] for all targets used, as an example, the spectra due to La targets are shown in Fig. 2. As could be observed in Fig. 2, the LPP x-ray spectra contain a continuous bremsstrahlung component as well as discrete K_α- and K_β-characteristic lines. The continuous component is approximately independent of the target composition and extended to high energies with no evident cutoff energy below 100 keV. The shape of the continuous bremsstrahlung spectrum is best described by $exp(-E/kT_e)$, where T_e was the hot electron temperature. We estimated that hot electrons' temperature in these experiments ranged from 30keV to 50 keV. The x-ray focal spot size was controlled by the laser beam focusing optics and the laser pulse duration. It ranged from 13 to 50 microns. The object contrast, C, vs. Iodine concentration, due experimentally obtained LPP x-ray spectra, was calculated. It was defined as $C=(N_o-N_b)/N_b$, where N_o and N_b is the integrated over 10 keV- 100 keV range primary x-ray photon flux that traversed the object and the background, respectively. In this simple model the scatter was neglected. It could be justified by relatively small size of the investigated objects (not exceeding 2 cm in diameter). Two extreme cases were considered: (i) broad band imaging utilizing Ba and La K_α- and K_β - characteristic lines along with entire bremsstrahlung spectrum and (ii) narrow band imaging utilizing only the narrow energy bandwidth (FWHM = 1 keV) centered around the La or Ba K_α characteristic lines. In DESA the important parameter is the contrast difference between the high energy and the low energy beams. In Fig. 4 the contrast difference for both types of imaging is shown. We observe that the contrast difference due to the narrow band imaging is an order of the magnitude higher than due to the broad band imaging. The measured contrast and contrast difference for the broad band laser-based DESA system is shown in Fig. 5. For comparison, the contrast difference obtained using a dedicated angiography unit in DSA mode is also included. Laser-based DESA images of rats with opacified vessels (see Sec. 2.2) as well as standard x-ray tube-based DSA were also obtained.

4. CONCLUSIONS

As a result of this study, we confirm that the laser-based DESA imaging with properly selected targets offers better contrast than a standard x-ray tube-based angiography operated in DSA mode, see Fig. 5. Moreover, as can be seen in Fig. 4, a further significant contrast improvement can be achieved by using narrower high and low energy bands. This can be accomplished via utilization of thin (as compared to the hot electrons range) laser targets or inserting a crystal monochromator between the laser x-ray source and the imaged object. In addition, we have demonstrated feasibility of laser-based DESA imaging by acquiring a DESA image of rats with opacified vessels.

In conclusion, a laser-based x-ray source has promise for angiography in DESA regime providing that sufficient x-ray flux can be delivered by the laser (minimum 40 J per frame with two frames acquired within 250 ms to avoid motion artifacts).

ACKNOWLEDGMENT

This work was supported in part by NIH/NHBLI grant RO1 HL52643-01 A2.

REFERENCES

1. W.R. Dix, "Intravenous coronary angiography with synchrotron radiation," *Prog. Phys. Biol.* **63**, 159-191, 1995.
2. B. Jacobson, "Dichromatic absorption radiography-Dichromatography," Acta Radiolog. **89**, 437 (1953).
3. J.-C. Kieffer, M. Chaker, J. P. Matte, C. Y. Cote, Y. Beaudoin, Z. Jiamg, C. Y. Chien, S. Coe, G. Nourou. O. Peyrrusse, and D. Gilles, "Ultrafast x-ray emission from ultra-short plasmas," *SPIE Proc.* **1860**, 127-132, 1993.
4. Hypaque (Diatrizoate Meglumine),60% @ 141 mg iodine/milliliter.
5. A. Krol, A. Ikhlef, J.-C. Kieffer, D.A. Bassano, C.C. Chamberlain, Z. Jiang, H. Pepin, and S.C. Prasad, Laser-based microfocused x-ray source for mammography: Feasibility studies," *Medical Physics* **24** **(5)**, pp. 725-733 (1997).
6. X-ray Generator: Electromed International, Model EDEC-100A, high frequency, constant potential with automatic voltage adjustment. X-ray Tube: Varian, Model G1582TRI, Tri-focal (0.3 mm,0.6 mm, 1.0 mm), and an Anode angle of 10°.

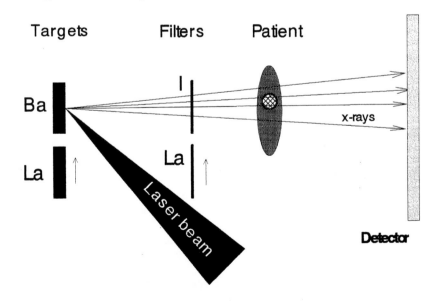

Fig. 1. Laser-based angiography set-up.

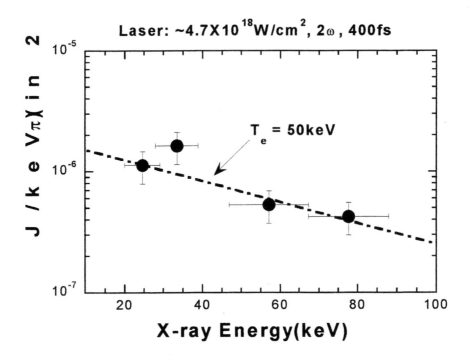

Fig. 2. LPP x-ray spectrum obtained using La target.

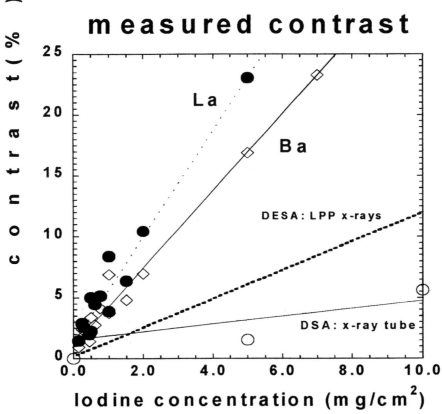

Fig. 3. Measured contrast difference: solid circles -- LPP with La
target; open diamonds -- LPP with BaF$_2$ target; open circles -- standard
DSA angiography; broken line -- predicted DESA contrast due to La
and BaF$_2$ targets.

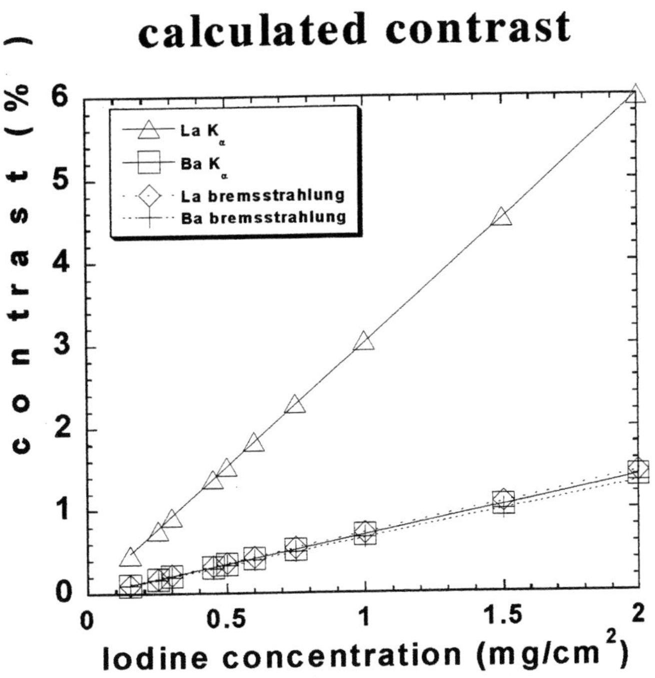

calculated contrast

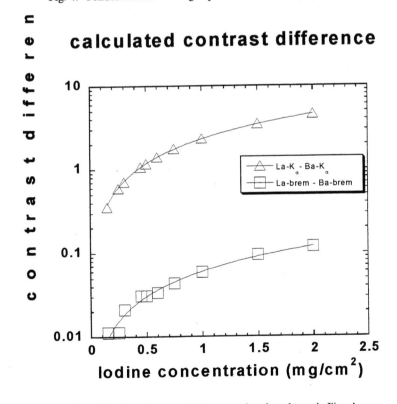

Fig. 4. Contrast obtained using experimental LPP x-ray spectra.

calculated contrast difference

Fig. 5. Predicted contrast difference using data shown in Fig. 4.

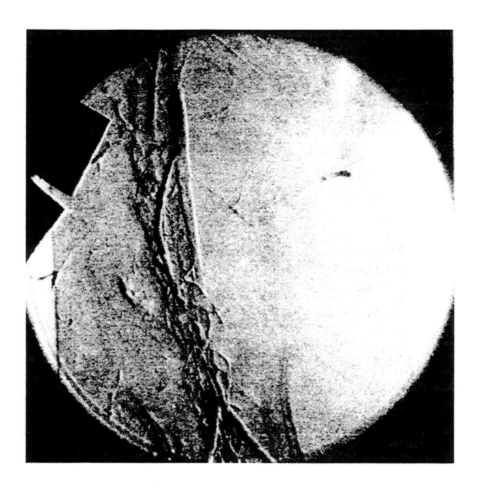

Fig. 6. Laser-based DESA image of a rat, with vascular structures opacified with Ba contrast agent, obtained using a Nd filter with the Nd target and a Gd target with a Nd filter

LROC analysis of human detection performance in PET and time-of-flight PET

H. C. Gifford, R. G. Wells, and M. A. King

Division of Nuclear Medicine
Univ. of Massachusetts Medical School
55 Lake Ave. N, Worcester, MA 01655

ABSTRACT

Previous investigations into time-of-flight positron emission tomography (TOFPET) have shown that stochastic noise in images can be reduced when the reconstruction process accounts for the differences in detection times of coincidence photons. Among the factors that influence this reduction are the sensitivity and the spatial and temporal resolutions of the TOFPET detectors. Within the framework of a simplified time-of-flight imaging model, we have considered the effect of these factors on task performance for human observers. The task was detection of mediastinal "hot" tumors in simulated images of the chest. There were 14 simulated TOFPET systems and 2 simulated PET systems considered. Image reconstruction was performed using filtered backprojection (FBP) for PET and a modified FBP for TOFPET. Localization receiver operating characteristic (LROC) methodology, in which the observers must detect and locate the tumors, was used. The LROC study gives insight into how TOFPET detector characteristics might improve in order to make possible observer task performance on a par with PET. A comparison of our results to a theoretical result from the literature was also conducted.

Keywords: image quality, objective task assessment, signal-to-noise ratio (SNR), receiver operating characteristic (ROC) study, localization ROC (LROC), positron emission tomography (PET), time-of-flight PET (TOFPET).

1. INTRODUCTION

In positron emission tomography (PET), radioactive tracer levels within the body are determined by coincidence detection of photon pairs emitted by positron annihilation events. Each detected (unscattered) photon pair defines a line along which an annihilation occured. In time-of-flight PET (TOFPET), the point of annihilation is located on the line by measuring the difference in detection times of the photon pair. The potential imaging advantages of TOFPET have been well-documented.[1-3]

The ability of a TOFPET system to resolve differences in photon detection times is quantified by its temporal resolution. Existing systems have temporal resolutions on the order of 0.5 nanoseconds (nsec) FWHM,[4] which translates to an uncertainty of 7.5 cm in the positioning of the annihilation event. Since this uncertainty is nearly twenty times the spatial resolution routinely achieved with today's standard PET systems, TOFPET systems do not attain greater spatial resolutions by virtue of the time-of-flight data. Instead, the main advantage is realized in the reconstruction process, as algorithms adapting for time-of-flight data can produce images with reduced levels of stochastic noise. This is because noise in the data influences smaller areas of the image.[5]

The fast timing resolution of TOFPET detectors also makes them superior to PET detectors for rejecting random coincidences.[2] However, this temporal resolution comes at a price. The accuracy of the timing data is heavily dependent on the scintillator material, as well as the size and shape of the scintillator crystals. Crystals used for PET are evaluated based on sensitivity, defined as the square of the probability that a gamma ray will be absorbed, and photon emission rate. For TOFPET, a short decay time for the light emission is more important than the emission rate.[3] The most common material used for PET is bismuth germanate (BGO), which has a high sensitivity and a moderate emission rate but also has a decay time that is too long for TOFPET application. For example, the decay time of BGO is 300 nsec, whereas one TOFPET scintillator, cesium fluoride (CsF), has a decay time of

---

Further author information: (Send correspondence to H.C.G.)
H.C.G.: E-mail: gifford@wachusett.ummed.edu
R.G.W.: E-mail: wells@wachusett.ummed.edu
M.A.K.: E-mail: king@wachusett.ummed.edu

Part of the SPIE Conference on Image Perception and Performance
San Diego, California • February 1999
SPIE Vol. 3663 • 0277-786X/99/$10.00

5 nsec.[6] The drawback with the available TOFPET scintillators, CsF and barium fluoride (BaF_2), is their low stopping power for 511-keV photons. The sensitivity is given as 0.88 for BGO, but only 0.53 for CsF and 0.58 for BaF_2.[2] This difference results in poorer counting statistics for TOFPET in comparison to PET, especially with the small crystal sizes required for high spatial resolution. The sensitivity problem can be alleviated by increasing crystal thickness, but at a cost of diminished spatial resolution.

The combined effects of TOFPET detector sensitivity and the detector spatial and temporal resolutions on image quality have been examined in previous studies.[5, 7-9] The figure of merit in these analyses was signal-to-noise ratio (SNR) of reconstructed pixels, although Parra and Barrett also considered the SNR for a model observer[10] applied to a "signal-known-exactly" (SKE) ROC task. Our work investigated how incremental changes in TOFPET detector properties would influence image quality from the standpoint of human-observer task performance. The task considered was detection of "hot" tumors in the chest. Both PET and TOFPET systems were simulated, and reconstruction was carried out using filtered backprojection (FBP) for PET and a modified FBP for TOFPET. Observer performance was evaluated using localization receiver operating characteristic (LROC) studies.[11] In LROC studies, an observer must detect and locate the tumors. This methodology provides a closer approximation to actual clinical detection tasks than is offered by the more common SKE-ROC study. LROC also offers increased statistical power for evaluating differences between study variables.

2. THEORY

2.1. PET and TOFPET Data

A comparison of PET and TOFPET data can be understood with reference to the imaging system geometry shown in Fig. (1a). Function f is the two-dimensional (2D) distribution of radioactivity within a thin slice of the body. For a specified projection angle θ, an arbitrary point $\mathbf{r}$ in the body is expressed in terms of rotated coordinates u and v obtained from the original coordinates x and y. An annihilation event occurs at $\mathbf{r}' = (u', v')$, and the resulting photon pair is recorded by detectors. For the moment, we ignore the sampling process inherent in real imaging systems, and assume that the detectors have perfect resolution. In PET, the photons' arrival at the detector is measured for the coordinates v' and θ, which define the projection line as the set of points $\mathbf{r}$ such that $(\mathbf{r} - \mathbf{r}') \cdot \hat{\mathbf{v}} = 0$. With TOFPET, the difference in photon detection times, Δt, also allows measurement of u'. If the detectors are equidistant from the v-axis, then one photon travels a distance $2u'$ farther than the other, and

$$u' = \frac{c\Delta t}{2},\tag{1}$$

where c is the speed of light. This relation will also be used to express the TOFPET temporal resolution in units of length.

We refer to the 3D space $\Omega = \Re^2 \times [0, \pi]$ spanned by the coordinates $(\mathbf{r}, \theta)$ as detection space. A "detector" should be considered the camera and electronic circuitry necessary to make a measurement in this space. In our mathematical modeling, we shall assume that Ω applies to both PET and TOFPET. Normally, the 2D Radon space $\Re \times [0, \pi]$ is assumed for PET. From our point of view, a PET system is treated as a TOFPET system with very poor temporal resolution.

2.2. The Imaging System Model

The relation between the imaging system data and f is defined by the equation

$$g_m = [\mathcal{H}f]_m + n_m, \; m = 1, \ldots, M,\tag{2}$$

where g_m is the photon count from the mth detector, and $[\mathcal{H}f]_m$ is the mth output of the continuous-to-discrete operator $\mathcal{H}$ acting on f that characterizes the deterministic aspects of the photon emission and detection.[12] Measurement noise is represented by n_m. The datum g_m is considered to be a Poisson process[13] with mean $[\mathcal{H}f]_m$, so n_m is a zero-mean Poisson variable that is a function of f.

Assume that $\mathcal{H}$ has the form

$$[\mathcal{H}f]_m = \int_0^\pi \int_{\Re^2} D_m(\mathbf{r}, \theta) P(\mathbf{r} \cdot \hat{\mathbf{v}}, \theta) f(\mathbf{r}) d\mathbf{r} d\theta\tag{3}$$

where function D_m defines the properties of the mth detector and the function P models the attenuation of photons emitted from the point $\mathbf{r}$ and detected along the line $\mathbf{r} \cdot \hat{\mathbf{v}} = v$. Photon scatter is not considered in this paper. We define the product

$$\lambda(\mathbf{r}, \theta) = P(\mathbf{r} \cdot \hat{\mathbf{v}}, \theta) f(\mathbf{r}) \tag{4}$$

as the photon density[13] at points $(\mathbf{r}, \theta) \in \Omega$. It is worthwhile to emphasize how this TOFPET model differs from the typical projection model for PET that uses the Radon transform[14] to express the photon density as

$$\lambda_{\text{PET}}(v, \theta) = P(v, \theta) \int_{\Re^2} f(\mathbf{r}') \delta(\mathbf{r}' \cdot \hat{\mathbf{v}} - v) d\mathbf{r}'. \tag{5}$$

at a point (v, θ) in Radon space. The delta function is nonzero only for points along the line $(\mathbf{r} - \mathbf{r}') \cdot \hat{\mathbf{v}} = 0$.

A transformation from the continuous coordinates of detection space to the discrete coordinates representing detectors occurs in Eqn. (3) through the integration over Ω. In our model, D_m is factored into a detector blur function $b(\mathbf{r})$ and a sampling function $p_m(\mathbf{r}, \theta)$ that defines the detector geometry. In terms of b, p_m, and $\lambda(\mathbf{r}, \theta)$,

$$[\mathcal{H}f]_m = \int_0^\pi \int_{\Re^2} p_m(\mathbf{r}, \theta) \int_{\Re^2} b(\mathbf{r} - \mathbf{r}') \lambda(\mathbf{r}', \theta) d\mathbf{r}' d\mathbf{r} d\theta. \tag{6}$$

For a make-believe TOFPET system that can continuously sample in detection space with perfect resolution, delta functions let us write a sampling function as $p_m(\mathbf{r}, \theta) = \delta(\theta - \theta_m)\delta(\mathbf{r} - \mathbf{r}_m)$, where $(\mathbf{r}_m, \theta_m) \in \Omega$. When attenuation is ignored, Eqn. (6) gives

$$[\mathcal{H}f]_m = [b(\mathbf{r}) ** f(\mathbf{r})]_{(\mathbf{r}_m, \theta_m)}, \tag{7}$$

where the double asterisks denote a 2D convolution, and the subscript indicates that the convolution is sampled at $(\mathbf{r}_m, \theta_m)$. Thus, data from this "ideal" TOFPET system are points of a blurred version of f.

A more realistic detector consists of a rectangular pixel in the $\hat{\mathbf{u}}$–$\hat{\mathbf{v}}$ plane, with widths w_u and w_v [see Fig. 1b]. We parameterize the mth detector by an angle θ_m and coordinates $\mathbf{r}_m = (u_m, v_m)$ that are the center points of the pixel. With the definition[15]

$$\text{rect}(\frac{x_1 - x_2}{k}) = \left\{ \begin{array}{ll} 1 & |x_1 - x_2| < \frac{k}{2} \\ 0 & \text{otherwise,} \end{array} \right. \tag{8}$$

for scalars x_1, x_2, and k, we have the sampling function

$$p_m(\mathbf{r}, \theta) = \delta(\theta - \theta_m)\text{rect}(\frac{u - u_m}{w_u})\text{rect}(\frac{v - v_m}{w_v}). \tag{9}$$

The choices for w_u and w_v are not arbitrary. To minimize aliasing, the pixel widths must satisfy Nyquist conditions[16] set by the spectral properties of the detector blur function b. In our model, Gaussian blurring is applied in both the u and v coordinates, with standard deviations σ_u and σ_v, respectively, so that

$$b(\mathbf{r}) = \frac{1}{2\pi\sigma_u\sigma_v}\exp[-\frac{1}{2}(\frac{u^2}{\sigma_u{}^2} + \frac{v^2}{\sigma_v{}^2})]. \tag{10}$$

The Gaussian full-width, half-maximum (FWHM) in (e.g.) the $\hat{\mathbf{u}}$-direction is $2\sigma_u\sqrt{2\ln 2}$. According to Sorenson and Phelps,[17] the pixel width w_u should satisfy

$$w_u \leq \frac{\text{FWHM}}{3}. \tag{11}$$

For a PET system, σ_u is quite large, and nothing is gained by having w_u smaller than the width of the field of view.

2.3. FBP Reconstruction

Our reconstructions were performed using FBP methods. For PET data, standard rho-filtered FBP[14, 18, 19] was applied. For TOFPET, a modified FBP routine[7] utilizing the timing data was used. This method approaches rho-filtering as the temporal resolution of a system decreases.

The mathematical theory of FBP assumes noise-free, continuous sampling in the 2D Radon space coordinates v and θ. A reconstructed function is created through an additive process, built up from weighted lines of projection.

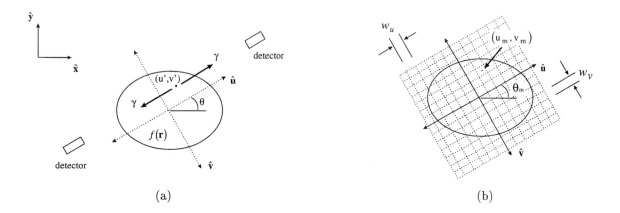

(a)
(b)

Figure 1. a) PET and TOFPET data. For a projection angle θ, rotated coordinates u and v are obtained from x and y. In PET, (v', θ) are determined for the annihilation event. In TOFPET, measurement of the timing differential leads to placement of the annihilation event at (u', v'). b) Discretization of 3D detection space. The mth detector is a rectangular pixel in the $\hat{\mathbf{u}}$–$\hat{\mathbf{v}}$ plane. The pixel widths are w_u and w_v. The detector is parameterized by an angle θ_m and the center coordinates (u_m, v_m) of the pixel.

A point (v, θ) in Radon space is associated with the line $\mathbf{r} \cdot \hat{\mathbf{v}} = v$. Each line is weighted by its associated projection datum. A point spread function is determined for the projection-backprojection with the assumption of no attenuation. From Eqn. (5), the projection datum of a point source $\delta(\mathbf{r})$ is 1 for projection lines through the origin and 0 for all other projection lines. We use the delta function $\delta(\mathbf{r} \cdot \hat{\mathbf{v}})$ to represent a line through the origin in the backprojection integral

$$\text{PSF}_{\text{FBP}}(\mathbf{r}) = \int_0^{\pi} \delta(\mathbf{r} \cdot \hat{\mathbf{v}}) \mathrm{d}\theta, \tag{12}$$

which reduces to $\text{PSF}_{\text{FBP}}(\mathbf{r}) = \|\mathbf{r}\|^{-1}$. The backprojection obtained from a source f is

$$f_b(\mathbf{r}) = f(\mathbf{r}) * *\text{PSF}_{\text{FBP}}(\mathbf{r}), \tag{13}$$

and the distribution f is recovered by inverse filtering f_b with the 2D Fourier transform of PSF_{FBP},

$$\widehat{\text{PSF}}_{\text{FBP}}(\boldsymbol{\rho}) = \|\boldsymbol{\rho}\|^{-1}. \tag{14}$$

For the modified FBP, we again consider the 3D detection space Ω. The point spread function is altered in two ways. First, there is the blurring in the forward projection. Second, a backprojected line associated with the point $(\mathbf{r}', \theta) \in \Omega$ should be heavily weighted in the neighborhood of $\mathbf{r}'$ to account for the time-of-flight measurement. According to our imaging model, a point source at the origin projects to the 2D Gaussian function $b(\mathbf{r})$ [see Eqn. (7)]. In Wong $et~al.$,[8] time-of-flight FBP that considers this 2D blur is presented. Here, only the temporal blurring is modeled in the reconstruction, and the projection of the point source is taken to be

$$w(\mathbf{r}, \theta) = \frac{\delta(\mathbf{r} \cdot \hat{\mathbf{v}})}{\sqrt{2\pi}\sigma_u} \exp[\frac{-\mathrm{u}^2}{2\sigma_{\mathrm{u}}^2}] \tag{15}$$

For backprojecting $w(\mathbf{r}, \theta)$, we associate a point $(\mathbf{r}', \theta)$ with the shifted 1D Gaussian $w(\mathbf{r} - \mathbf{r}', \theta)$ scaled by its projection datum. The Gaussian provides time-of-flight weighting. The superposition of the backprojected lines for a fixed angle θ is the 1D convolution

$$\begin{aligned} h(\mathbf{r}, \theta) &= \frac{\delta(\mathbf{r} \cdot \hat{\mathbf{v}})}{2\pi\sigma_{\mathrm{u}}^2} \int_{\Re} \exp[\frac{-(\mathrm{u}')^2}{2\sigma_{\mathrm{u}}^2}] \exp[\frac{-(\mathrm{u} - \mathrm{u}')^2}{2\sigma_{\mathrm{u}}^2}] \mathrm{du}' \tag{16} \\ &= \frac{\delta(\mathbf{r} \cdot \hat{\mathbf{v}})}{2\pi\sigma_{\mathrm{u}}^2} \exp[\frac{-\mathrm{u}^2}{4\sigma_{\mathrm{u}}^2}]. \tag{17} \end{aligned}$$

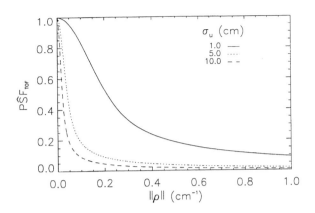

Figure 2. Profiles of the 2D function $\widehat{\mathrm{PSF}}_{\mathrm{TOF}}(\rho)$ for standard deviations σ_u=1.0, 5.0, and 10.0 cm of the Gaussian weighting function b. Each profile has been normalized to 1.0 at $\|\rho\|$=0.

The fact that $h(\mathbf{r}, \theta)$ is nonzero only when $\mathbf{r} \cdot \hat{\mathbf{v}} = 0$ allows us to replace the variable u with $\|\mathbf{r}\|$, and the point spread function is found from the integration

$$\mathrm{PSF}_{\mathrm{TOF}}(\mathbf{r}) = \frac{\exp[\frac{-\|\mathbf{r}\|^2}{4\sigma_u^2}]}{2\pi\sigma_u^2} \int_0^\pi \delta(\mathbf{r} \cdot \hat{\mathbf{v}}) d\theta \tag{18}$$

$$= \frac{\exp[\frac{-\|\mathbf{r}\|^2}{4\sigma_u^2}]}{2\pi\sigma_u^2\|\mathbf{r}\|} \tag{19}$$

The backprojection for a source f is

$$f_b(\mathbf{r}) = \frac{1}{2\pi\sigma_u{}^2} f(\mathbf{r}) ** \frac{\exp[-\frac{\|\mathbf{r}\|^2}{4\sigma_u{}^2}]}{\|\mathbf{r}\|}, \tag{20}$$

and the appropriate TOF-adjusted FBP inverse filter is

$$\widehat{\mathrm{PSF}}_{\mathrm{TOF}}(\rho) = \pi^{\frac{3}{2}}\sigma_u \exp(-2\pi^2\sigma_u{}^2\|\rho\|^2) I_0(2\pi^2\sigma_u{}^2\|\rho\|^2), \tag{21}$$

where I_0 is the zeroth-order modified Bessel function.[20] Plots of $\widehat{\mathrm{PSF}}_{\mathrm{TOF}}(\rho)$ for several values of σ_u are shown in Fig. 2. Note that the FWHM of $\widehat{\mathrm{PSF}}_{\mathrm{TOF}}(\rho)$ grows as σ_u decreases (temporal resolution improves). Thus, noise in the higher frequencies will be amplified less as a result of increased temporal resolution. For large values of σ_u, $\widehat{\mathrm{PSF}}_{\mathrm{TOF}}(\rho)$ has an asymptotic expression that is proportional to $\|\rho\|^{-1}$.

2.4. LROC Methodology

In an SKE-ROC study, the observer response for an image consists of a confidence rating that quantifies observer certainty that a tumor is present or absent at a specified image location. In an LROC study, the observer supplies the rating, but also must point to the most likely tumor location. With the addition of this search component, the task in the LROC study more closely approximates clinical detection tasks than does SKE ROC. Furthermore, by incorporating the observer's choice of tumor location, LROC improves on the statistical accuracy of ROC for measuring detection performance.[11] Thus, LROC offers greater statistical power for resolving differences between psychophysical study variables.

The LROC curve is a parametric plot similar to the ROC curve. For ROC, the true-positive fraction (TPF) of an observer's responses is plotted against the false-positive fraction (FPF) as a function of the decision threshold of the observer.[21] In LROC, true-positive responses are subdivided according to whether a correct tumor localization was made. The LROC curve plots the fraction of true-positive responses with correct localization against the FPF. Observer performance is classified by two figures of merit associated with the LROC curve. One is the area under the LROC curve A_L. The other is the probability of correct location (p_{CL}), the probability that the observer will correctly locate the tumor irrespective of confidence rating.

If the tumor location data supplied by the observer are ignored, then the LROC study can be analyzed as a "location-unknown" ROC study, with an area under the ROC curve of[11]

$$A_Z = \frac{1}{2}(A_L + 1).$$ (22)

3. METHODS

3.1. Projection Data Simulation

The observer studies used simulated images of the chest area of the 3D mathematical cardiac-torso (MCAT) phantom.[22] The phantom outline is elliptical, with a major axis length of 36 cm, and a minor axis length of 25 cm. For convenience, The relative concentrations of radioactivity within the phantom were set to be the same as those used in a similar SPECT detection study of Ga-67-avid lymphoma.[23] A single spherical tumor 1 cm in diameter was used. This was considered the smallest likely to be rated as "abnormal" in clinical CT images. The soft-tissue-to-tumor activity ratio was set at 4.5:1. The tumor placements in the phantom were randomly selected from a three-dimensional (3D) mask of "most probable" locations. A total of 75 sites were used, examples of which are given in the noise-free images of Fig. 3.

There were 14 TOFPET and 2 PET systems modeled. For TOFPET, the resolutions used were (all FWHM): spatial resolutions of 4, 8, and 16 mm with temporal resolutions of 0.8, 2.0, 4.0, and 7.5 cm, and spatial resolutions of 4 and 8 mm with a temporal resolution of 10.0 cm. The temporal resolutions were selected to window the currently available resolution of 7.5 cm. As the spatial resolution of current PET systems is approximately 4 mm, TOFPET spatial resolutions of 8 and 16 mm were considered in order to investigate the extent to which time-of-flight data could overcome poor spatial resolution. This is of interest since it might be necessary to trade off spatial resolution for temporal resolution in system design. Each data set for the TOFPET systems consisted of 1.28 million counts. Both PET systems had 4 mm spatial resolution, one with twice (2.56 million counts) and the other with six times (7.68 million counts) the sensitivity of the TOFPET systems. The choice of the TOFPET count level was intended, in conjunction with the soft-tissue-to-tumor activity level, to generate average observer areas under the ROC curve in the range of 0.70 to 0.85.[24]

Simulated PET projections with time-of-flight information were produced for 511-kev photons from 256×256 discretized slices of the MCAT phantom, using a ray-driven analytical projector[25] that modeled attenuation and detector response but ignored scatter. Each slice cut through the center coordinates of a tumor location. The dimensions of the projection sets in θ, u, and v were $128 \times 256 \times 256$, yielding square pixels of width 0.1585 cm in the $\hat{u}$–$\hat{v}$ plane. Sums over the index for u were taken to give PET projection sets with dimensions 128×256.

Noise was added to the data sets prior to reconstruction by using the analytical projection values as means of independent Poisson variables. No allowance was made within our simple analytical projection model for random coincidences in the data. Thus, TOFPET's improved ability to distinguish randoms was not a factor in this investigation.

3.2. Image Reconstruction

The dimensions of the reconstructed images were 256×256. PET images used FBP, while the TOFPET images used the modified FBP outlined in Section 2.3. Post-filtering for the purpose of smoothing high frequencies was done for all the images, using a 5th-order Butterworth filter with a cut-off frequency of 0.1 pixel^{-1} FWHM. This choice of filter cut-off was based on an observer study for a similar detection task using FBP-reconstructed SPECT images.[23] Attenuation correction was performed using the same attenuation map for 511-keV photons as was used for creating the projections, and in that sense represented an ideal attenuation correction.

Post-reconstruction processing also included the truncation of negative pixels, and an upper thresholding of pixel greyscale values. An adaptive method was applied independently to the images of each imaging system. The method considered the maximum tumor-pixel value ψ_i of the ith tumor-present image. From the set of all ψ_i, the maximum

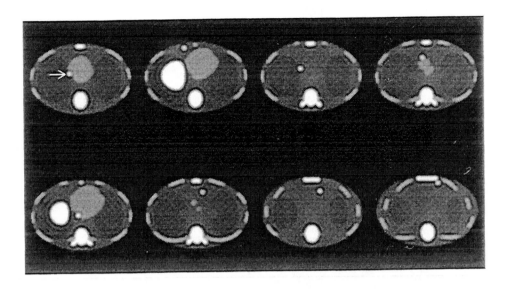

Figure 3. Noise-free images showing examples of the tumor locations used in the observer study.

$\psi_{\max}$ was selected and a standard deviation calculated. The upper limit of the greyscale for the images was set to $\psi_{\max}$ plus 1 standard deviation.

Some of the tumor-present images read by the observers are shown in Fig. 4. Each of the imaging systems is represented for two of the tumor locations.

3.3. Observer studies

Observer performance was measured through an LROC study with 5 members of our medical physics research group, all but one of whom had substantial experience in observer studies. A set of 150 images was generated for each of the imaging systems, representing the 75 tumor locations with one noise realization each of the tumor-present and tumor-absent images.

These image sets were divided into training subsets with 25 tumor locations (50 images), and study subsets with 50 locations (100 images). An observer's reading of the training images from a particular imaging system immediately preceeded the reading of the study subset for the same system. The image reading order in all subsets was randomized, and the order in which each observer read the sets was varied.

The observer data for an image consisted of a confidence rating regarding tumor presence that was selected from a 6-level scale, along with the selection of image coordinates of the most likely tumor site. Coordinates were chosen even if the observer was confident that no tumor was present. Only the results from the study subsets of 100 images were analyzed. A family of LROC curves was produced for each observer, one curve per imaging system, using analysis given in Swensson.[11] Observer performance for an imaging system is given as an average area under the LROC curve, $\overline{A}_L$, obtained from the A_L's of the individual observers. The average of the individual observers' probability of correct localization for each imaging system was correlated with $\overline{A}_L$ (rank correlation coefficient=0.997), so results are reported solely in terms of $\overline{A}_L$.

4. RESULTS

The one observer without much previous viewing experience showed statistically significant differences at levels of $p < 0.025$ with each of the other observers. When this observer's A_L values were scaled upwards by a constant derived from the average A_L's of the other observers, these differences disappeared. This suggests that the significance was due to the magnitudes of the A_L's, and not to a radically different ranking of the imaging systems. No significant differences below $p = 0.20$ were found among the other observers.

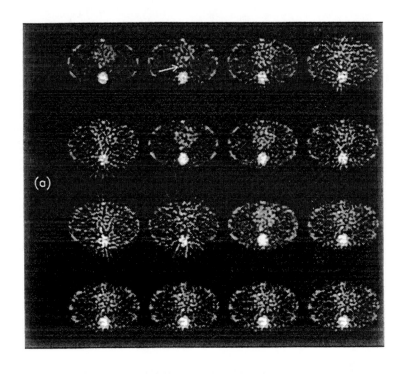

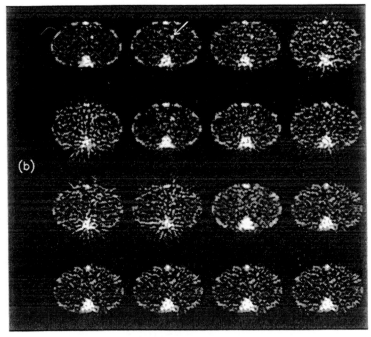

Figure 4. Examples of the study images used. In both (a) and (b), a single tumor location (indicated by arrow) is shown for all 16 imaging systems. The ordering of the systems is (from left to right, and top to bottom): TOFPET systems with 4 mm spatial resolution with 0.8, 2.0, 4.0, 7.5, and 10.0 cm temporal resolution; 8 mm spatial resolution with 0.8, 2.0, 4.0, 7.5, and 10.0 cm temporal resolution; 16 mm spatial resolution with 0.8, 2.0, 4.0, and 7.5 cm temporal resolution; the PET systems with low and high sensitivity.

In Fig. 5, TOFPET system $\overline{A}_L$ as a function of temporal resolution is shown along with horizontal lines depicting $\overline{A}_L$ for the two PET systems. These results indicate that a TOFPET system with a spatial resolution of 4 mm requires a temporal resolution between 5.0 and 5.5 cm to match the performance of the high-sensitivity PET system. By comparison, the TOF systems with temporal resolution of 7.5 cm and spatial resolutions of 4 and 8 mm outperform the low-sensitivity PET system. Fig. 5 also shows that time-of-flight data can overcome poor (16 mm) spatial resolution, but this requires temporal resolutions on the order of twice what is now available.

In considering how the trade-off of spatial and temporal resolutions affected human performance with TOFPET imaging, we see from these results that there is an equivalence in the effects that spatial resolution and temporal resolution had on performance. For example, the human performance with the TOFPET system with 4 mm spatial and 7.5 cm temporal resolution was roughly equivalent to the performance with the TOFPET system with half the spatial resolution (8 mm) but nearly twice the temporal resolution (4 cm). In our imaging model, the spatial and temporal resolutions in the data took the identical form of Gaussian blur. As a consequence, this equivalence in the trade-off would be expected. The equivalence should not be exact, however, because the modified FBP for TOFPET accounted for the temporal resolution of the forward projection but not the spatial resolution.

The increase in $\overline{A}_L$ with improved temporal resolution that is demonstrated by the TOFPET-related curves in Fig. 5 is in qualitative agreement with studies in the literature[5, 8, 9] that considered the SNR of reconstructed pixels or of model observers applied to SKE tasks. This agreement is to some extent due to the particular detection task chosen. In a previous work[26] that considered Ga-67 imaging of tumors in the chest, human performance measured through an LROC study correlated with a SNR figure of merit obtained by averaging model observer SKE-ROC performance over tumor location. Detection tasks in other parts of the body may not show this correlation.

Of interest was whether the improvement in human task performance as a function of TOFPET resolution is well described by the theory. To check this, we considered an expression for mean SNR of reconstructed image pixels that is given by Budinger.[5] Given a field-of-view width of L, a TOFPET temporal resolution of ϵ_t, and a PET-to-TOFPET ratio s of mean counts per pixel, the ratio of the mean reconstructed pixel SNR's for TOFPET and PET systems with the same spatial resolution is

$$\frac{\text{SNR}_{\text{TOF}}}{\text{SNR}_{\text{PET}}} = \sqrt{\frac{L}{s\epsilon_t}}. \tag{23}$$

The imaging systems used for the comparison were the two PET systems and the TOFPET systems with 4 mm spatial resolution. Our calculations based on Eqn. (23) used $L=30$ cm, count ratios of $s=2$ (the sensitivity ratio between the low-sensitivity PET system and the TOFPET systems), and $s=6$ (the sensitivity ratio between the high-sensitivity PET system and the TOFPET systems), and the FWHM temporal resolutions listed in Section 3.1. To transform the averages of the observer performances from areas under the LROC curve to SNR's, we first converted $\overline{A}_L$ to an average area under the ROC curve ($\overline{A}_z$) with Eqn. (22), and then applied the equation[27]

$$\text{SNR}_{\text{human}} = 2\,\text{erf}^{-1}(2\overline{A}_z - 1), \tag{24}$$

where $\text{erf}^{-1}(\cdot)$ is the inverse of the error function,

$$\text{erf}(z) = \frac{2}{\sqrt{\pi}} \int_0^z e^{-t^2} dt. \tag{25}$$

The results of the comparison are shown in Fig. 6. The solid line represents the predicted ratio of pixel SNR's as a function of temporal resolution for the low-sensitivity PET system, while the dashed line is the predicted pixel-SNR ratio using the high-sensitivity PET system. The human observer SNR ratios are plotted as points. For the comparison of TOFPET to the high-sensitivity PET, the human results are in agreement with the prediction curve, while for low-sensitivity PET, the improvement due to time-of-flight information is greater than that predicted by Eqn. (23). This shows that the adverse effect on the observers from nonuniformities in the low-sensitivity PET images is mitigated by the addition of time-of-flight data in a way that is not addressed by the average reconstructed pixel SNR.

5. CONCLUSIONS

In this work we have used LROC studies to investigate the promise of future improvements in TOFPET imaging systems on the basis of human observer task performance. We found from the observer results that incorporating

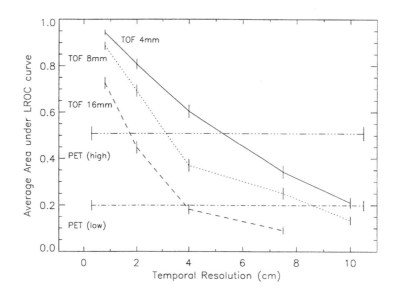

Figure 5. Mean areas under the LROC curve for the 16 imaging systems described in the text. For the TOFPET systems, the areas are plotted as a function of temporal resolution. Separate lines are shown for each spatial resolution. The areas for the PET systems are indicated as horizontal lines. Error bars represent the standard errors for the average observer.

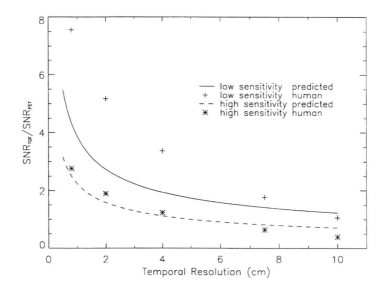

Figure 6. A comparison of the predicted ratio of TOFPET-to-PET SNR's to the ratio computed from the human observer results. The two PET systems and the TOFPET systems with 4 mm spatial resolution are considered.

time-of-flight data in the reconstruction could compensate for poor detector spatial resolution. A comparison of the observer results to theory indicated that task performance improvement can be greater than what is predicted using a reconstructed-pixel SNR figure of merit. A very basic level of imaging system model was used in this work, and important aspects of TOFPET detection such as superior rejection of random coincidences were excluded. Further work with a realistic Monte-Carlo projector, an array of different detection tasks, a more extensive range of detector sensitivities and resolutions, and other reconstruction methods will help us evaluate the merit of future development in TOFPET design.

ACKNOWLEDGMENTS

We thank Manoj V. Narayanan and P. Hendrik Pretorius for their participation in the observer studies. This work was supported by the National Cancer Institute (NCI) under grant number CA-42165. Its contents are solely the responsibility of the authors and do not necessarily reflect the official views of the NCI.

REFERENCES

1. N. A. Mullani, J. Markham, and M. M. Ter-Pogossian, "Feasibility of time-of-flight reconstruction in positron emission tomography," *J. Nucl. Med.* **21**, pp. 1095–1097, 1980.
2. G. Muehllehner and J. S. Karp, "Positron emission tomography imaging—technical considerations," *Seminars in Nuclear Medicine* **16**, pp. 35–50, 1986.
3. M. M. Ter-Pogossian, N. A. Mullani, D. C. Ficke, J. Markham, and D. L. Snyder, "Photon time-of-flight-assisted positron emission tomography," *Journal of Computer Assisted Tomography* **5**, pp. 227–239, 1981.
4. W. W. Moses and S. E. Derenzo, "Prospects for time-of-flight PET using LSO scintillator," *IEEE Trans. Nucl. Sci.* , 1998 [submitted].
5. T. F. Budinger, "Time-of-flight positron emission tomography: Status relative to conventional PET," *J. Nucl. Med.* **24**, pp. 73–78, 1983.
6. R. Allemand, C. Gresset, and J. Vacher, "Potential advantages of a cesium fluoride scintillator for a time-of-flight positron camera," *J. Nucl. Med.* **21**, pp. 153–155, 1980.
7. D. L. Snyder, L. J. Thomas, Jr., and M. M. Ter-Pogossian, "A mathematical model for positron-emission tomography systems having time-of-flight measurements," *IEEE Trans. Nucl. Sci.* **28**, pp. 3575–3583, 1981.
8. W.-H. Wong, N. A. Mullani, E. A. Philippe, R. Hartz, and K. L. Gould, "Image improvement and design optimization of the time-of-flight PET," *J. Nucl. Med.* **24**, pp. 52–60, 1983.
9. L. Parra and H. H. Barrett, "List-mode likelihood: EM algorithm and image quality estimation demonstrated on 2-d PET," *IEEE Trans. Med. Imaging* **17**, pp. 228–235, 1998.
10. H. H. Barrett, J. Yao, J. P. Rolland, and K. J. Myers, "Model observers for assessment of image quality," *Proc. Natl. Acad. Sci. USA* **90**, pp. 9758–9765, 1993.
11. R. G. Swensson, "Unified measurement of observer performance in detecting and localizing target objects on images," *Med. Phys.* **23**, pp. 1709–1725, 1996.
12. H. H. Barrett, J. L. Denny, R. F. Wagner, and K. J. Myers, "Objective assessment of image quality II: Fisher information, Fourier crosstalk, and figures of merit for task performance," *J. Opt. Soc. Am. A* **12**(5), pp. 834–852, 1995.
13. H. H. Barrett and W. Swindell, *Radiological imaging, The theory of image formation, detection, and processing*, Academic Press, New York, 1981.
14. H. H. Barrett, *The Radon transform and its applications*, vol. 21 of *Progress in Optics*, pp. 219–285. North-Holland, Amsterdam, 1984.
15. J. Gaskill, *Linear Systems, Fourier Transforms, and Optics*, Wiley, New York, 1978.
16. R. J. Marks, *Introduction to Shannon Sampling and Interpolation Theory*, Springer-Verlag, New York, 1991.
17. J. A. Sorenson and M. E. Phelps, *Physics in Nuclear Medicine*, Grune & Stratton Inc., Orlando, second ed., 1987.
18. G. T. Herman, *Image Reconstructions from Projections: The Fundamentals of Computerized Tomography*, Academic Press, New York, 1980.
19. S. R. Deans, *The Radon Transform and some of its Applications*, John Wiley and Sons, New York, 1983.
20. M. Abramowitz and I. A. Stegun, *Handbook of Mathematical Functions*, Dover, New York, 1965.

21. H. L. Van Trees, *Detection, Estmation, and Modulation Theory*, vol. I, Wiley, New York, 1968.

22. B. M. W. Tsui, X. D. Zhao, G. K. Gregoriou, J. Li, D. L. Lalush, and R. L. Eisner, "Quantitative cardiac SPECT reconstruction with reduced image degradation due to patient anatomy," *IEEE Trans. Nucl. Sci.* **41**, pp. 2838–2848, 1994.

23. R. G. Wells, P. Simkin, P. Judy, M. A. King, P. H. Pretorius, and H. C. Gifford, "The effect of filter cut-off frequency and dimensionality on the localization and detection of small lesions in FBP reconstructed SPECT images," *J. Nucl. Med.* **39**, p. 79P, 1998 [abstract].

24. C. E. Metz, "Some practical issues of experimental design and data analysis in radiological ROC studies," *Invest. Radiol.* **24**, pp. 234–245, 1989.

25. T.-S. Pan, D.-S. Luo, and M. A. King, "Design of an efficient 3-D projector and backprojector pair for SPECT," in *Proc. Fully 3D Image Reconstruction in Radiology and Nuclear Medicine (Aix-les-Bains)*, pp. 181–185, 1995.

26. H. C. Gifford, R. G. Wells, and M. A. King, "A comparison of human observer LROC and numerical observer ROC for tumor detection in SPECT images," *IEEE Trans. Nucl. Sci.* , 1998 [submitted].

27. A. E. Burgess, "Comparison of receiver operating characteristic and forced choice observer performance measurement methods," *Med. Phys.* **22**, pp. 643–655, 1995.

Diagnostic performance and image quality assessment in teledermatology

Elizabeth A. Krupinski*[a], Ben LeSueur[b], Lansing Ellsworth[b], Norman Levine[b], Ronald Hansen[b],
Nancy Silvis[b], Peter Sarantopoulos[b], Pamela Hite[b], James Wurzel[b],
Ronald S. Weinstein[a], Ana Maria Lopez[a]

[a]Arizona Telemedicine Program University of Arizona, Tucson, AZ 85724
[b]Section of Dermatology University of Arizona College of Medicine, Tucson, AZ 85724

ABSTRACT

Digital photography is available for use in telemedicine using commercially available compact digital cameras. The goal of this study was to compare and evaluate the diagnostic accuracy of dermatological diagnoses based on photos obtained with a digital camera versus in-person diagnoses. 308 subjects were recruited from a university dermatology clinic. Patients were examined in-person by one of three dermatologists who provided the clinical diagnosis. Digital photos were then obtained on all patients. The three dermatologists reviewed the images on a computer monitor and provided a diagnosis and confidence rating. There was 80% agreement between in-person versus digital photo diagnoses. Intra-dermatologist agreement averaged 84%. Decision confidence was rated as very definite to definite 70% of the time using the photo images. Monitor reading agreement with biopsy results averaged about 75%. Image resolution and color were rated as good to excellent 83% and 93% of the time respectively. The use of digital photography for store and forward teledermatology yields high quality images and diagnostic accuracy rates which correlate well with in-person clinical diagnoses and biopsy results.

Keywords: teledermatology, image quality, digital photography, diagnostic accuracy

1. INTRODUCTION

Telemedicine services are rapidly becoming an integral part of many hospitals and rural clinics around the world, providing the potential for accessing underserved populations.[1-5] In many programs teledermatology comprises the most frequently used specialty within a telemedicine service, accounting for over 50% of consultations.[6-7] For the Arizona Telemedicine Program (ATP) teledermatology constitutes 47% of referrals. Two basic systems are typically used in telemedicine: real-time, live-interaction video, and store-forward. Which system maintains the highest degree of diagnostic accuracy when compared to the gold standard, the physical exam, is the subject of many investigations. Most of the evaluative studies in teledermatology have focused on real-time video images.[8-13] In general, the results have been positive when comparing video with in-person diagnosis. Agreement rates between video and in-person diagnoses range from 75%[10] to 97%.[13] Other studies [14-21] have evaluated the use of photographic slides, video capture still images, and digitally scanned versions of slides displayed on a CRT monitor. The results have been mixed. Given the equivocal results of digitized color slides, other methods of obtaining still photos need to be investigated.[22-23] The goal of the present study was to compare the diagnostic accuracy of a dermatologic diagnosis based on in-person physical exam versus a diagnosis based on still photo images acquired using a digital camera.

Part of the SPIE Conference on Image Perception and Performance
San Diego, California ● February 1999
SPIE Vol. 3663 ● 0277-786X/99/$10.00

199

2. MATERIALS AND METHODS

2.1. In-Person Examinations

Three-hundred-eight consecutive patients, referred by either primary care providers or other dermatologists, to the Dermatology Clinic at the University of Arizona Health Sciences Center participated in the study. The patients were examined in the clinic by one of three board-certified dermatologists. Each dermatologist examined approximately one-third of the patients and recorded the clinical diagnosis in each case. Two-hundred-thirty (75%) were given a single diagnosis, and 78 (25%) had two or three differential possibilities listed. Table 1 shows the variety of cases acquired for the study.

Table 1. Types of cases acquired during the study (n = 308).

Clinical Diagnosis	Number of Cases
Malignant or Premalignant	91
Benign Proliferations	74
Eczema/Dermatitis	36
Pigmented Lesions	32
Infections/Infestations	20
Papulosquamous Disorders	12
Urticarial & Allergic	5
Collagen/Vascular	1
Miscellaneous	37

2.2. Digital Image Acquisition and Presentation

After a clinical examination, each of the patient's skin lesions was photographed with the Canon PowerShot600. The Canon PowerShot600 has a 570,000-pixel CCD image sensor with 24-bit color resolution, a 7 mm f/2.5 lens, built-in flash, and a shutter speed of 1/30 - 1/500 sec. It is a relatively small (159.5 mm (w) x 92.5 mm (h) x 58.8 mm (d)) and light camera, weighting only 420 g. The camera has three resolution settings: fine (832 x 608 pixels), normal (640 x 480 pixels) and economy (320 x 240 pixels), corresponding to file sizes of 150 kB, 75 kB and 43 kB respectively. Changes in resolution are accomplished by compressing the image files. Up to five photographs were obtained from each area in question to maximize the information available for image analysis. All photos were taken using the fine resolution setting.

The images were transferred to a Gateway 2000 computer (Gateway, North Sioux City, SD) with a Gateway CrystalScan color monitor (1024 x 768 resolution). The software program PhotoImpact Album v. 3.0 (ULead Systems, Inc., Torrance, CA) was used to arrange the images for each case into a separate file for presentation. A brief patient history derived from the patient file was inserted into each case folder on the computer using the same software program. Care was taken to include only patient history information and exclude any reference to actual diagnosis, patient name, or the identity of which dermatologist had examined the patient. The 308 cases were randomized and numbered for presentation order during the study.

The dermatologists who examined the patients in person also examined the digital images for each case presented on the computer. For each case, the dermatologists had to respond to a four-part questionnaire. A diagnosis was rendered with an associated degree of confidence. The following scale was used to record decision confidence: very definite, definite, probable, possible, no decision. After the diagnosis and confidence were reported, image resolution and color were rated using a 4-level scale: 1 = excellent, 2 = good, 3 = fair, 4 = poor. Additional comments could be recorded if desired. Viewing time was recorded (by a study coordinator using a stopwatch) as the dermatologists read each case. Viewing time began when the first image of a case appeared on the computer monitor, and ended when the dermatologist gave the diagnosis. The time to provide decision confidence, color and resolution ratings was not included in viewing time. The 308 cases were randomly grouped into 14 sets of 22 cases each. Dermatologists were restricted to one-hour sessions for viewing cases. Each dermatologist evaluated all 308 digital records, which included the one-third of images obtained from patients whose in-person evaluation he/she had performed.

2.3. Data Analysis

For purposes of analysis, the in-person diagnoses were defined as the correct diagnoses ("truth"). Diagnostic decisions based on the digital photos were divided into five classifications. Exact matches were those diagnostic decisions where the digital photo and in-person diagnoses matched exactly. Matches were diagnostic decisions in which the digital photo diagnosis matched one of the differential diagnoses provided during the in-person examination, but did not match exactly the single most likely in-person diagnosis. If the digital photo diagnosis did not match the in-person single or one of the differential diagnoses, the diagnosis was reviewed by the senior dermatologist. If the diagnosis made by the reviewing dermatologist did not differ significantly from the differential diagnoses actually listed by the in-person review, cases were classified as a match with a minor difference. If the diagnosis made by the reviewing were significantly different, cases were classified as a mismatch (i.e., incorrect decision). Those cases where the dermatologist could not provide a diagnosis were classified as no decision.

Biopsies were taken in 104 cases from the original 308. This subset of 104 cases was used in a second series of analyses on the data where the biopsy result was the definitive diagnosis. Table 2 shows the distribution of the types of lesions biopsied for the 104 cases.

Table 2. Distribution of the types of lesions (n = 104) biopsied.

Lesion Type	Number	Percent
Infection/Infestation	3	3%
Pigmented Lesions	26	25%
Malignant/Premalignant	49	47%
Dermatitis/Eczema	4	4%
Benign Proliferations	12	11%
Miscellaneous	10	10%

3. RESULTS

3.1. Diagnostic Accuracy

As described above, there are five categories of diagnostic decisions: exact match (EM), match (M), match with a minor difference (MMD), mismatch (MM) and no decision (ND). Combining the EM, M and MMD categories (correct decisions), the correspondence between the in-person and digital photo diagnoses, was 80%. The MM category accounted for 16% of the decisions; and 4% of the decisions fell in the ND category. Analysis of Variance (ANOVA), revealed no statistically significant differences (F = 0.011, df = 2, p = 0.989) between dermatologists for the percentage of decisions falling into each category. Dermatologists 1, 2 and 3 had 81%, 82% and 78% correct decisions, with 15%, 15% and 18% mismatches respectively. The remainder of the decisions were ND. If the "no decisions" are removed, the percentages increase to 84%, 85% and 81% respectively.

Overall, 61% of the decisions had a 1 = very definite or 2 = definite confidence rating, 22% had 3 = probable, 13% had 4 = possible, and 4% had 5 = no decision ratings. An ANOVA analysis revealed a significant difference in confidence ratings (F = 39.76, df = 2, p < 0.0001) between the three dermatologists. Dermatologists 1 (mean = 1.92, sd = 1.21) and 3 (mean = 1.97, sd = 1.07) did not differ significantly (p > 0.05), but dermatologist 2 (mean = 2.64, sd = 1.07) differed from the other two dermatologists (p < 0.001). Overall the correlation between diagnostic accuracy and confidence was r = 0.39. If the data are divided into those cases where only a single diagnosis was rendered during the in-person examination versus those where two or more differential diagnoses were rendered, the correlations between accuracy and confidence are r = 0.43 and r = 0.38 respectively.

Inter-observer variation was analyzed to determine the degree to which the three dermatologists agreed with each other on the diagnoses made viewing the 308 cases on the computer monitor. The decision category data were analyzed by collapsing the data into correct and incorrect decisions as defined above. The data were then analyzed using the kappa statistic. The kappa statistic[24] for dermatologists 1 and 2 was 0.82, for 1 and 3 it was 0.81 and for dermatologists 2 and

3 it was 0.80. Kappa values greater than 0.80 are considered to indicate a high degree of correlation or agreement. Intra-observer variation was analyzed to determine the degree to which each dermatologist's diagnosis using the digital images agreed with their own in-person diagnosis. The data were analyzed in two ways. For the first analysis, only the EM and M decisions were considered. For the second analysis, the MMD decisions were included. For the first analysis dermatologists 1, 2 and 3 had agreement between original and digital diagnoses 66%, 65% and 62% of the time. For the second analysis, agreement levels increased significantly to 90%, 85% and 76% for dermatologists 1, 2 and 3 respectively.

3.2. Image Quality
On average each case had 1.9 digital images (sd = 0.73): 27% had 1 image, 60% had 2, 9% had 3, 3% had 4, and 1% had 5 images. Overall, 83% of the cases were rated as having excellent or good image resolution, with only 1% being rated as poor. When tested with an ANOVA, there was a significant main effect due to dermatologist (F = 119.38, df = 2, p < 0.0001). All three dermatologists differed significantly from one another (p < 0.05). Dermatologists 1, 2 and 3 had mean ratings of 1.7 (sd = 0.87), 2.2 (sd = 0.04), and 1.3 (sd = 0.04) respectively. Recall that 1 = excellent and 4 = poor. Overall, 93% of the images were rated as excellent (1) or good (2) with respect to color. The ANOVA again showed significant differences between dermatologists (F = 323.26, df = 2, p < 0.0001), with all three dermatologists differing significantly from one another (p < 0.05). Dermatologists 1, 2 and 3 had mean color ratings of 1.3 (sd = 0.58), 2.1 (sd = 0.03), and 1.2 (sd = 0.03) respectively. Correlation analyses were also performed on the color and resolution rating data. Overall there was a high positive correlation (r = 0.73) between color and resolution ratings. Images with excellent or good resolution ratings generally received excellent or good color ratings. There were relatively low correlations between color (r = 0.48) and resolution (r = 0.47) ratings and the decision confidence values. Decision confidence was not affected significantly by the overall quality of the image in terms of resolution or color.

3.3. Viewing Time
On average, dermatologists took 22.66 sec (sd = 22.34) to read each case from the monitor and provide their diagnosis. The ANOVA showed a significant difference between dermatologists (F = 113.38, df = 2, p < 0.0001). Dermatologists 1 (mean = 16.34 sec, sd = 10.32) and 3 (mean = 14.96 sec, sd = 12.00) did not differ significantly from each other, but dermatologist 2 (mean = 36.67 sec, sd = 30.87) differed significantly (p < 0.0001) from the other two. Viewing time did not correlate highly with color ratings (r = 0.35), resolution ratings (r = 0.24), diagnostic confidence (r = 0.54), or diagnostic accuracy (r = 0.21). The minimum viewing time was 3 sec and the maximum was 167 sec. Overall, 80% of the cases were diagnosed in less than 30 sec. An additional 14% were diagnosed in less than 60 sec, and 6% took longer than 60 sec to diagnose. Viewing time did not correlate highly (r = 0.15) with whether the original diagnosis had a single diagnosis or multiple alternatives.

3.4. Comparison With Biopsy Results
Sixty of the 104 biopsied cases (58%) were given only a single diagnosis during the in-person examination, and 44 (42%) had two or more differential diagnoses provided. For the original 308 cases, 170 had a single diagnosis and 34 had two or more differential diagnoses. A Chi-Square analysis of the number of single versus differential cases for those sent to biopsy and those that were not revealed a statistically significant difference (X^2 = 25, df = 1, p < 0.001). A significantly higher number of cases with multiple diagnostic options provided during the in-person exam were sent to biopsy than those that were not sent to biopsy. For the analyses of the decision results associated with the biopsy data, the biopsy results were definitive. The same categories for diagnostic decisions were used as in the previous analyses. The first analysis looked at the rates of decision agreement for the three readers for the various conditions: in-person diagnosis versus biopsy results, photo diagnosis versus biopsy results, and in-person versus photo diagnoses. The in-person versus biopsy rates can only be derived for each dermatologist for the cases that they saw in-person. The other two conditions include all the cases. The results, in terms of percent agreement can be found in Table 3. Those cases for which a diagnostic decision was not made are not included in the analyses. A Friedman test (X^2 = 4.667, df = 2, p = 0.097) indicates that there were no statistically significant differences between the in-person vs biopsy, photo vs biopsy and photo vs in-person % agreement rates.

Table 3. Rates (%) of agreement (EM + M + MMD) for the three readers for the various conditions. Numbers in parentheses indicate number of cases (ND cases excluded).

Reader	In-Person vs Biopsy	Photo vs Biopsy	Photo vs In-Person
1	80% (40)	78% (99)	87% (99)
2	97% (34)	76% (102)	79% (102)
3	90% (30)	73% (99)	85% (99)

Contingency analyses, which measure rates of agreement in a similar manner to a correlation analysis, between the photo vs biopsy and photo vs in-person decisions reflect this moderate level of agreement between the two comparisons for each of the three readers (reader 1 C = 0.798; reader 2 C = 0.780; reader 3 C = 0.794). If the contingency analysis is done for each observer using only those cases which the reader saw in-person, the results are C = 0.764, C = 0.655, C = 0.819, for readers 1 (n = 40), 2 (n = 34) and 3 (n = 30) respectively.

An Analysis of Variance (ANOVA) was done on the confidence levels (given during the photo interpretations sessions) from the entire data set (308 cases), using whether or not a biopsy was performed as the independent variable. This analysis revealed that the confidence levels given on those cases that went to biopsy were significantly different (F = 3.948, df = 1,922, p = 0.047) than those that did not go to biopsy. Overall, the biopsy cases received confidence ratings in the definite range, while those that did not go to biopsy received confidence ratings in the very definite range.

The decision time data were also analyzed with an ANOVA. The ANOVA revealed that the decision time (for the photo interpretation) for cases sent to biopsy (mean = 24.82 sec, sd = 25.08 sec) was significantly longer (F = 4.445, df = 1,922, p = 0.035) than that for cases not sent to biopsy (mean = 21.55 sec, sd = 20.74 sec).

4. DISCUSSION

Teledermatology can be conducted using a variety of technologies with varying levels of image quality and cost. Each system has specific advantages and disadvantages; therefore, the choice of a system must be tailored to the needs and goals of the individual site. In many cases, video-capture or digitization of photographs may provide the necessary clinical data. The present investigation demonstrated that direct digital photography can reliably capture dermatology images. The cameras are compact, lightweight and can be maneuvered easily around the patient to obtain the desired views of the lesion. Once the image is acquired, it is easily downloaded to a personal computer and transmitted to a consulting site. Data transmission may employ the simplest of methods – modem and phone. The data from the present study support the use of the digital camera for acquiring teledermatology images. Diagnostic accuracy, how well diagnostic decisions based on digital images correspond to those based on in-person examination, was quite high for all three dermatologists. Although agreement rates between in-person and telemedicine consult diagnoses are likely to differ by sub-specialty, it is interesting to note that the present teledermatology findings are not that different from two other image-based sub-specialties: pathology [25-27] and radiology [28]. Agreement between direct viewing of pathologic slides versus viewing static images via telepathology tends to be quite high, generally greater than 85%[26] and can be greater than 90%.[27] In radiology, agreement rates between film on a viewbox and teleradiology viewing of radiographic images on a CRT monitor also tend to be greater than 85%,[28] depending on the imaging modality.

In the present study, inter-observer and intra-observer variability were relatively low and in line with variabilities noted by other investigators.[18,25] Contributing partly to the observed variability is the case mix found in a tertiary medical center where diagnostic dilemmas are often referred. Clinical dermatologic examination may not be sufficient to render a single definitive diagnosis. In this study, approximately one-third of the patients required biopsy assessment. Cases for which differential diagnoses were given at the time of in-person review had a lower correlation between diagnostic accuracy and decision confidence (r = 0.38), than those cases that had only a single diagnosis in-person (r = 0.43).

Image quality, in terms of resolution and color, were generally rated as excellent to good. One interesting finding was that neither diagnostic decision accuracy or diagnostic confidence was highly correlated with ratings of color or resolution or with viewing time. Dermatologist 2 consistently rated the images lower on resolution and color, had longer viewing times and lower decision confidences than dermatologists 1 and 3, but had essentially the same level of diagnostic accuracy. This finding demonstrates how subjective image quality ratings can be and how they often may not affect diagnostic performance.

The average time for viewing the images on the computer monitor and reaching a diagnostic decision averaged only 23 sec. The range of viewing times was from 3 sec to 167 sec. None of the cases took more than 3 min to diagnose from the monitor, and diagnostic accuracy was still quite high. The results indicate that the dermatologists did not experience any major difficulties in reading dermatologic images from the monitor. Although most telemedicine suites are not likely to have as well-controlled viewing situations, which may result in longer viewing times, it is unlikely that viewing time would increase to the length of a clinical encounter. Use of a digital camera to acquire images for teledermatology appears to represent a useful and reliable new technology.

The value of teledermatology services appears to be considerable. A recent study surveying patients' opinions about direct access to dermatologic specialty care[34] revealed that only 24% of the patients surveyed were very satisfied with previous care by a non-dermatologist, but 89% were very satisfied with a dermatologist's care. Only 6% of those surveyed believed that a generalist could adequately treat their skin disease, and 87% indicated that direct access to a dermatologist was very important to their health care. Using teledermatology to reach patients who would not otherwise be able to easily access specialty care not only fills a gap in health care services in rural areas, it also may serve as a useful tool in improving patient satisfaction and trust in the care they are receiving.

ACKNOWLEDGMENTS

This work was supported by: U.S. Department of Agriculture, Rural Utilities Service Distance Learning and Telemedicine Grant; U.S. Department of Commerce, National Telecommunications and Information Administration TIIAP Grant; Office of Rural Health Policy, HRSA Department of Health and Human Services Rural Telemedicine Grant Program

REFERENCES

1. S.A. Norton, A.E. Burdick, C.M. Phillips, B. Berman. "Teledermatology and underserved populations," *Arch Dermatol* **133**, pp.197-200, 1997.

2. R. McGee, E.G. Tangalos. "Delivery of health care to the underserved: potential contributions of telecommunications technology," *Mayo Clin Proc* **69**, pp.1131-1136, 1994.

3. D.A. Perednia, N.A.Brown. "Teledermatology: one application of telemedicine," *Bull Med Libr Assoc* **83**, pp.42-47, 1995.

4. D.A. Perednia. "Fear, loathing, dermatology, and telemedicine," *Arch Dermatol* **133**, pp. 151-155, 1997.

5. A.E. Burdick, B. Berman. "Teledermatology," *Advances in Dermatology* **12**, pp. 19-45, 1997.

6. A. Allen, D. Allen. "Telemedicine programs. Second annual review reveals doubling of programs in a year," *Telemedicine Today* **3**, pp.10-20, 1995.

7. J. Tichenor, D. Balch, S. Gustke, et al. "Operational issues at the East Carolina University School of Medicine," *Telemedicine Today* **4**, pp. 28-29, 1996.

8. M.A. Loane, H.E. Gore, R. Corbett, K. Steele, et al. "Effect of camera performance on diagnostic accuracy: preliminary results from the Northern Ireland arms of the UK Multicentre Teledermatology Trial," *J of Telemedicine and Telecare* **3**, pp. 83-88, 1997.

9. M.A. Loane, H.E. Gore, R. Corbett, K. Steele, et al. "Preliminary results from the Northern Ireland arms of the UK Multicentre teledermatology Trial: effect of camera performance on diagnostic accuracy," *J of Telemedicine and Telecare* **3**, pp. 73-75, 1997.

10. A.M.M. Oakley, D.R. Astwood, M. Loane, M.B. Duffill, M. Rademaker, R. Wootton. "Diagnostic accuracy of teledermatology: results of a preliminary study in New Zealand," *New Zealand Medical Journal* **28 Feb**, pp. 51-53, 1997.

11. S.G. Burgiss, C.E. Julius, H.W. Watson, B.K. Haynes, E. Bounocore, G.T. Smith. "Telemedicine for dermatology care in rural patients," *Telemedicine Journal* **3**, pp. 227-233, 1997.

12. C.M. Phillips, W.A. Burke, A. Shechter, D. Stone, D. Balch, S. Gustke. "Reliability of dermatology teleconsultations with the use of teleconferencing technology," *J of the American Academy of Dermatology* **37**, pp. 398-402, 1997.

13. P.A. Solomon, M.J. Torma, R.M. Strickland, P.S. Martin, et al. "Dermatology screening with telemedicine," *The J of Family Practice* **42**, pp. 84-85, 1996.

14. C. Sneiderman, R. Schosser, T.G. Pearson. "A comparison of JPEG and FIF compression of color medical images for dermatology," *Computerized Medical Imaging and Graphics* **18**, pp. 339-342, 1994.

15. D.A. Perednia, J.A. Gaines, T.W. Butruille. "Comparison of the clinical informativeness of photographs and digital imaging media with multiple-choice receiver operating characteristic analysis," *Arch Dermatol* **131**, pp. 292-297, 1995.

16. C.A. Sneiderman, A.F. Hood. "A comparison of video and photographic display of skin lesions for morphology recognition," *JBC* **18**, pp. 22-25, 1991.

17. R.H. Schosser, C.A. Sneiderman, T.G. Pearson. "How dermatologists perceive CRT displays and silver halide prints of transparency-based images: a comparison study," *J of Biological Photography* **62**, pp. 135-137, 1994.

18. D.A. Perednia, J.A. Gaines, A.C. Rossum. "Variability in clinician assessment of lesions in cutaneous images and its implications for skin screening and computer-assisted diagnosis," *Arch Dermatol* **128**, pp. 357-364, 1992.

19. B. Gerbert, T. Maurer, T. Berger, S. Pantilat, et al. "Primary care clinicians as gatekeepers in managed care," *Arch Dermatol* **132**, pp. 1030-1038, 1996.

20. R.L.H. Murphy, T.B. Fitzpatrick, H.A. Haynes, K.T. Bird, T.B. Sheridan. "Accuracy of dermatologic diagnosis by television," *Arch Dermatol* **105**, pp. 833-835, 1972.

21. B.D. Zelickson, L. Homan. "Teledermatology in the nursing home," *Arch Dermatol* **133**, pp. 171-174, 1997.

22. C.C. Lyon, P.V. Harrison. "A portable digital imaging system in dermatology: diagnostic and educational applications," *J of Telemedicine and Telecare* **3**, pp. 81-83, 1997.

23. J.C. Kvedar, R.A. Edwards, E.R. Menn, M. Mofid, E. Gonzalez, J. Dover, J.A. Parrish. "The substitution of digital images for dermatologic physical examination," *Arch Dermatol* **133**, pp. 161-167, 1997.

24. J.L. Fleiss. *Statistical Methods for Rates and Proportions. 2nd Ed.* John Wiley and Sons, New York, 1981.

25. B.E. Halliday, A.K. Bhattacharyya, A.R. Graham, J.R. Davis, et al. "Diagnostic accuracy of an international static-imaging telepathology consultation service," *Hum Pathol* **28**, pp. 17-21, 1997.

26. R.S. Weinstein, A.K. Bhattacharyya, A.R. Graham, J.R. Davis. "Telepathology: a ten-year progress report," *Hum Pathol* **28**, pp. 1-7, 1997.

27. R.S. Weinstein. "Static image telepathology in perspective," *Human Pathology* **27**, pp. 99-101, 1996.

28. E.A. Krupinski, L. Hopper. "Teleradiology in rural Arizona: user's perspective," *SPIE Medical Imaging* **3035**, pp. 350-354, 1997.

*Correspondence: Elizabeth Krupinski, PhD Department of Radiology, University of Arizona 1609 N. Warren Bldg 211 Rm 112 Tucson, AZ 85724   520-626-4498 (ph) 520-626-4376 (f) krupinski@radiology.arizona.edu

Classification of Mammographic Patterns:
Beyond Fraction of Dense Tissue

Philip F. Judy, Richard Nawfel, Francine Jacobson, Darrell Smith, Steven E. Seltzer

Brigham and Women's Hospital
and
Harvard Medical School

Boston, MA

ABSTRACT

Women with mammograms that radiologists classify as dense have been found to have an increased risk of breast cancer. The purpose to this investigation was to determine whether human readers are willing and able to make reliable comparisons of five attributes of pairs of mammograms matched by a quantitative estimate of the fraction of dense tissue (FDT).

Forty pairs of CC projections were digitized and presented using a computer workstation. The 40 pairs of mammograms had the same FDT as measured by a visual threshold procedure. Each breast image was from a different woman. The difference in the following 5 attributes were rated: (i) fraction of dense tissue, (ii) fraction of homogeneous of the dense tissue, (ii) fraction of ductal dense tissue, (iv) prominence of scalloping of dense tissue, and (v) prominence of subareolar structures. The rating were replicated to evaluate their reliability.

Spearman rank-order correlations of replicated measurements ranged from 0.89 to 0.65 (p was less than 0.0001). Homogeneous dense tissue ratings were negatively correlated with ductal dense tissue ratings (-0.59, p=0.0001). The prominence of scalloping rating was not significantly correlated with other attributes. The ratings of the attributes, except scalloping, were significantly correlated to differences mean gray level of breast parenchyma.

Readers can make reliable judgments regarding the differences in attributes of mammograms that are matched by FDT. The negative correlation between the homogeneous dense and the ductal dense tissue ratings suggest that homogeneous dense and ductal dense tissues contend for perceived dense breast area. The absence of correlation between scalloping and other image attributes suggests further investigation of scalloping as an independent, breast-cancer risk factor is warranted.

Keywords: breast cancer, risk, mammography

1. INTRODUCTION

The numerous programs using mammography to detect breast cancer have provided many opportunities to study the variations of the breast cancer risk that are associated with the variations of mammographic parenchymal patterns. In 1976, Wolfe reported strong associations of 4 categories of mammographic parenchyma patterns with breast cancer risk (1). Prompted by such large effects, many subsequent studies have in general reproduced Wolfe's results (2,3). Yet, the consensus of the subsequent studies is that while these risk variations are large from an epidemiology perspective, the risks predicted for the high-risk mammography categories are much less than Wolfe's original results.

Wolfe classified the images of breast parenchyma in 4 categories that have been approximately related to fraction of area dense tissue projected onto the image (FDT). Dense tissue is any non-fat tissue in parenchyma. Yet, Wolfe discussed image attributes of the parenchymal pattern beyond density to describe his 4 categories. The long-term goal of our research is to assess the breast cancer risk information present on a mammogram that is independent of FDT. Ultimately, we plan to determine whether the recent investigations have focused too much on the FDT component of Wolfe's classifications and ignored the other attributes of the parenchymal patterns that may also be associated with risk. If these attributes of the parenchymal patterns beyond the FDT are associated with breast cancer risk then any study ignoring these attributes might produce lower risk estimates than Wolfe's, if he actually used these non-density attributes to classify mammograms.

2. METHODS

2.1 Perceptual Studies

This investigation determined whether humans (readers) are willing and able to make reliable comparisons (ratings) of attributes of pairs of mammograms matched by a quantitative estimate of the FDT (4). The stimuli were digitized mammograms in a PowerPoint presentation. Each image was a pair of CC projections of the breast having the same fraction of dense tissue (Figure 1). The images were scaled such that the breast had the same axilla to sternum dimension.

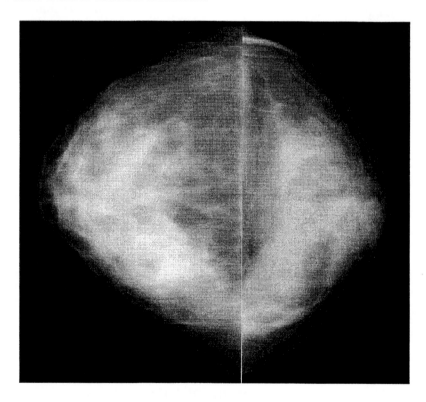

Figure 1 – Images of two breasts with same FDT (52%, 51%)

Readers were provided paper sheets to record their ratings. Each sheet had 40 pairs of boxes representing the left and right images in the image set. Readers rated their level of confidence on a scale 1 to 4 (1 meaning low confidence to 4 meaning high confidence) in the box representing the breast image with most of the specified attribute. This scheme provided at 8-category scale of the magnitude of difference between the specified attribute.

The readers were given the following written description of each specific rating task. The specific task description was printed on each answer sheet.

Task: Compare the pairs of mammograms
  i. Which breast has the larger fraction of dense tissue?
  ii. Which breast has the larger fraction of homogeneously dense tissue?
  iii. Which breast has more ductal density?
      The term, ductal density, means serpentine, beaded, or nodule features. Use of ductal density does not imply that these features are ducts.
  iv. Which breast has more scalloping?
  v. Which breast has the more prominent subareolar structure?

Two readers rated the 40 pairs of mammographic images on two occasions. These mammograms were obtained from 80 different women. The reliability of the rating was estimated using the Spearman rank order correlation of the replicated ratings.

2.2 Image Calculations

The difference of FDT between image pairs was always less than 0.04. This value is less than the reproducibility of FDT measurement.

The mean gray level of breast parenchyma was calculated from the digitized mammograms. The breast parenchyma was defined as the portion of breast image on mammogram that does not include the subcutaneous fat. This region was determined using the same threshold-histogram procedure that was used determine the dense area in breast parenchyma. This procedure uses the visually selected threshold that was the transition between the subcutaneous fat and the breast parenchyma. The procedure to estimate the FDT selects the transition between dense and fat tissue within the breast parenchyma.

3. RESULTS

Readers reliably reported differences of all attributes. Spearman rank-order correlations of replicated measurements (Table 1.) ranged from 0.89 to 0.66 (p was less than 0.0001). There was no significant correlation between reader ratings and calculated differences of FDT between image pairs. The ratings of the attributes, except scalloping, were significantly correlated to differences mean gray level of breast parenchyma of the pairs of mammograms (ΔGL).

Attribute	Reliability	Correlation with Δ GL	
		Value	P-value
Fraction of dense tissue	0.842	0.483	0.0013
Homogeneous density	0.892	0.514	0.0006
Ductal density	0.657	-0.401	0.0097
Scalloping	0.868	-0.115	0.4831
Subareolar density	0.784	0.415	0.0072

Table 1   Reliabilities and Correlations

Homogeneous dense tissue rating was negatively correlated with ductal dense tissue ratings (-0.59, p was less than 0.0001). The ratings of differences of the prominence of scalloping were not significantly correlated with other ratings.

4. CONCLUSIONS

Readers can make reliable judgments regarding the differences in attributes of mammograms that are matched by fraction of dense tissue. The high reliability may in part be an artifact to not matching the breast parenchymal gray levels of the pairs of mammograms.

The negative correlation between the homogeneous dense and the ductal dense tissue ratings suggest that homogeneous dense and ductal dense tissues contend for the dense breast area as perceived by the reader. A threshold method of estimating the FDT does not make a distinction in types of dense tissue that a human can reliably make. This is a distinction that Wolfe discussed. The absence of correlation between scalloping (an attribute noted by Wolfe to be associated with "dense" breasts) and other attributes suggests further investigation of scalloping as an independent breast cancer risk factor is warranted.

REFERENCES

1. J.N. Wolfe, "Mammographic parenchymal patterns and breast cancer risk," Cancer, 37, pp146-174, 1976.

2. C. Byrne, C. Shaired, J. Wolfe, N. Parekh, M. Salane, L.A. Brinton, R. Hoover, R Haile,"Mammographic features and breast cancer risk: effects with time, age, and menopause status," JNCI, 87, pp. 1622-1629, 1995.

3. N.F. Boyd, G.A. Lockwood, J.W. Byng, D.L. Tritchler, M.J. Yaffe, " Mammographic densities and breast cancer risk," Cancer Epidemiology, Biomarkers & Prevention , 7, pp. 1133-1144, 1998.

4 J.W. Byng, M.J. Yaffe, R.A. Jong, R.S. Shumak, G.A. Lockwood, D.L. Tritchler, N.F. Boyd, "Analysis of Mammographic Density and Breast Cancer Risk from Digitized Mammograms," RadioGraphics, 18, pp. 1587-1598, 1998.

SESSION 6

Technology Assessment and Observer Performance II

Effect of monitor luminance on the detection of solitary pulmonary nodule : ROC analysis

Koun-Sik Song[*], Jin Seong Lee, Hyae Young Kim, Tae-Hwan Lim

Dept. of Diagnostic Radiology, Asan Medical Center, Univ. of Ulsan College of Medicine,
Seoul, 138-736, South Korea

ABSTRACT

We compared the detectability of solitary pulmonary nodule(SPN) in chest radiographs displayed on different gray-scale monitor luminance. From the long-term archive of Asan Medical Center PACS 40 normal chest PA images and 40 chest PA images with SPN were fetched into the short-term storage. All Chest PA images were acquired using Fuji FCR 9501 or 9500 HQ and down-sampled from 4k to 2k pixel resolutions, and archived to ODJ with 10:1 compression ratio. Mean diameter of the nodules were 12mm ranging in size from 8 to 20mm. Nodules were located within the free lung fields(10 cases), overlapped with rib(13 cases), and overlapped with hilum, heart, or subphrenic areas(17 cases). Gray-scale monitors compared in our study were Image Systems M21P2KHBMAX monitor with 100 fL brightness and M21PMAX monitor with 65 fL brightness. After randomization, eight board-certified radiologists determined the presence or absence of nodules independently using worksheet. All radiologists interpreted the images displayed on low-brightness monitors, then after 10 days interpreted the images displayed on high-brightness monitors. Data were gathered using five rating categories, and ROC analysis was performed. Area under the ROC curve was compared for low and high brightness monitors. Mean area under the ROC curve for low-brightness monitor was 0.8597 and high-brightness monitor was 0.8734. Although high-brightness monitor is slightly superior to low-brightness monitor, there was no statistically significant differences between low-brightness and high-brightness monitors($p=0.3$). Further studies are required for various other subtle lung diseases, long-term physiologic effect.

Keywords: Monitor luminance, ROC analysis, chest radiography, solitary pulmonary nodule, soft-copy image presentation, perception, PACS

1. INTRODUCTION

When we select the monitors for soft-copy reading in a PACS environment, we usually consider many physical parameters of the monitors such as physical size, spatial resolution, vertical refresh rate, luminance intensity, gray levels, monitor characteristic curve, and so on[1-4]. Among these parameters the prices of the monitor mostly depends on the luminance intensity. Although the prices of the high-resolution gray-scale monitors are becoming cheaper, it is still expensive especially for high-brightness gray-scale monitors. High-brightness monitors are generally twice the prices of low-brightness monitors. Moreover most of the monitor companies produce only portrait models for high-resolution high-brightness monitors, which is an another factor for increasing the unit price of the diagnostic display workstations, because expensive special display controllers are required when we use portrait monitors. For the cost-effective installation of the PACS we can make much cheaper diagnostic display workstations using medium-resolution low-brightness monitor of landscape model and general purpose display controller, but radiologists generally wants to view the images with portrait type monitors especially when they interprets the plain radiographic images either using computed radiography(CR) or direct digital radiography(DR). If reading performance of radiologists using low-brightness monitors are comparable to high-brightness monitors, significant cut-off of diagnostic display workstations may be possible by using medium-resolution low-brightness monitors with or without special display controllers.

The purpose of this study was to compare the detectability of solitary pulmonary nodule in chest radiographs displayed on high-resolution gray-scale monitors with different luminance intensity, high-brightness and low-brightness under the PACS environment.

2. MATERIALS AND METHODS

From the long-term archive of Asan Medical Center(AMC) PACS, 40 normal chest PA images and 40 chest PA images with solitary pulmonary nodule were fetched into the personal folder in short-term storage unit. Chest PA images were acquired with the patient in an erect position at a source-to-patient distance of 180cm. The studies were phototimed at 150 kVp, and 10:1 grid was used to reduce scattered radiation. Chest PA images were acquired using Fuji FCR 9501 or 9500 HQ and down-sampled from its original 4k pixel resolution to 2k pixel resolution, and archived into the optical disk jukebox after 10:1 JPEG lossy compression. Only brightness and contrast settings are changed from the acquired images. Other image processing were not done. Retrieved all 80 images were decompressed from 10:1 to 2:1 compression ratio and stored in personal folder, then randomized. After randomization each radiologist interpreted the images independently using the worksheet. The presence or absence of solitary pulmonary nodule was determined by consensus of two radiologists after reviewing the CT scans obtained within one week when chest PA images were taken. They determined the most optimal brightness and contrast levels for detection of solitary pulmonary nodule and saved the above brightness and contrast settings. Above two radiologists did not participated in the image interpretation session. All solitary pulmonary nodules did not contain any calcifications. Solitary pulmonary nodules were pathologically confirmed as bronchogenic carcinoma(17 cases), solitary pulmonary metastasis(11 cases), pulmonary hamartoma(2 cases), and inflammatory granuloma(10 cases). Mean diameter of the nodules were 12mm ranging in size from 8mm to 20mm. The number of cases according to the diameter of the nodule was as follows. Twenty nodules were diameter between 8-10mm, sixteen nodules between 10-15mm, and four nodules between 15-20mm. All nodules larger than 15mm in diameter were located within the lung parenchyma overlapped with pulmonary hilum, heart, or subphrenic lung zones. Nodules were located within the free lung fields(10 cases), overlapped with rib(13 cases), and overlapped with hilum, heart, or subphrenic areas(17 cases). Gray-scale monitors compared in our study were Image Systems M21P2KHBMAX monitor with 100 fL brightness and M21PMAX monitor with 65 fL brightness. Because the maximum resolution of the M21PMAX monitor is 1.2 x 1.6k and the maximum resolution of the M21P2KHBMAX monitor is 2.0 x 2.5k, we displayed all images with 1.2 x 1.6k display pixel resolution(Table 1). Workstation used in our study consists of SUN Ultrasparc 167 MHz, 256 RAM, Gxtra graphics display card with 1,280 x 1,600 display pixel resolution.

Table 1. Specifications for the ImageSystems Monitors

Parameters	M21P2KHBMAX	M21PMAX
CRT screen size	21" Flat Square	21" Flat Square
Deflection angle	90	110
Glass transmission	48%	34%
Phosphor	P104	P104
Brightness	100 fL	65 fL
Resolution	1,728 x 2,304	1,200 x 1,600
Vertical refresh	70 Hz	70 Hz

Eight board-certified radiologists participated in this study. Two radiologists(observer 4 and 5) specialize in thoracic imaging with 15 and 4 years of experience, but had little experience in soft-copy reading. Three radiologists(observer 3, 7, 8) are fellows with some experience in soft-copy reading, and the other three radiologists(observer 1, 2, 6) are fellows with little experience in soft-copy reading. We did not provided the preliminary reading sessions for radiologists who had had little experience in soft-copy reading. Each radiologist determined the presence or absence of the nodules independently using worksheet. All radiologists interpreted the images displayed on low-brightness monitors at first session. After 10 days eight radiologists interpreted the same set of images displayed on high-brightness monitors at second session. Observers were allowed to change the brightness and contrast settings of the displayed images, but not allowed to change the brightness and contrast settings of the monitors. Reading room brightness was not strictly controlled, so each observer selected the most comfortable reading room brightness individually. All radiologists turned off the direct fluorescent illumination from the ceiling and film alternators. All radiologists used only indirect dimming illumination from the ceiling.

Data were gathered using five rating categories, and ROC analysis was performed using ROCFIT program. Area under the ROC curve was compared for low and high-brightness monitors.

3. RESULTS

Area under the ROC curve for each eight radiologists was shown in Table 2. Mean area under the ROC curve for low-brightness monitor was 0.8597 and high-brightness monitor was 0.8734. Although high-brightness monitor was slightly superior to low-brightness monitor, there was no statistically significant differences between low-brightness and high-brightness monitors($p=0.3$ by student's t-test). Figure 1 is an actual ROC curve generated from the pooled data. Two thoracic radiologists(observer 4 and 5) performed best instead of little experience in soft-copy reading and difference between low-brightness and high-brightness monitors was smaller than other radiologists. Performance using low-brightness monitor was much lower than high-brightness monitor in 3 fellow radiologists(observer 1, 2, 6) who had no experience in soft-copy reading. There was little performance differences between low-brightness and high-brightness monitors in the other three fellow radiologists(observer 3, 7, 8) who had had some experience in soft-copy reading. Performance using low-brightness monitors was higher than performance using low-brightness monitors in one thoracic radiologist(observer 5) and two fellow radiologists(observer 3 and 8).

Table 2. Area under the ROC curve(Az) for different gray-scale monitor luminance

Observer	Low-brightness monitor	High-brightness monitor
1	0.8372 ± 0.0495	0.8970 ± 0.0430
2	0.8425 ± 0.0458	0.8848 ± 0.0378
3	0.8566 ± 0.0424	0.8461 ± 0.0456
4	0.8865 ± 0.0376	0.8904 ± 0.0401
5	0.9185 ± 0.0356	0.9105 ± 0.0401
6	0.8446 ± 0.0461	0.8677 ± 0.0514
7	0.8458 ± 0.0474	0.8493 ± 0.0479
8	0.8461 ± 0.0466	0.8410 ± 0.0449
Mean	0.8597 ± 0.0283	0.8734 ± 0.0261

P=0.3 by Student's t-test

4. DISCUSSION

One of the reasons why number of hospitals installing the PACS is smaller than previously expected is its high initial investment. It is generally accepted that clinical review workstations need not be high-end, so personal computer with general-purpose color monitor is enough. But in case of diagnostic workstations used in radiology department more powerful display workstations equipped with more than one pair of high-resolution monitors and special display graphic controller cards are generally required. As far as spatial resolution is concerned there are tools such as magic glass function to display original plain radiographic images with 2k pixel resolution on a medium resolution monitor(1.2k x 1.6k). Moreover if we display these radiographic images on a landscape type monitors, expensive special display controllers are not needed so prices of the diagnostic display workstations can be significantly lowered. Most of monitor companies produce high-brightness monitors for high-resolution(2k x 2.5k) monitors only. If reading performances using low-brightness monitors are comparable to high-brightness monitors, significant cut-off of diagnostic display workstations may be possible by using medium-resolution low-brightness monitors with or without special display controllers. There is an influence at least maximum luminance since the combination of CRT-human observer is a cascade system. And much of the light emitted by the CRT is not collected by the human eye due to the small numerical aperture of the eye-lens and the low quantum efficiency of the retina of the eye[3]. As a result there will be a quantum sink with respect to luminance and observer performance will degrade[4].

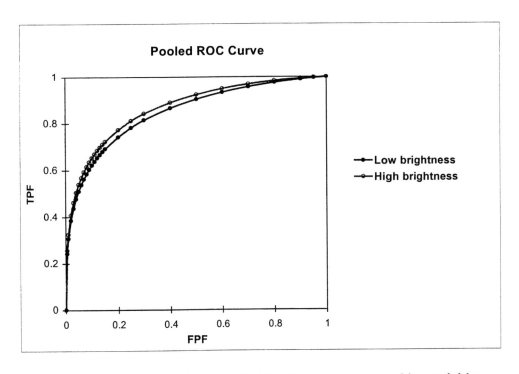

Figure 1. ROC curve for low-brightness and high-brightness monitors generated from pooled data.

Overall, performance using high-brightness monitor was slightly higher than that of low-brightness monitors, but this performance difference was statistically not significant($p=0.3$). There was an individual performance differences between much experienced thoracic radiologists and fellow radiologists with less clinical experience, between fellow radiologists with or without experience of soft-copy reading. These individual differences in performance suggest that some adaptation periods are required for soft-copy reading under the PACS environment in radiologists with little clinical experience. In case of much experienced thoracic radiologists there was no differences in performance between low-brightness and high-brightness monitors in detection of solitary pulmonary nodule, so it may not be necessary to have an adaptation period before soft-copy reading in PACS environment.

The interval between the two reading sessions was only 10 days, so some memory effects might have affected our study results. But because first reading session was designed to interpret the soft-copy chest PA images with low-brightness monitors, even if some memory effects actually existed, it might not have favorably affected for performances with low-brightness monitors. Limitation of our study is that because we did not absolutely control the reading room environment, effect of environmental illumination might have influenced on our study results.

In conclusion, low-brightness gray-scale monitor is not inferior to high-brightness monitor in the detection of solitary pulmonary nodule under the usual reading room illumination conditions. Further studies are required for various other subtle lung diseases and long-term physiologic effect on human observer.

ACKNOWLEDGEMENTS

This work was supported by Grant from the Health Technology Planning & Evaluation Board, Ministry of Health and Welfare, Korea.

REFERENCES

1. H. Roehrig, H. Blume, T. Ji, and M. Browne, Performance Tests and Quality Control of Cathode Ray Tube Displays," *Journal of Digital Imaging*, vol. 3(3), pp. 134-145, August, 1990.
2. G. Spekowius, M. Weibrecht, P. Quadflieg, and H. Blume, Image quality assessment of monochrome monitors for medical soft copy display", *SPIE Proceedings, Medical Imaging*, vol. 3031, 232-244, 1997.
3. H. Roehrig, H. Blume, T. Ji, et al., Noise of CRT display systems", *SPIE Proceedings*, vol. 1897, 232-245, 1993.
4. Albert Macovski, *Medical Imaging Systems*, Englewood Cliffs, NJ, Prentice-Hall Inc, 1993.

* Correspondence: Email: kssong@www.amc.seoul.kr; Telephone: 822 2224 4369; Fax: 822 476 4719

Observer performance using CRT monitors with different phosphors

Hans Roehrig, Elizabeth A. Krupinski, Mahesh Sivarudrappa

Department of Radiology University of Arizona, Tucson, AZ 85724

ABSTRACT

The goal of this study was to compare observer performance on two monitors – one with a P45 and the other with a P104 phosphor. Phosphors have distinctly different physical properties that, among other things, affect the noise properties of the display. Differences in noise have an effect on the signal-to-noise ratio, and hence may have a significant affect on observer's detection performance. A complete physical analysis was done on the 2 monitors. A JND study was conducted to measure observer performance. A series of grating patterns was generated for display on the 2 monitors. Observers were instructed to report whether the pattern was vertical, horizontal or blank. Observer performance with the P45 was better than with the P104 phosphor. This result was supported those found in the physical evaluation, that showed poorer results on various parameters. The results indicate that the type of phosphor does affect the physical aspects, which in turn affects observer performance. Two clinical areas in particular that might be affected by phosphor differences are nodule detection in chest images and mass detection in mammograms, since low contrast targets will be most affected by the noise differences (SNR) in different monitor phosphors.

Keywords: CRT displays, phosphor, observer performance

1. INTRODUCTION

The practice of radiology is increasingly changing from a film and light box-based to a computer and CRT monitor-based display medium. Although this transition may seem straightforward and easy to some, it is actually a rather involved and sensitive process.[1-3] There are many differences between film and monitor displays. Our group at the University of Arizona has conducted a number of studies to assess the differences between film and monitor displays, from both the physical and psychophysical perspectives. For example, we have found in general that although observer performance tends to be equivalent for film and monitor viewing,[4-5] there are distinct and often significant differences in search behaviors as reflected in longer viewing times and differences in scanning patterns as measured by eye-position recording. Dwell times are longer and the number of fixation clusters generated for all types of decisions are longer with a monitor than with film. Differences in the physical properties of monitors have also been shown to affect detection and search performance. When monitor luminance is decreased (80 ft-L vs 140 ft-L), detection performance for microcalcifications and masses in mammograms does not change significantly, but search behaviors do.[6] Decision dwell times increase, more fixation clusters are generated and viewing times increase. The choice of tone scale also affects performance.[6] Detection performance was found to be significantly worse with a non-perceptually linearized display curve (calibrated with the SMPTE pattern), compared to a perceptually linearized display (Barten) curve. Eye-position parameters were not affected as much as with changes in display luminance, but the same trend towards longer dwells, more clusters and longer total viewing times were observed with the non-linearized display.

Another important physical parameter of CRT monitors that might affect detection and search performance is the phosphor used. Phosphors have many different properties (e.g., grain size) which

Part of the SPIE Conference on Image Perception and Performance
San Diego, California • February 1999
SPIE Vol. 3663 • 0277-786X/99/$10.00

217

certainly affect the physical properties of the display (e.g., noise) and thus have potential to affect the performance of observers using the display. The goal of this experiment was to assess both physically and psychophysically the effects of two different commonly used monitor phosphors (P45 and P104). The results of these measurements should help us determine which type of phosphor is more appropriate for viewing medical images on a CRT monitor. As noted previously, monitors are becoming more prevalent in radiology departments for viewing clinical images. It is therefore, extremely important that we understand these digital displays and how observer performance might be affected by various physical characteristics.

2. MATERIALS AND METHODS

2.1. Physical Evaluation

Evaluations[7-8] were done on two ImageSystems monochrome monitors in the mid-resolution range (1600 x 1200 pixels). The physical performance characteristics evaluated include: (1) display function, (2) dynamic range, (3) veiling glare, and (4) maximum signal-to-noise ratio per pixel. The display function was measured with a spot-photometer determining the luminance in the ten gray-steps of the SMPTE pattern displayed on the monitor. The dynamic range was found from the ratio of the luminance in the 100% video signal field and the 0% video field of the SMPTE pattern. For measuring veiling glare, a black disk (0% video signal) of variable diameter was displayed on a white background (100% video signal). Using a spot photometer, the luminance in the center of the black disk was measured for different disk diameters and related to the luminance of the white background.

Noise and signal-to-noise ratio were determined with the aid of a CCD camera using the setup shown in figure 1. Here a portion of the CRT is imaged under large optical magnification onto the CCD such that there are approximately 6 to 8 CCD pixels per CRT pixel ("oversampling"). Flat fielding has to be applied in order to eliminate spatial noise of the CCD camera. The CCD camera was a high-performance one. It features cooling to -20°C, read out at 500 kHz and 14 bits contrast resolution. The pixel matrix was 1317 x 1035, the pixel size was 0.0068 mm. The imaging optics was a Nikon Macro lens with a focal length of 55 mm. The f/stops of the lens ranged from f/2.8 to f/16. The magnification can go up to m = 1:1 We will most likely use a magnification which permits oversampling of the CRT at 8 CCD pixels per CRT pixel. An iris in front of the lens served as baffle and assured optimum rejection of stray light and consequently assured reduction of veiling glare by the lens. At an f/16 contrast ratios of 65:1 have been measured.

The camera software permits imaging with flatfielding, where a "flat" image is taken using a integrating sphere to compensate ("normalize") for CCD pixel non-uniformity and vignetting of the lens.

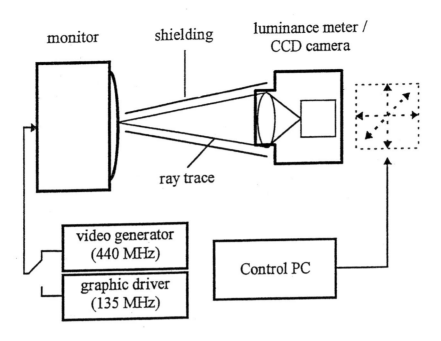

Figure 1. Setup for measurements with the CCD camera.

2.2. Observer Performance Evaluation

The psychophysical study used stimuli consisting of grating (bars) patterns consisting of 7 pixels on and 7 pixels off (2 cm x 2 cm). There were 11 bars total. The bar gray levels ranged from 512 to 517, corresponding to a luminance of about 20 ft-L on a 10 bit scale. There were 10 horizontal and 10 vertical renditions of each stimuli, complimented with 42 blank (no bars) stimuli for a total of 162 images in the test set. The stimuli were displayed once on the P45 and once on the P104 ImageSystems monitor, operated at 1600 x 1200 pixels. Nine undergraduate students participated as observers in each viewing condition. Viewing distance was 50 cm (targets subtended 2.3 deg visual angle) and the room lights were turned off. Observers had to indicate whether each target was vertical, horizontal or blank on a pre-formatted answer sheet.

3. RESULTS

3.1. Physical Evaluation

A number of physical parameters of the two monitors (P45 and P104) were characterized as described above. Many of the graphs presented below contain data from other types of monitors (e.g., a 1600 x 1200 pixel color CRT, a 2048 x 2560 pixel monochrome flat panel) for comparison purposes. The display functions of the monochrome monitors are shown in figure 2 together with the display functions of a color monitor and a monochrome flat panel display. Maximum luminance and dynamic range values are listed in Table 1.

Table 1. Maximum luminance and dynamic range of CRTs and a monochrome flatpanel.

	Pixel Size [mm]	Maximum Luminance (ft-L)	Dynamic Range When SMPTE Pattern Is Displayed
Monochrome P104	0.245	47.7	129
Monochrome P45	0.245	39.8	120
Color Monitor	0.245	43.0	18.6
Monochrome Flatpanel	0.147	228	228
Film Light Box		500	800

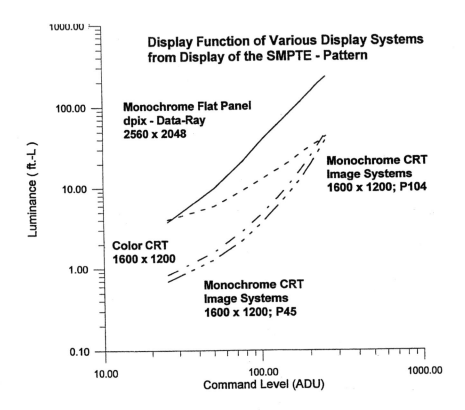

Figure 2. Display function of various display systems from display of the SMPTE pattern.

Maximum luminance and dynamic range of the CRTs as well as that of the flat panel are much smaller than those of the film/light box combination (about 500 ft-L and about 800:1).

The spread of light by way of scatter from one location of the display to another one is described by veiling glare. Monochrome CRTs suffer from scatter of light in the usually 3 to 4 mm thick glass face plate. Color CRTs suffer from electron scatter between the faceplate and the shadow mask. Figure 3 presents veiling glare for all four displays. Note that the color monitor is the one with the largest amount of veiling glare, while the monochrome flat panel has the lowest amount of veiling glare.

There are commonly two noise sources in CRT systems:
- Temporal noise, caused by the bandwidth of the electronics, the electron beam shot noise and light photon shot noise,
- Spatial noise, caused by the phosphor granularity.

Commonly, temporal noise is negligible except at very low luminance.
Spatial noise is best evaluated with the aid of a CCD camera. In addition, the raster lines of the CRT has to be eliminated by defocusing of the CRT.

Figure 4 presents the SNR per pixel for the two monochrome CRTs as a function of the CRT luminance. Notice that the SNR for the P45 is larger than that for the P104, indicating that the P104 phosphor exhibits larger phosphor noise than the P45 phosphor. It is interesting that the signal-to-noise per pixel is independent of the luminance at high luminance, while it is dependent on the luminance at low luminance value. Furthermore, notice that maximum values of signal to noise ratio per pixel are in the order of 60 to 120.

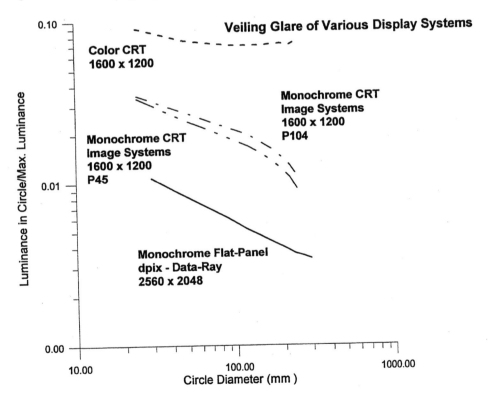

Figure 3. Veiling glare of various display systems.

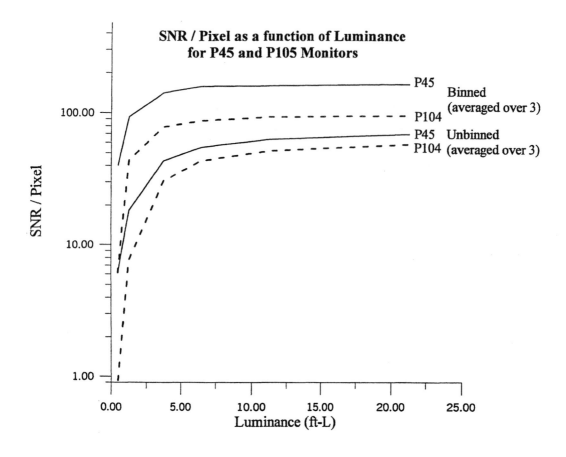

Figure 4. SNR/pixel as a function of luminance for P45 and P104 monitors.

3.2. Observer Performance

For both the P45 and P104 monitors there were no significant differences in percent correct decisions for horizontal vs vertical stimuli. There were, however, significant differences at all gray levels for P45 versus P104 (F = 28.55, df = 23, p < 0.0001). The percent correct decisions for the two viewing conditions can be found in figure 5. The JND or 50% correct point for the P45 monitor was at gray level 513, and the JND for the P104 monitor was at gray level 514.

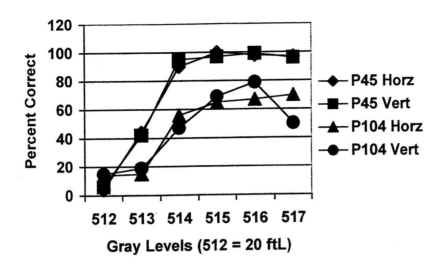

Figure 5. Percent correct decisions for P45 vs P104 monitors for the horizontal (horz) and vertical (vert) stimuli. The dark vertical lines indicate the 50% correct JND points for P45 versus P104.

4. DISCUSSION

The threshold contrasts for the CRT's at high luminance are significantly larger than those found for a noise free display i.e., the limits of the human observer. The implication is that there is a potential for improvement in the perceived dynamic range by almost a factor of 10, if the phosphor noise can be made smaller. It is also interesting to know that over a wide range of luminance levels the threshold contrast is inversely proportional to the spatial signal-to-noise ratio. With respect to color monitors, the maximum luminance is even smaller than that of monochrome monitors, even though the dynamic range can be similar to that of the monochrome monitor. The spatial resolution of color monitors is clearly poorer than that of the monochrome monitor.

The physical measurements done on the two monitors indicate that in almost every respect the P45 phosphor monitor out performs the P104 monitor. Perhaps the most important finding is the fact that the SNR/pixel is higher for the P45 monitor than for the P104 monitor. This would suggest that the noise characteristics of the P45 monitor are better than the P104, which should result in better observer performance with the P45 monitor. Indeed, this is exactly what was found in the observer performance study. Percent correct decisions were significantly higher at all gray levels for the P45 than the P104 monitor, and the JND point was significantly lower. Naturally there are many other physical parameters tat contribute to whether a monitor displays images in such a way as too promote good observer performance, but the SNR is one of the most important.

These results are important because they suggest that monitor phosphor not only makes a difference in the physical characteristics of a CRT monitor, but it also affects observer performance. The present observer performance study was purely psychophysical using simple grating patterns. Further studies with real clinical images will have to be conducted to determine if the results generalize to the clinical situation. However, given the importance of SNR and noise characteristics in general on the perception of subtle targets in noisy stimuli, it will not be surprising if monitot phosphor affects performance with clinical images.

ACKNOWLEDGMENTS

This work was supported by: Toshiba Medical Systems, Tokyo Japan.
as well as by Image Systems Inc.

REFERENCES

1. H. Roehrig, "Image quality assurance for CRT display systems", *J Digital Imaging* **12**, pp. 1-2, 1999.
2. H. Blume, S. Bergstrom, J. Goble, "Image pre-hanging and processing strategies for efficient work-flow management with diagnostic radiology workstations", *J Digital Imaging* **11**, pp. 66, 1998.
3. T. Mertelmeier, "Why and how is soft copy reading possible in clinical practice?", J Digital Imaging 12, pp. 3-11, 1999.
4. Comparison of conventional and computed radiography: assessment of image quality and reader performance in skeletal extremity trauma", *Acad Radiol* **4**, pp. 570-576, 1997.
5. E. Krupinski, K. Maloney, S.C. Bessen, et al., "Receiver operating characteristic evaluation of computer display of adult portable chest radiographs", *Invest Radiol* **29**, pp. 141-146, 1994.
6. E. Krupinski, H. Roehrig, "Influence of monitor luminance and tone scale on observers' search and dwell patterns", *Proc SPIE Medical Imaging*, 1999, In Press.
7. H. Roehrig, H. blume, T.L. Ji, M. Browne, "Performance tests and quality control of cathode ray tube displays*", *J Digital Imaging* **3**, pp. 134-145, 1990.
8. H. Roehrig, "Image quality control of displays for the PACS environment", in H.U. Lemke, M.W. Vannier, K. Inamura, A.G. Farman (eds*), *Computer Assisted Radiology and Surgery '98*, Elsevier, New York, 1998, pp. 337-342.

*Correspondence: Hans Roehrig, PhD Department of Radiology, University of Arizona
1609 N. Warren Bldg 211 Tucson, AZ 85724   520-626-7965 (ph) 520-626-4376 (f)
hans@radiology.arizona.edu

A Web based tool for Subjective Observer Ranking of Compressed Medical Images

Steve G. Langer, Brent K Stewart, and Rex K Andrew

University of Washington, Seattle WA 98195.

1. ABSTRACT

In the course of evaluating various compression schemes for ultrasound teleradiology applications, it became obvious that paper based methods of data collection were time consuming and error prone. A method was sought which allowed participating radiologists to view the ultrasound video clips (compressed to varying degree) at their desks. Furthermore, the method should allow observers to enter their evaluations and when finished, automatically submit the data to our statistical analysis engine. We have found the World Wide Web offered a ready solution. A web page was constructed that contains 18 embedded AVI video clips. The 18 clips represent 6 distinct anatomical areas, compressed by various methods and amounts, and then randomly distributed through the web page. To the right of each video, a series of questions are presented which ask the observer to rank (1-5) his/her ability to answer diagnostically relevant questions. When completed, the observer presses "Submit" and a file of tab delimited text is created which can then be imported to an Excel workbook. Kappa analysis is then performed and the resulting plots demonstrate observer preferences.

Keywords: ROC, World Wide Web, Image Analysis

2. INTRODUCTION

The gold standard for evaluation of any new imaging advance, and how it will interact with human observers, has been the Receiver/Operator Curve (ROC) study (1, 2). However, such studies are typically expensive and time consuming, because they demand a large number of trials to produce results with any statistical significance and power (3, 4). Typically, a tradeoff is made: either using fewer subjects and several sessions to get the required number of trials, or using fewer trials per subject but many more subjects. The second method is preferable from the standpoint of the subject, but worse for the study coordinator who must find and compel the cooperation of more observers.

In the course of our ultrasound research, we have found that the World Wide Web offered a ready solution to the problem (5, 6, 7). A page was constructed which can contain an arbitrary number of embedded AVI video clips. In the current study this happens to be 18 clips representing 6 anatomical areas, compressed by various methods and amounts, and then randomly distributed through the page. To the right of each video, a series of questions are presented which ask the observer to rank (1-5) his/her ability to answer diagnostically relevant questions. When completed with all clips, the observer presses "Submit" and a file of tab delimited text is created which can then be imported to an Excel workbook. Kappa analysis is then performed and a series of plots generated which demonstrate the mean observer rankings.

3. METHODS

Our design goal was to keep the page as uncluttered and simple to navigate as possible. Since the purpose of our page was to display a series of video clips, each one coupled to a group of questions, we strove to

Part of the SPIE Conference on Image Perception and Performance
San Diego, California • February 1999
SPIE Vol. 3663 • 0277-786X/99/$10.00

225

"bind" video and text together within the browser's window. Many WWW pages are not designed to do this. Typically, a page is designed with "static" content placed in the page, but when the video is launched, a "helper" application (which is not part of the browser) is called to run the video clip. This "helper" application may be capable of playing QuickTime or MPEG (Motion Picture Experts Group) video, but will not respect the borders of the browser. Also, each time the reader would finish with one clip and start another, another video player would be created. With 18 video clips, the unprepared subject of our test page could be faced with up to 18 separate video players! The following HTML (Hypertext Markup Language) sample shows this method of authoring (8).

```
<center>
  <img src=sagmov01.gif> <br>
  <a href=sagmov.mov> Launch cine </a>
</center>
```

Figure 1: HTML for a helper based video page.

However, Microsoft offers a solution via their ActiveX and ActiveMovie technologies (Microsoft, Redmond WA). ActiveX is the Application Programming Interface (API) to the Distributed Common Object Model (DCOM) which is Microsoft's alternative to Sun's Java (Sun Microsystems, Palo Alto CA). What this really means is that it's a set of functions and graphical objects (buttons, labels, text entry areas, etc.) which permit a browser user to have an interactive session with the WWW server. ActiveMovie is the object implementation to play video within the client browser (9, 10). An example of the HTML is shown below.

```
<object id="ActiveMovie1"
        classid="CLSID:05589FA1-C356-11CE-BF01-00AA0055595A"

        align="baseline" border="3" width="352" height="300">
  <param name="FileName" value="2video06.mpg">
  <param name="AutoStart" value="0">
  <param name="ShowDisplay" value="0">
</object>
```

Figure 2: The HTML/ActiveX coding for playing a video in the page.

Note that in this example, we define Object and Class IDs. The Object ID is just a unique identifier within the page, but the Class ID defines all the attributes of the ActiveMovie player, and the parameters provide defaults for the player's controls. ActiveX objects permit a great deal more functionality than generic HTML, but it should be noted that this is gained at a cost. Namely, using ActiveX classes severely limits the portability of WWW pages as not all browsers support it natively, and even for those that do, the Classes that a page relies on may not be available on all operating systems (11).

After settling the video issue, the page still needs to accept user input such as: first and last name, and the responses for every question in the survey. For this we relied on generic HTML form support, but the CGI (Common Gateway Interface) program responsible for collecting and writing the data to disk was generated automatically by using the "SaveResults WebBot" function of Microsoft's FrontPage '97.

After acquiring the data from several subjects, the data file is harvested for input to a spreadsheet based statistical analysis tool using the Kappa model (12, 13).

4. RESULTS

A WWW page was constructed that contains 18 embedded AVI video clips. The 18 clips represent 6 distinct anatomical areas, compressed by various methods and amounts, then randomly distributed through the web page. To the right of each video, a series of questions are presented which ask the observer to rank (1-5) his/her ability to answer diagnostically relevant questions. When completed, the observer presses "Submit" and a file of tab delimited text is created which can then be imported to an Excel workbook. The following figure shows an example of a single clip.

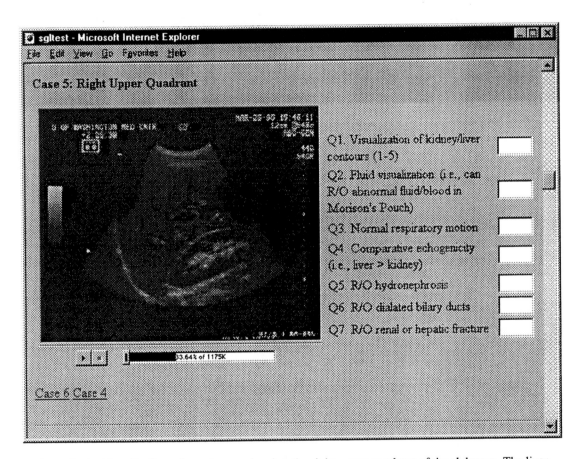

Figure 3: A video clip from the web page showing the right upper quadrant of the abdomen. The liver, right kidney and diaphragm are demonstrated.

As the reader will have noticed, each video is accompanied by one or more questions. Each question is in turn accompanied by a text field to enter the subject's rating. In the case of the the right upper quadrant scan shown in Figure 3, there are a total of seven. Figure 4 shows four curves (Q1-Q4) generated from responses to those questions (unfortunately the Q1 curve is obscured by Q2).

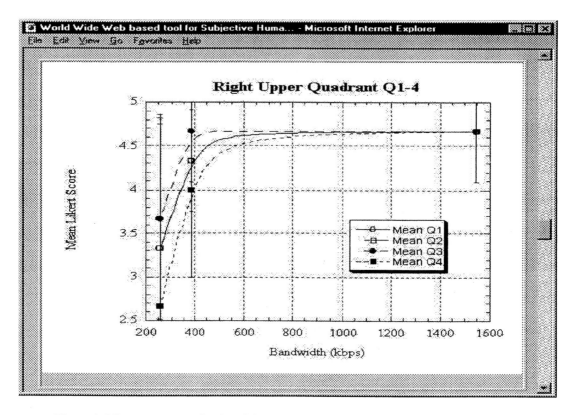

Figure 4: Likert assessment for the Right Upper Quadrant data, questions 1-4.

A casual inspection of the plots shows that for the Right Upper Quadrant, diagnostic utility approaches asymptotically approaches maximum diagnostic value (4~5 on our Likert scale) at an effective bandwidth of 384 Kbps (kilo bits/second). This corresponds to a compression of about 105:1 for the commercial compressor evaluated in this study. Interestingly, this value proved to be relatively constant among the other anatomical sites as well.

5. CONCLUSIONS

While we have not used the survey instrument yet in a ROC type study, one can easily envision how this would be possible. For instance, one could use video clips of similar anatomic regions, compressed to various amounts, and ask observers to rank their confidence in identifying abnormality. The same survey template could be used, and by altering the questions and the statistical analysis performed by the spreadsheet, a ROC would be performed. Furthermore, the study shown in this paper made use of a commercially available compression tool for which we now have an established baseline. The WWW page will now be refitted to evaluate our in-house wavelet compressor (5, 6).

The WWW based survey page has proven to be a boon to our research, for rather than taking the participating observers away from their clinical duties, they can participate from their office or reading room - anywhere where a Windows based PC is available. Consequently, it has proven easier to get radiologists to participate which in turn leads to more participants and less work per observer. It can be argued that from a scientific rigor point of view, this method is flawed since the observer's ambient viewing conditions are not held constant. That is ameliorated somewhat with the observers in our studies since the PCs available to them have similar monitors, although ambient lighting is problematic. We try to compensate by asking participants to use lighting levels similar to that in our reading rooms, even if they view the survey in their office.

In sum, this method permits centralized and automated data collection, remote observer participation, and is readily modified for new studies. We recommend this approach to others who need to perform human observer studies.

6. REFERENCES

1. el-Saden SM, Hademenos GJ, Zhu W, et. al. "Assessment of intraaxial and extraaxial brain lesions with digitized computed tomographic images versus film: ROC analysis." Acad-Radiol. 1997; 4(2):90-95.
2. Kheddache S, Angelhed JE, Mansson LG, et. al. "Digital chest radiography: comparing two types of CRT monitors in a ROC experiment with a chest phantom." Eur J Radiol. 1996; 22(3):236-240.
3. Sorenson JA, Wang X. "ROC methods for evaluation of fMRI techniques." Magnetic Resonance in Medicine 1996; 36(5):737-744.
4. Hassard TH. Understanding Biostatistics. St. Louis MO. Mosby Year Book, 1991; 167-181.
5. Andrew RK., Stewart BK, Langer SG, and Stegbauer KC. "Wavelet Compression of Ultrasound Video Streams for Teleradiology." Washington, D.C. IEEE EMB society special topic conference on Information Technology Applications in Biomedicine (ITAB) - 1998.
6. Andrew RK, Stewart BK, Langer SG, and Stegbauer KC. "A Novel Wavelet- compression codec for pre-scan-converted diagnostic ultrasound video." Chicago IL. RSNA 1998.
7. Stewart BK, Carter SJ, Langer SG and Andrew RK. "Compressed Ultrasound Video Image Quality Evaluation Using a Likert Scale and Kappa Statistical Analysis." San Diego CA. SPIE Proceedings 1998;365-377.
8. Langer SG and Berger RM. "Goals and Methods for Radiology Teaching Files." RSNA-EJ 1997;1 .
9. Breedlove RF. Web Programming Unleashed. Indianapolis IN. Sams Publishing, 1996; 117-655.
10. Walther S. Active Server Pages Unleashed. Indianapolis IN. Sams Publishing 1998; 118-628.
11. Langer SG and Stewart BK. "World Wide Web based Quality Assurance, Problem Reporting and Information Management in Radiology Departments." RSNA-EJ 1998; 2.
12. Altman DG. Practical Statistics for Medical Research. London England. Chapman and Hall, 1991; 396-439.
13. Fleiss L. Statistical Methods for Rates and Proportions. New York NY. John Wiley and Sons, 1981; 213-235.

SESSION 7

Modeling Visual Signal Detection I

Evaluation of Keyhole MR Imaging with a Human Visual Response Model

Kyle A. Salem[a], Jeffrey L. Duerk[a,b], Michael Wendt[a,b] and David L. Wilson[a,b]

[a]Department of Biomedical Engineering
Case Western Reserve University
Cleveland, OH 44106

[b]Department of Radiology
University Hospitals of Cleveland &
Case Western Reserve University
2074 Abington Road
Cleveland, OH 44106

ABSTRACT

As a first step toward developing a methodology suitable for optimizing the many parameters in keyhole and other fast imaging techniques, we applied an accepted human visual system (HVS) perceptual difference model to simulated keyhole images. A series of "gold-standard" full k-space images were acquired during the insertion of a needle into ex vivo bovine liver. Keyhole imaging, a method by which image frame rate is increased due to sub-sampling k-space, was simulated from this image data. A perceptual difference HVS model was used to create a map of the likelihood of visible differences between a simulated keyhole image and the corresponding full k-space acquisition. Visible difference degradation was compared with a mean squared error (MSE) metric for both entire images and regions of interest around the needle tip. The output of the HVS model was a spatial map of perceptual differences. This map proved useful since it provided an accurate tool for finding the location of image differences. According to the perceptual model, the quality of the entire image is preserved most favorably with a stripe parallel to the direction of insertion. For a region of interest surrounding the needle, a perpendicular stripe resulted in the lowest level of image error. The HVS model agreed favorably with anecdotal human inspection. For example, while high frequency noise in the image produces effective changes in the MSE metric, the visual model and inspection show no true perceivable image difference. Additionally, inspection verified the importance of the direction of the k-space sub-sampling. Examination of rotated stripes of k-space show that a step of 45 degrees is preferred. Larger steps caused high initial error, while smaller steps took too long to traverse k-space. Experience indicates that the HVS model is an objective, promising tool for the automated evaluation and optimization of keyhole imaging sequences. Hopefully, it will provide a rational method for optimizing the large number of potential techniques and infinite number of parameters in fast MR imaging.

Keywords: Interventional MRI, medical imaging, image perception, quantitative image quality, visual difference modeling, mean squared error

1. INTRODUCTION

We use a low-field, interventional MRI (iMRI) system to guide diagnostic biopsies and minimally invasive ablation cancer therapies. With regard to ablation, we have the most experience with radio frequency (RF) thermal ablation of liver tumors.[1] Not only is iMRI used to guide the insertion of the RF electrode into the tumor, it is also used to monitor tissue destruction. While in diagnostic MR, the goal is to obtain the highest possible image quality within a reasonable, but relatively long-duration, in iMRI there are severe time constraints. By limiting the total time of the procedure, one reduces patient discomfort and risk. Also, fast image updates are required for reliable, safe insertion of a needle. Currently, we image at 0.5-0.75 frames/sec for clinical needle guidance. We want to increase this rate to 2-4 images/sec using a variety of emerging techniques. One also needs to easily visualize the target tumor and to accurately localize the needle tip in order to place the

232

Part of the SPIE Conference on Image Perception and Performance
San Diego, California • February 1999
SPIE Vol. 3663 • 0277-786X/99/$10.00

needle properly. There are additional imaging issues for iMRI monitoring of tissue destruction. In this paper, we will focus on the problem of iMRI guidance.

There are a variety of ways to speed imaging including the use of alternative spatial encoding schemes, such as wavelets and the singular value decomposition. In this report, we will focus on keyhole MR imaging. In MR imaging, data is acquired in the frequency domain, also known as k-space, and then transformed to create an image in spatial coordinates. In keyhole, one starts with a full k-space acquisition and transforms to create an output image. The time for subsequent image acquisitions is reduced by sampling only a portion of k-space. There is no limit to the number of strategies for k-space sampling. For example, one can sample the same portion of k-space over the entire set of images, sample different portions throughout the acquisitions, or even vary the pattern used to sample k-space. Moreover, each strategy might have many different parameters such as the amount of k-space acquired or the MR sequence used to sample that information. Given the very large number of variables at the disposal of the MR imaging engineer, a strategy for optimizing the imaging techniques becomes very important.

The requirements of iMRI necessitate a departure from traditional detectability methods of image quality analysis. Detectability measurements and models have been applied in nuclear medicine imaging,[2] image compression,[3] x-ray fluoroscopy sequences,[4-6] and various synthetic images with lumpy backgrounds.[7] In these cases, medical image quality is measured using detection experiments like receiver operating characteristic curves or forced choice experiments.[8] The determination of image quality in iMRI, however, cannot be accomplished through detection experiments for several reasons. First, in iMRI there are various structures of interest throughout the image such as the target tumor, the treatment needle, and blood vessels. It is unclear as to what one should use as the target for a detection task. Second, important, critical structures should always be easily seen. They must be well above the threshold for detection. Third, detection of a needle is not nearly as important as the ability to localize the tip. Likewise, detection of a tumor is not as important as determining its border allowing a needle for thermal ablation to be appropriately positioned. Fourth, in MR imaging contrast can be maximal for one object of interest, such as a tumor, and minimal for others with different tissue characteristics, such as blood vessels. Similarly, the needle having very different MR properties must be easily seen. Fifth, iMRI needle guidance requires a sequence of images. Sixth, keyhole imaging sometimes creates image artifacts that should be minimized. In general, it is difficult to map all the issues in iMRI image quality to the experiments and models that have been used in the past for detection tasks.

Human perception experiments are very costly, especially for problems like fast iMRI imaging where there are literally an infinite number of variable values. Computer evaluation is desirable. One criterion for optimality is a minimum visual difference between a fast technique and a very slow, high quality MR image. Hence, we use a mechanistic perceptual difference model similar to the class of models first described by Wilson and Bergen.[9;10] Such models have been validated by comparing model output with human observer subjective quality ratings for a number of processes that degrade image quality such as blur, increased image noise, decreased gray scale resolution.[11;12] These models have been applied to evaluate image compression techniques as well as tumor detection in medical images.[10;12] Essentially, they are used to determine when a human can see a difference between an original, high quality image and a degraded image after the application of some degrading process. Experimentally, we will create this situation in fast iMRI imaging. We will acquire high quality images with full k-space acquisitions and simulate the results of reduced k-space acquisitions, creating visually degraded images for comparison. A full k-space acquisition is the very best image that we can achieve with the fast techniques.

2. BACKGROUND

1. Keyhole MR Imaging

In keyhole MR imaging, imaging frame rate is increased by decreasing the time allowed for acquisition per frame. This is accomplished by decreasing the number of points that are sampled in k-space, often only selecting those points which will contain the most information. Different methods for selecting this information have been described in detail by Busch et al.[13] and Duerk et al.[14] Various new applications of keyhole MR imaging have also been proposed, such as in functional MRI,[15] active tip tracking,[16] and breast imaging.[17] Many have attempted to evaluate the quality of keyhole acquisitions and set limitations on how the acquisitions should be performed, suggesting that the maximum allowable improvement in imaging speed is 16 times the current frame rate.[13;14;18] Others have attempted to model the errors created by keyhole imaging through the use of a priori knowledge or representations of the point spread function simulating both spatial and contrast distortions caused by keyhole imaging.[18;19] A drawback of some previous evaluations is the use of the mean square error (MSE) measure of image quality, which has been shown to be deficient when determining subjective image quality.[12;20]

For this study, two different keyhole methods were simulated. The first used a static stripe of k-space oriented in one of four directions as shown in Figure 1. After an initial full k-space image was acquired, a stripe was sampled from subsequent images and used to replace "stale" data from the initial full acquisition. This "sample-and-replace" process was repeated with the stripe in the exact same position for every new image over time. In this case, the same portion of k-space, one quarter of a full acquisition, was updated, and the outer three fourths never changed after the initial acquisition. The four different directions used in this study are horizontal and vertical with respect to the image and parallel and perpendicular to the needle. Since most of the spatial frequency content of a line is located perpendicular to that line in k-space, one expects that the perpendicular orientation will be best for imaging the needle.

The second strategy consisted of rotating the "update" stripe through the sequence of images. In this method, no portion of k-space was allowed to become too "stale;" most, if not all of k-space was updated at some point during the acquisition sequence. We examined the effect of rotation rate on image quality. By moving the stripe through 18, 30, 45, and 90 degrees per frame, we hope to determine if there are limits that dictate minimum or maximum rotation step size. In these studies 1/16th of k-space was sampled for each frame, regardless of the rotation step. This implies that the same image frame rate was maintained for each different keyhole strategy. At 18 degrees, all of k-space is updated. At larger steps, portions of k-space are not updated.

2. Perceptual Models of the Human Visual System

The goal of a perceptual difference model is to mimic the human visual system (HVS) and produce an output representing what a human observer would perceive as the difference between two images. The HVS processes information in an image by creating a composite of shapes, edges, and textures. For this reason, a simple subtraction is insufficient to determine what a human observer will view as the difference between two images. This effect can be observed by examining two fields of gray, one pixel different in gray value. The HVS is not able to distinguish the difference between these two fields, yet a simple subtraction will show a small difference at all points in the image. Another example highlights the human attention to edges. Blurring the edges of an object will cause a human observer to note tremendous differences between the two images while a simple subtraction may only show slight image differences, especially if averaged over the entire image.

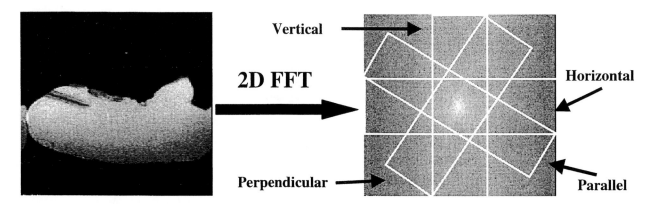

Figure 1. Static keyhole stripe acquisition orientations. The right-hand image shows the two-dimensional Fourier transform of the sample insertion image on the left. There are four orientations used in this study: vertical, horizontal, perpendicular, and parallel. The horizontal and vertical stripes are taken with respect to the image, and the parallel and perpendicular stripes are taken with respect to the direction of insertion of the needle as seen in the left-hand image.

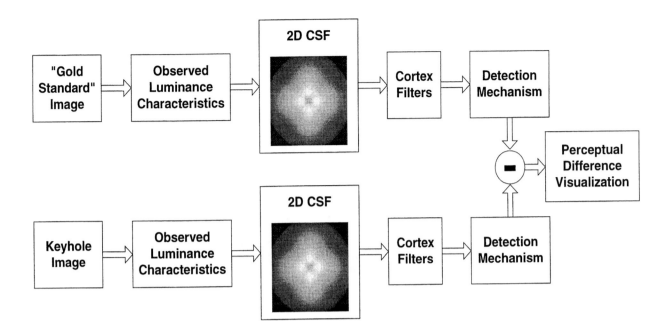

Figure 2. Block diagram of the components of the perceptual difference human visual system model. The layout and ordering of components of the perceptual difference model used in this study are represented above. The four primary components of the model, from observed luminance characteristics through detection mechanisms, are carried out on each input image separately and then the differences are combined and visualized as either a grayscale map or a single value of total perceptual error.

Many use the same basic architecture necessary to build a mechanistic model of the human visual system.[21] The mechanistic perceptual model used in this study is a modified version of the models developed by Lubin[11] and Daly[22] and was designed to represent the functional anatomy of the visual pathway. For this reason, it contains components that model the optics and sensitivity of the retina, the contrast sensitivity function, the channels of spatial frequency as found in the visual cortex, and visual masking. A block diagram showing the major components of the perceptual difference model used in this study is shown in Figure 2. The output of the model was a spatial map representing the likelihood that a human observer would perceive a difference between the two images at that point. We summed the map, or a region of interest in the map, to provide a scalar value representing the total perceptual error between the two images.

3. METHODS

Keyhole MR imaging was simulated from a series of full k-space acquisitions of ex vivo bovine liver. The image series were acquired using True FISP (16/8/1/90, TR/TE/Nacq./FA) and Turbo Spin Echo sequences (2000/102/1/90), both sequences that could be used to acquire portions of k-space in actual keyhole imaging experiments. During each image sequence, twenty images were acquired while a needle was inserted at an angle of thirty degrees north of the horizontal axis over a distance of approximately 4 cm. 20 images were taken in the plane of the needle while the needle was advanced approximately 1.5 mm between each frame. This series of full k-space acquisitions was designated as the "gold standard" by which the keyhole methods would be evaluated. Each image of the 20-frame sequence was converted to k-space by taking the two dimensional Fourier transform, and then the first image was designated as the initial full k-space acquisition. Its reconstruction, through the inverse two dimensional Fourier transform, is an exact match of the first image in the "gold standard" series, since the k-space maps for the two images are identical. To simulate a keyhole technique, values from the full acquisition were selected and used to replace the appropriate portion of k space. The process continued through the entire sequence of twenty images. In the case of the static keyhole simulations, several k-space values were never replaced through the 20-frame sequence.

For each test scenario, the twenty simulated keyhole images were compared to their corresponding images in the "gold standard" sequence using both the perceptual difference model and a simple mean square error (MSE) metric. The MSE metric was calculated by finding the mean value of the magnitude of the difference in gray level at each pixel location. The perceptual metric and MSE metric were also applied to a region of interest that encompassed the needle. The outputs from both the perceptual model and the MSE metric were displayed in a plot of image error versus frame number. The perceptual difference map was examined as a confirmation that differences in the input images, found by visual inspection, matched qualitatively with the model output.

4. RESULTS

The keyhole simulations produced a number of visible image artifacts. In some cases the needle track, clearly defined in the full k-space acquisitions, disappeared or shrunk in the keyhole acquisitions. Other images showed the needle tip expanding beyond the expected susceptibility artifact. In the rotated stripe simulations only 1/16th of k-space was sampled, as suggested by Busch[13] and Spraggins,[18] and these small stripes produced noticeable rotating banding artifacts. In all cases the keyhole simulations decreased the conspicuity of the true needle in the images. Figure 3 shows this degradation; the needle is indistinguishable from the susceptibility artifact surrounding it. Keyhole images are noisier than full k-space acquisitions due to both the blurring of edges and the discontinuity created by replacing a portion of k-space. In the right-most panel there is a sample perceptual difference map. By examining such output maps, the areas of image quality degradation could be easily identified.

The mean output of the perceptual model for the static stripe scenarios is presented for whole image comparison in Figure 4(a). The error for all stripe orientations is zero for the first image since it is an exact copy of the first image in the "gold standard" sequence. The error then rises over approximately the first five images to a near steady state level, where variations in error are equally reflected in all sequences. The results point to a parallel acquisition as having the least perceptual error for all images after the first. Figure 4(b) shows the results from the MSE metric for the same images. In this case, the metric rises almost immediately to a steady state level and then maintains a vertical acquisition as most like the "gold standard". Evaluation of the images only in the region of interest by the perceptual model show results opposite to those of the whole image, selecting a perpendicular stripe as having the highest perceptual quality. These results, shown in

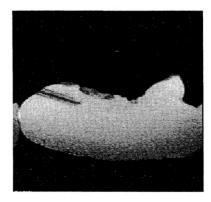 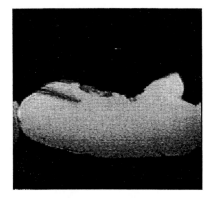 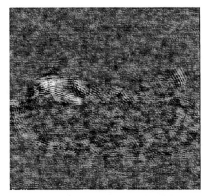

Figure 3. Keyhole simulation results and perceptual difference output. The left-most image is a "gold standard", full k-space acquisition showing a needle being inserted into ex vivo liver. The gray area surrounding the black needle is the susceptibility artifact of the needle. The center image, a keyhole acquisition, shows the approximate location of the needle, but the actual needle track has been blurred into the susceptibility artifact, and the image is noisier. The perceptual difference map, on the right, shows that the perceptual errors occur in the region of the needle with the area of maximal change along the shaft and at the entry point.

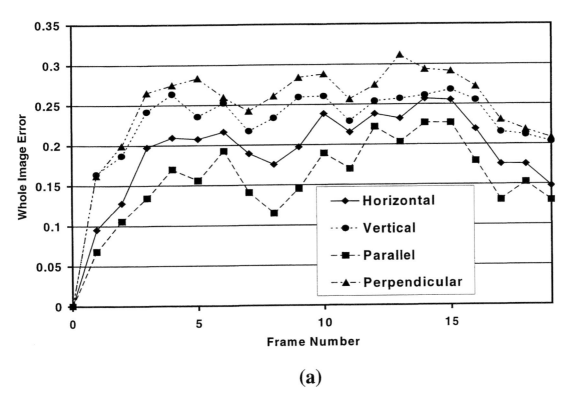

(a)

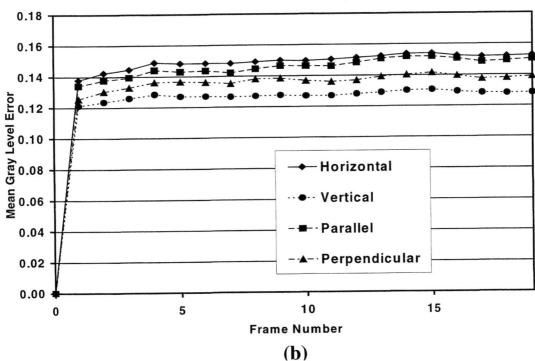

(b)

Figure 4. Image differences as determined by both the perceptual difference model and the MSE metric. The perceptual difference model results are shown in (a) and the MSE results are in (b). The errors from the perceptual metric are described as the mean error per pixel in the image. While the error changes from frame to frame, the error curves never cross.

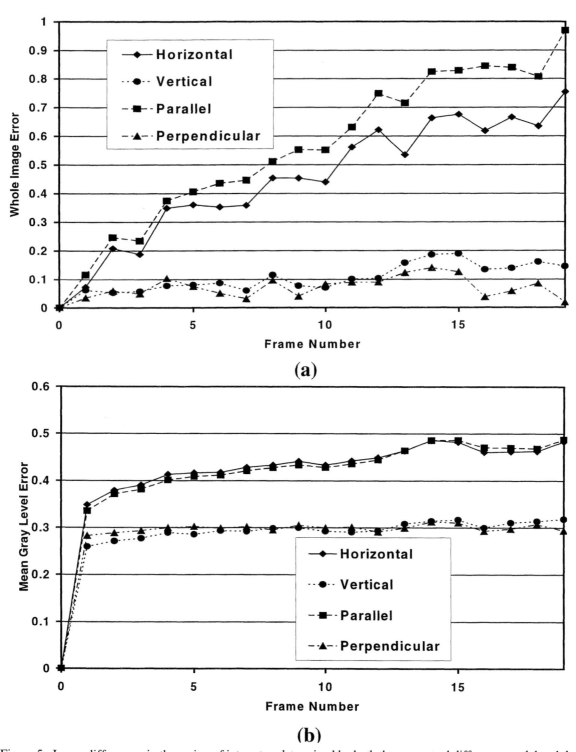

(a)

(b)

Figure 5. Image differences in the region of interest as determined by both the perceptual difference model and the MSE metric. The perceptual difference model results are shown in (a) and the MSE results are in (b). The errors from the perceptual metric are described as the mean error per pixel in the image. While the error changes from frame to frame, the ordering of the orientations remains constant. These results show error in the region of the needle tip. This area contains a higher mean error than the entire image. The perceptual model results selects the perpendicular orientation as preferred, while the MSE metric, where error is described as mean gray level difference selects the vertical stripe.

Figure 5(a), are relatively constant for perpendicular and vertical stripes but show an increasing trend for the parallel and horizontal orientation. The MSE results for the ROI are shown in Figure 5(b). The MSE measure for the parallel and horizontal orientations increase approximately 33% over the sequence of 20 images, while the perceptual model shows a 600% increase in error. A summary of error metric results is presented in Table 1. The perceptual model disagrees with the MSE technique for both analysis regions. The MSE selected the same orientation for both whole image and ROI analyses, while the perceptual model was able to discriminate between the two different areas of analysis. Additionally, while the perceptual model shows increasing error for the horizontal and parallel orientations, the MSE model shows a constant error. Human inspection results for both the entire image and the ROI support the output of the perceptual difference model selecting the parallel and perpendicular orientations, respectively, as creating the least perceptual error.

Table 1. Rankings for the four different static keyhole stripe methods. The output from the two different error models for both whole image and ROI analysis were ranked according to the total amount of reported error. For example, the parallel orientation produced the lowest error in the entire image according to the perceptual difference model. The horizontal orientation resulted in the second lowest amount of error, followed by vertical and perpendicular.

Image Quality Ranking (1 = best quality/least error, 4 = worst quality/most error)	Evaluation Method			
	Perceptual Model (Whole Image)	Mean Squared Error Technique (Whole Image)	Perceptual Model (ROI)	Mean Squared Error Technique (ROI)
1	Parallel	Vertical	Perpendicular	Vertical
2	Horizontal	Perpendicular	Vertical	Perpendicular
3	Vertical	Parallel	Horizontal	Parallel
4	Perpendicular	Horizontal	Parallel	Horizontal

Figure 6 shows the average image error for each of the three rotated stripe imaging schemes. The data show error at a minimum when the angular rotation is 45 degrees. All comparisons have only one independent variable, rotation step. Since the error increases both above and below the 45-degree step, there must be a relationship between the k-space covered in that sequence and image quality. In comparison to the static stripe simulations, the rotated data have mean error values similar to the two worst static orientations, vertical and perpendicular. The rotated schemes, however, reached this error level sampling only 1/16th of k-space, as opposed to 1/4th in the static stripe case. This suggests that rotating the keyhole stripe can produce equivalent error at four times the acquisition rate. Alternatively, one could expect that if the rotated scheme was used at an equivalent frame rate and sampled more k-space, the image quality would be increased, as compared to the static stripe acquisition strategies.

5. DISCUSSION

The usefulness of perceptual difference modeling of the HVS is evidenced by its ability to agree with human observer inspection.[12;22] It allows for the evaluation of a number of different possible iMRI sequences in a relatively quick and inexpensive manner. Computer-assisted image evaluation, performed prior to perceptual testing, ensures that a maximal amount of information will be learned from well-designed experiments. This type of study provides the information necessary for that design process. In addition, the perceptual difference map provided quantitative results allowing the identification and localization of areas change in images.

In retrospect, the perceptual difference model output can be related to the strongest, changing edge in the image. For example, in the whole image, the parallel stripe shows the least error. This is because a stripe perpendicular to the tissue edge, the strongest dynamic edge in the image, was sampled. Likewise, the strongest edge in the ROI is the needle, and a

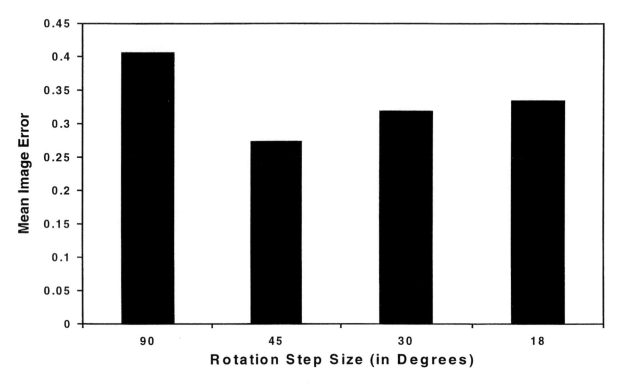

Figure 6. Mean image error according to the perceptual difference model for rotating keyhole stripes with variable rotation step size. The mean image error for each of the four different rotation step sizes shows that a step of 45 degrees produces the highest quality images. Moving both below and above 45 degrees increases perceptual error and decreases image quality.

stripe perpendicular to it produces the least error. For this reason, static keyhole acquisitions should be acquired perpendicular to the edge of interest.

The results from the MSE method were particularly insensitive to relevant changes in the image. The image changes very little from frame one to frame two. The MSE shows a large increase in error between these two frames but then only increases approximately 40% of that original increase. Inspection shows that the large increase is due to random noise and the small effect from frames 2 through 20 are due to the needle movement. The perceptual difference model increases linearly with needle displacement for the parallel orientation. By discriminating between simple noise and actual image differences, the perceptual difference model is superior to the MSE metric for evaluation image changes.

Finally, the tradeoff of rotation step and central k-space coverage revealed by the rotating stripe simulations shows that there must be important information contained in the stripe 45 degrees from the horizontal axis of the image. This information is also sampled when the angular step size is less than 45 degrees, but decreasing the angular step below 45 degrees also causes image error to increase. In this instance, the quality decreases because small degree steps, below 45 degrees, sample information that is relatively unimportant for image quality. These small degree steps sample more k-space with each revolution at the expense of sampling the most important portions of k-space less often than an optimal step.

This work is probably the first in which quantitative image quality modeling has been applied to fast MR imaging, and shows that the HVS model is an objective, promising tool for the automated evaluation and optimization of keyhole imaging sequences. Hopefully, this will present a rational method for optimizing the large number of potential techniques and infinite number of parameters in fast MR imaging.

6. ACKNOWLEDGEMENTS

This work was supported by a Whitaker Foundation student fellowship to KAS, NIH grant R01-HL48918, and a Whitaker Special Opportunity Grant to JLD .

7. REFERENCES

1. Lewin, JS, Connell, CF, Duerk, JL, Chung, YC, Clampitt, ME, Spisak, J, Gazelle, GS, and Haaga, JR. Interactive MRI-guided radiofrequency interstitial thermal ablation of abdominal tumors: Clinical trial for evaluation of safety and feasibility. Journal of Magnetic Resonance Imaging 8(1), 40-47. 1998.

2. Barrett, HH, Yao, J, Rolland, P, and Myers, KJ. Model observers for assessment of image quality. Proceedings of the National Academy of Science USA 90, 9758-9765. 1993.

3. Whiting J, Eckstein M, Morioka C, Staffel B, Eigler N: Lossy image compression has insignificant effect on the accuracy and precision of quantitative coronary angiography. *Circulation* 1993;88:652-652.(Abstract)

4. Jabri, KN and Wilson, DL. Detection improvement in spatially filtered x-ray fluoroscopy image sequences. Journal of the Optical Society of America A 16(3), 742-749. 1999.

5. Wilson, DL, Xue, P, and Aufrichtig, R. Perception in x-ray fluoroscopy. Kundel, HL. 2166, 20-23. 1994. Bellingham, WA, SPIE. Proceedings of SPIE Medical Imaging 1994: Image Perception.

6. Xue, P, Thomas, CW, Gilmore, GC, and Wilson, DL. An adaptive reference/test paradigm with applications to pulsed fluoroscopy perception. Behavior Research Methods, Instruments, and Computers 30(2), 332-348. 1998.

7. Burgess, A. E., Wagner, R. F., and Jennings, R. J. Human signal detection performance for noisy medical images. 99-105. 1982. New York, IEEE. Proceedings of IEEE Computer Society International Symposium on Medical Imaging and Image Interpretation.

8. Burgess AE: Comparison of receiver operating characteristic and forced choice observer performance measurement methods. *Med.Phys.* 1995;22:643-655.

9. Wilson, HR and Bergen, J. A four mechanism model for threshold spatial vision. Vision Research 19, 19-32. 1979.

10. Jackson, WB, Said, MR, Jared, DA, Larimer, JO, Gille, JL, and Lubin, J. Evaluation of human vision models for predicting human-observer performance. Kundel, HL. 3036, 64-73. 1997. Bellingham, WA, SPIE. Proceedings of SPIE Medical Imaging 1997: Image Perception.

11. Lubin J: *Sarnoff JND Vision Model: algorithm description and testing*, 1997; Unpublished.

12. Lubin J: A visual discrimination model for imaging system design and evaluation, in Peli E (ed): *Vision Models for Target Detection and Recognition*. River Edge, NJ, World Scientific; 1995:245-283.

13. Busch, M, Bornstedt, A, Wendt, M, Duerk, JL, Lewin, JS, and Gronemeyer, D. Fast "real time" imaging with different k-space update strategies for interventional procedures. Journal of Magnetic Resonance Imaging 8(4), 944-954. 1998.

14. Duerk, JL, Lewin, JS, and Wu, DH. Application of keyhole imaging to interventional MRI: a simulation study to predict sequence requirements. Journal of Magnetic Resonance Imaging 6(6), 918-924. 1996.

15. Gao, JH, Xiong, J, Lai, S, Haacke, EM, Woldorff, MG, Li, J, and Fox, PT. Improving the temporal resolution of functional MR imaging using keyhole techniques. Magnetic Resonance in Medicine 35(6), 854-860. 1996.

16. Wendt, M, Busch, M, Wetzler, R, Zhang, Q, Melzer, A, Wacker, F, Duerk, JL, and Lewin, JS. Shifted rotated keyhole imaging and active tip-tracking for interventional procedure guidance. Journal of Magnetic Resonance Imaging 8(1), 258-261. 1998.

17. Bishop, JE, Santyr, GE, Kelcz, F, and Plewes, DB. Limitations of the keyhole technique for quantitative dynamic contrast-enhanced breast MRI. Journal of Magnetic Resonance Imaging 7(4), 716-723. 1997.

18. Spraggins, TA. Simulation of spatial and contrast distortions in keyhole imaging. Magnetic Resonance in Medicine 31(3), 320-322. 1994.

19. Oesterle, C and Henning, J. Improvement of spatial resolution of keyhole effect images. Magnetic Resonance in Medicine 39(2), 244-250. 1998.

20. Girod B: What's wrong with mean-squared error?, in Watson A (ed): *Digital Images and Human Vision*. Cambridge, MA, MIT Press; 1993:207-220.

21. Lubin J: The use of psychophysical data and models in the analysis of display system performance, in Watson A (ed): *Digital Images and Human Vision*. Cambridge, MA, MIT Press; 1993:163-178.

22. Daly S: The Visual Differences Predictor: an algorithm for the assessment of image fidelity, in Watson A (ed): *Digitial Images and Human Vision*. Cambridge, MA, MIT Press; 1993:179-206.

The effect of image compression in model and human performance

Miguel P. Eckstein[*], Craig K. Abbey, François O. Bochud,
Jay L. Bartroff, James S. Whiting
Department of Medical Physics & Imaging, Cedars Sinai Medical Center, Los Angeles,
CA 90048-1865

ABSTRACT

We applied three different model observers (non-prewhitening matched filter with an eye filter, Hotelling and channelized Hotelling) to predict the effect of JPEG image compression on human visual detection of a simulated lesion (clinically known as thrombus) in single frame digital x-ray coronary angiograms. Since the model observers' absolute performance is better than human, model performance was degraded to match human performance by injecting internal noise proportional to the external noise. All three model-observers predicted reasonably well the degradation in human performance as a function of JPEG image compression, although the NPWEW and the channelized Hotelling models (with internal noise proportional to the external noise) were better predictors than the Hotelling model.

Keywords: signal detection, model observers, image compression, image quality, structured backgrounds

1.INTRODUCTION

The use of digital angiographic cardiac catheterization laboratories in clinical practice is eminent. The digital format allows for image-manipulations that might improve image quality including filtering techniques, feature motion stabilization[1], and variable rate playback of image sequences as well as computer analysis. However, one of the practical limitations in the archival storage and retrieval of digital images is the excessive size of the patient images. An individual cardiac catheterization procedure can occupy up to ~ 1 Gigabyte.[2] In addition, very high data transfer rates for display (512 x 512 x 8 bits at 30 frames/sec) are required for dynamic display of image sequences. Lossy image compression algorithms provide a means for reducing storage and communication requirements. However, maximum levels of image compression without degradation in diagnostic decisions need to be established.

A number of studies have evaluated the effect of JPEG image compression on diagnostic decision in x-ray coronary angiograms. Rigolin et al.[3] have examined the effect of compression on quantitative angiographic analysis of phantom coronary stenosis. Other studies have examined the effect of JPEG compression on human visual detection of morphologic features.[4-6] In general these studies seem to agree that JPEG compression ratios of up to 12:1-15:1 do not significantly degrade image quality. As the number of new and different compression algorithms available increases more psychophysical studies are required to evaluate them. If the number of algorithms is rather high a full psychophysical evaluation of all algorithms and compression ratios becomes time consuming. One attractive possibility is to develop a metric of image quality that can reflect the degradation in the compressed images for any arbitrary compression algorithm and ratio. This metric of image quality could then be used for automated optimization of parameters of the compression algorithm.

The root mean square error (RMSE) between an uncompressed and compressed image has been commonly used to measure image quality as a function of compression ratio.[7-9] However, studies have shown that image quality evaluation based on RMSE can lead to erroneous conclusions.[10] A different approach to quantifying image quality would be to use image discrimination models developed in the field of human vision.[11-13] Image discrimination models often consist of a contrast sensitivity function, a set spatial frequency and orientation-tuned channels, non-linear compressive channel response curves and divisive inhibition across channels with similar spatial frequency and orientation. These models quantify

---

[*] Correspondence: 8700 Beverly blvd. D-6065, 90048-1865; email: miguel@medphysics.csmc.edu; Tel: (310) 967-8415, Fax: (310) 652-8338

Part of the SPIE Conference on Image Perception and Performance
San Diego, California ● February 1999
SPIE Vol. 3663 ● 0277-786X/99/$10.00

human visual discrimination between an uncompressed image and a compressed image. However, one severe limitation of these models is that it is unknown how the discrimination between a compressed and uncompressed image relates to performance detecting a lesion in the medical image.

On the other hand, there are number of models of human visual detection in noise that generate explicit predictions about the detectability of a signal embedded in a noisy background.[14-29] Previous investigators have compared these model observers' performance to human performance in computer generated noise including white noise[15-18], filtered white noise[19], backgrounds with random inhomogeneities[20] (lumpy backgrounds), and combinations of white and low-pass filtered noise[22] (2-component noise).

A very recent study investigated the effect of image compression on a model observer (non-prewhitening matched filter) in white noise.[23] They found that performance degradation for this model for increasing wavelet image compression varied with the signal contrast and size of the signal. However, model performance was not compared to human performance and the model observer results might not generalize from white noise to anatomic backgrounds.

Few studies have compared human and model performance in real anatomic backgrounds.[25,26] These latter studies present several difficulties including gathering of a large amount of clinical images, developing techniques to embed realistic computer simulated signals in clinical backgrounds, and estimating model observer performance from samples rather than from mathematically closed form expressions.[26]

The purpose of the present paper is to apply model observers in order to predict the effect of JPEG image compression on human performance. We apply three different model observers: non-prewhitening matched filter with an eye filter, Hotelling observer, and channelized Hotelling model.

2. MODEL OBSERVERS

2.1 Description of models

All of the models used in the current paper are linear models. These models compare a template with the data by computing the correlation at each of the possible signal locations. The observer then makes a decision based on the output correlation. For a multiple alternative forced choice (MAFC) task where the signal appears in one of M locations, the model observer is assumed to obtain the template output at each location and select the location that elicited the highest response. The general form for all models is as follows:

$$\lambda_e = \sum_{x=1}^{N} \sum_{y=1}^{N} w(x,y) g(x,y) \tag{1}$$

where λ_e is the model response or correlation output, w(x,y) is the 2-dimensional template, g(x,y) is the data at a given location.

Many authors have used the matrix formulation as a framework for model observers.[14,21] In this framework the N x N template and image-data at a given location is represented by a N^2 x 1 column vector. The correlation is then computed as follows:[14,21]

$$\lambda_e = \sum_{n=1}^{N^2} \mathbf{w}_n \mathbf{g}_n = \mathbf{w}^t \mathbf{g} \tag{2}$$

where $\mathbf{w}^t$ and $\mathbf{g}$ are vectors and the superscript t refers to the transpose.

The different model observers tested in the present paper differ in the template profile. The templates vary due to the amount of prior knowledge used to derive them. In addition the templates of the different models differ in the built-in components that attempt to reflect the constraints imposed by the human visual system (e.g. contrast sensitivity function or spatial frequency and orientation tuned channels). Following, we describe in more detail the three different model observers used in the present paper.

2.1.1. Non-prewhitening matched (to the uncompressed signal) filter with an eye filter (NPWEW)

The non-prewhitening matched filter model is perhaps one of the most well-known in medical imaging[15,28] and consists of a template that exactly matches the signal profile: $w(x,y)= s(x,y)$. The addition of an eye filter (NPWEW[†]; also known as the modified non-prewhitening matched filter) takes into account the differential human visual sensitivity to different spatial frequencies due to optical and neural sources. Ishida[29] and Burgess[30] have previously used this model to predict human performance. The effective template used by the observer is given by:

$$w(x,y)= FFT^{-1}[s(u,v) |E(u,v)|^2]$$ (3)

where FFT^{-1} is the inverse fast-Fourier transform, $s(u,v)$ is the signal amplitude in the frequency domain and $E(u,v)$ is the contrast sensitivity function and is given by:

$$E(f)= f^{\rho} \exp(-cf^{\gamma})$$ (4)

where $f = sqrt(u^2 +v^2)$ is the radial spatial frequency in cycles per degree, $c = 0.978$, $\gamma = 0.674$ and $\rho = 1.5034$. The eye filter is different from to that used by Burgess and some of our previous work.[30] That eye filter is based on detection of sinusoidal gratings at threshold. The current eye filter is based on contrast matching of sinusoidals after adaptation to power law noise[31] which might be more relevant to signals embedded in x-ray coronary angiograms (which have a $1/f^{3.4}$ power spectrum).

One source of inefficiency in the NPWEW model is its inability to undo correlations in the noise (a process often referred to as "prewhitening"). In the current paper, the NPWEW model uses the profile of the signal in the uncompressed images for all compression levels. However, since compression does affect the signal profile, a different version of the NPWEW model could use a signal template that matched the compressed version of the signal for each compression condition.[23] This approach was not taken in our current implementation of the NPWEW. Therefore our implementation assumes that as the image is compressed, the observer still searches the M alternatives for a signal that matches the uncompressed signal.

2.1.2. Hotelling observer (with square spatial windowing)

The template of the Hotelling observer takes into account knowledge about not only the signal profile but also the background statistics.[14,19,20-22] The Hotelling observer is the best linear observer when image statistics are approximately Gaussian. In white noise the Hotelling observer template is the signal profile itself and therefore is equivalent to the non-prewhitening matched filter. However, in correlated noise, the Hotelling observer derives a template that effectively decorrelates the noise prior to matched filtering. When the noise is computer generated then the covariance matrix is known in advance and the template for the Hotelling observer, w_h can be derived:[14,19,21]

$$w_h= K^{-1} [<s+b>-<b>]$$ (5)

where K^{-1} is the inverse of the image covariance matrix, a N^2 x N^2 matrix, $<s+b>$ is the mean signal plus background vector, and $<b>$ is the mean background vector.

Since samples of real x-ray angiographic backgrounds are used, the covariance matrix is not known and therefore has to be estimated from the data. There are different approaches to this problem. One is to assume that the anatomic background is stationary and therefore calculate the covariance matrix from the noise power spectrum. A second approach adopted in this paper is not to assume stationarity and calculate the covariance matrix directly from the images. However, estimating a covariance matrix for a 512 x 512 image becomes computationally intractable due to the large number of samples needed. In this paper, we reduce the dimensionality of the covariance matrix by using windows of 12 x 12 pixels centered at the possible signal locations. The calculation of the resulting 144 x144 covariance matrix was based on 300 images (1200 samples of 12 x 12 pixel regions). The images used to derive the template were different

---

[†] The common acronym for this model is NPWE. We have added a "W" to the acronym to emphasize, as will be seen later, that this version of the model uses an eye filter measured by Webster.[31]

from the 100 image testing set. Estimation of the Hotelling template through this windowing method restricts the template spatially and might result in systematic differences between the sample derived template and the population template. An alternative approach to reduce the dimensionality of the covariance matrix is using a set of basis functions such as Laguerre-Gauss.[32]

2.1.3. Channelized Hotelling (Gabor channels)

The channelized Hotelling observer consists of a set of spatial frequency channels that attempt to mimic some of the components in the human visual system.[33-35] The detection process is constrained by a reduction in information content by the processing through the channels. The channelized Hotelling template is the optimal template that can be derived from a linear combination of the channels. The channelized Hotelling is identical to the Hotelling except that it acts on the outputs of the channels rather than directly on the image-pixels. There are a number of different channelized Hotelling models in the literature including square channels,[33] difference of Gaussians,[21,27] difference of Mesa filters[30] and Gabor channels.[25,26] The Gabor channel mechanism is unlike most other channel models because it is not rotationally symmetric and has different channels tuned to different orientations. The Gabor mathematical functions were used by Marcelja[36] to model the response of cells in area V1 of the cat. Watson[37] used these functions for his model of spatial vision. The Gabor channels are given by:

$$G(x, y) = \exp[\frac{-4 \ln 2(x^2 + y^2)}{W_s^2}] \cos[2\pi f_c (x \cos \theta + y \sin \theta) + \beta] \qquad (6)$$

where f is the spatial frequency, θ is the orientation, W_s is the width and β is the phase. The Fourier transform of a Gabor channel is a Gaussian function centered at the center frequency f_c and with a half-height full width given by $W_f = 0.8825 W_s$. Another way of measuring the width in the frequency domain of the Gabor channel is in octave bandwidth defined as:

$$bandwidth = \log_2 \left[\frac{f_c + (W_f / 2)}{f_c - (W_f / 2)} \right] \qquad (7)$$

where f_c is the central frequency and W_f is as previously defined.

In this paper we used a 50 channel model with 5 spatial frequencies (central frequencies, 32, 16, 8, 4 and 2 cycles per degree), 5 orientations (0°, 72°, 144°, 210° and 284°), and two phases (odd and even). The spatial frequency bandwidth of the channels was approximately 0.9 octaves.

The channel weights for the best linear combination of the output of the channels (Hotelling combination rule) are given by:[26,33,34,35]

$$\mathbf{a} = \mathbf{K_V}^{-1} [<\mathbf{s_V} + \mathbf{b_V}> - <\mathbf{b_V}>] \qquad (8)$$

where $\mathbf{a}$ is a vector containing the optimal weights for each of the Gabor channels, $\mathbf{K_V}$ is a N x N matrix describing the covariance matrix of the output of the channels to the images. For our particular implementation the covariance matrix consisted of a 50 x 50 matrix. Also $<\mathbf{s_V} + \mathbf{b_V}>$ is a vector containing the mean signal plus background as seen by each channel and $<\mathbf{b_V}>$ is the mean background as seen by each channel. The best linear template that can be obtained from the channel weights and the channels profiles:

$$w(x, y) = \sum_{i=0}^{N} a_i \cdot V_i(x, y) \qquad (9)$$

where $V_i(x,y)$ is the two dimensional profile of the ith channel as given by Equation 6 and a_i is the weight for the ith channel.

2.1.4. Internal noise

One difficulty in the comparison of model and human performance is that the models often achieve a higher absolute performance level than the human. To quantitatively compare the variation of human and model performance as a function of an image property (noise power spectrum or image compression) it is desirable to scale model performance to human performance. A second option is to degrade model observer performance by injecting internal noise. In this paper internal noise was injected in to all model observers in order to match model and human performance in the uncompressed condition. The same level of internal noise was then used for the model in the compressed conditions.

For the Hotelling and channelized Hotelling models the templates can be derived taken into consideration or not the internal noise. In our implementation the template derivation was performed taking into account the external and internal noise. For the Hotelling model the total covariance is given by: $\mathbf{K} = \mathbf{K}_{ext} + \mathbf{K}_{int}$ where the internal noise is assumed to be proportional to the diagonal elements of the external noise covariance matrix, $\mathbf{K}_{int} = \alpha \text{Diag}(\mathbf{K}_{ext})$. The Diag function zeroes all off-diagonal elements of the covariance matrix and α is a proportionality constant. For the channelized Hotelling model the total covariance and internal noise are given by the same expressions as for the Hotelling model but where the covariance matrix is with respect to the channel outputs, $\mathbf{K}_v$. The templates are then derived from Equation 5 (Hotelling) and 8 (channelized Hotelling) for each model respectively.

For the calculation of model performance the internal noise was injected into the scalar decision variable as follows,[‡]

$$\lambda = \lambda_e + \varepsilon \tag{10}$$

where λ is the decision variable after injection of internal noise, λ_e is the decision variable due to the external noise (prior to internal noise injection, equation 1 and 2), and ε is a Gaussian random variable with zero mean and a variance proportional to the variance of the decision variable due to external noise, $\kappa \sigma_{\lambda_e}^2$. It can be shown that for the Hotelling and channelized model (with replacement of $\mathbf{K}$ by $\mathbf{K}_v$) that κ is related to α as follows,

$$\kappa = \frac{\mathbf{w}^t \alpha Diag(\mathbf{K}_{ext})\mathbf{w}}{\mathbf{w}^t \mathbf{K}_{ext}\mathbf{w}} \tag{11}$$

For the channelized Hotelling and Hotelling models α was iteratively changed so that the performance for the uncompressed model performance matched the human performance. For the NPWEW, which uses a fixed template irrespective of the internal noise, κ was iteratively changed so that performance for the uncompressed model performance matched the human performance.

2.2 Figures of merit for model observers in within-image M-AFC

An important issue is the method to quantify model observer performance. A method that makes no assumptions about the model internal response statistics nor background stationarity is to compute the probability of the model output to the signal location taking a larger value than the maximum output to the background only locations. One can estimate this probability from samples by tallying the number of trials where the model correctly identifies the signal location and divide it by the number of total trials. This can be mathematically expressed as:[27]

$$\hat{P}c = \frac{1}{J}\sum_{j=1}^{J} step\left(\lambda_{s,j} - \max_{i}(\lambda_{b,ij})\right) \tag{12}$$

[‡] Internal noise in the calculation of model performance in not injected directly into the covariance and calculated from d' due to correlations in the model observer responses to each location. Calculation of model performance with d' in the case internal response correlations can lead to erroneous estimates of the models' performance.[38]

where $\lambda_{s,j}$ is the model response to the signal plus background in trial j, $\lambda_{b,ij}$ is the model response to the background only at location i in trial j, J is the total number of trials. The *max* function takes the maximum model response among the responses to the background only locations, the *step* function is one when the argument is larger than zero and is zero when the argument is less than zero.

If the model responses are Gaussian distributed and statistically independent, then a convenient figure of merit is d', index of detectability defined as: [14,27]

$$d' = \frac{<\lambda_s> - <\lambda_b>}{\sqrt{\frac{1}{2}(\sigma^2_{\lambda s} + \sigma^2_{\lambda b})}} \tag{13}$$

where $<\lambda_s>$ is the mean model response to the signal plus background, $<\lambda_b>$ is the mean model response to the background only and $\sigma_{\lambda s}$ and $\sigma_{\lambda b}$ are the standard deviations of the model responses to the signal present background and background only locations respectively. For models that are linear, the index of detectability d' can also be directly calculated from the template/filter, signal profile and covariance matrix of the background.[14,19,27] Often, the detectability for a linear model performance in computer generated noise is often calculated using a continuous frequency domain equation.[20,22,28,30] Assumptions of stationarity inherent in this calculation might not be valid in real anatomic backgrounds (see Bochud et al, in this SPIE volume).

One important property of the task in the present paper is that the M possible signal locations are within an image and not in independent samples of anatomic background. Given the low-pass characteristics of the x-ray coronary angiograms, it is plausible that correlations between the model internal responses to the different locations might arise. Recent work has shown that this is the case for NPWEW model for task in the present paper.[38] When the model internal responses are correlated, use of the standard index of detectability might lead to erroneous estimates of model performance and comparisons across models.[38] This error occurs because the index of detectability assumes that the model internal responses to the signal plus background location and the background only location are statistically independent.

In this paper, we therefore compute model performance by first computing Pc (Equation 12). Model performance is then converted to a detectability metric with the use of the following equation: [39]

$$Pc(d_a,M) = \int_{-\infty}^{+\infty} \varphi(z - d_a)[\phi(z)]^{M-1} dz \tag{14}$$

where $\varphi(z) = \frac{1}{\sqrt{2\pi}}\exp\left(-\frac{1}{2}x^2\right)$, $\phi(z)$ is the cumulative Gaussian, M is the number of alternatives. In order to emphasize that this estimate of the index of detectability is a transformation of Pc, it is referred to as d_a (rather than d', Equation 13). For the case of Gaussian independent responses, d_a and d' are mathematically equivalent.

3.METHODS

3.1 Generation of simulated arteries and lesions

The test-images used in this study consist of simulated signals embedded in real x-ray coronary angiographic backgrounds. We have developed an algorithm to create the simulated arterial segments and lesions. The algorithm attempts to mimic the image generation process of x-ray coronary angiograms. It includes exponential attenuation, focal spot and image receptor blur, scattering and veiling glare. Details of the algorithm to generate the computer-simulated arteries and lesion (filling defect) are discussed in detail elsewhere.[40] For our test-images, the projected simulated arteries consisted of 3-D right circular cylinders with a diameter of 12 pixels (3.6 mm), a sinusoidally modulated narrowing in diameter toward the center (minimum diameter of 8 pixels), and a length of 50 pixels (15.0 mm). We generated four simulated arteries for each test-image and projected 32 pixels apart into 512 x 512 pixel images extracted from real patient digital x-ray coronary angiograms, acquired with a 7-in. image intensifier filed size (Advantx/DXC, General Electric Medical Systems), and with a resolution of 0.3 mm/pixel.

We set the attenuation coefficient μ, to 0.16/mm to produce simulated arteries with the same projected intensity as real angiograms of coronary arteries of the same diameter. The target was a simulated filling defect with an hemi-ellipsoidal shape (meant to simulate a thrombus) located at the vertical and horizontal center of one of the four simulated arteries with a diameter of 6 pixels. We simulated imaging system blur caused by the physical extent of the x-ray focal spot and image intensifier unsharpness by convolving the projected cylinders with an isotropic Gaussian point spread function with standard deviation of 1 pixel (0.3 mm).

3.2 JPEG compression of images

Images were compressed and decompressed with the 5th public release of the Independent JPEG Group's free JPEG software. Since a given quality level results in varying compression ratios for different images, a program (in IDL programming platform) was written to iteratively modify the quality level of the compression until the desired compression ratio was achieved (with a tolerance of up to 5 % error). We used five levels of JPEG compression: 7:1, 10:1, 15:1, 20:1, 30:1, 45:1. The actual achieved compression ratios for the 400 image-set were (averaged compression across all images ± standard deviation): 6.86 ± 0.14, 9.86 ± 0.2, 14.9 ± 0.39, 19.8 ± 0.75, 29.8 ± 0.93, 44.6 ± 0.56.

3.3 Psychophysical studies

The task of the observers was to detect the filling defect at the vertical and horizontal center of one of four simulated arteries (4 alternative forced choice). In each trial an image sequence was randomly sampled from the 400 image-set database. There were a total of 5 different compression conditions. Two observers participated in the experiment. Both observers were naïve observers (GR, CH) but with extensive training visually detecting simulated lesions in medical images. Observers first trained in 1 session of 100 trials for each experimental condition and then participated in 5 sessions of 100 trials per condition. Images were displayed on an Image Systems M17L monochrome monitor. The mean luminance was 16.0 cd/m^2. The luminance vs. gray level relationship was the default non-linear curve that would be used by the physicians in a clinic with this monitor. Observers viewed the images binocularly from a distance of 50 cm and had unlimited time to reach a decision. When a decision was reached they pressed the number 1, 2, 3 or 4 in the keyboard to indicate their choice for that trial.

3.4 Data Analysis of human performance

Accuracy for a given observer in a given experimental condition was quantified by computing the percent of trials (Pc) that the observer correctly detected the target. Pc was then transformed to an index of detectability (d_a) for a 4-alternative forced-choice given by Equation 14.

4. RESULTS AND DISCUSSION

Figures 1 and 2 shows human performance for two observers as a function of JPEG image compression. Error bars correspond to standard errors. The absolute performance level and the effect of compression are similar across both observers. Figure 3 shows human performance (d_a averaged across the two observers) and performance for the three models (non-prewhitening with an eye filter, Hotelling, channelized Hotelling) as a function of JPEG image compression. All three models seem to predict reasonably well the effect of JPEG compression on human performance. A simple root mean square error between the model predictions and the human data resulted in: 0.11 for the NPWEW model, 0.08 for the channelized Hotelling and 0.22 for the Hotelling model. These results suggest that the NPWEW and channelized Hotelling model predict the human data better than the Hotelling. However, some caution should be taken on the interpretation of these results due to the fact that there is some additional variability in model observer performance due to the injection of internal noise.

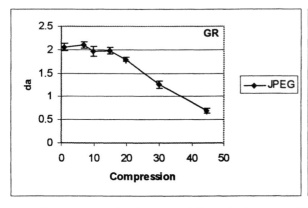 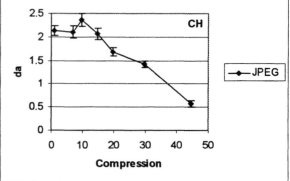

Figure 1 and 2. Performance d_a for both observers (CH and GR) as a function of JPEG image compression.

No sampling statistics are reported in the present paper but future work should establish the standard errors of the model performance and appropriate statistical testing. Our results are also dependent on the internal noise used to degrade model performance. For example, although not presented in this paper, some preliminary results show that if the internal noise is additive rather than proportional to the external noise, then the Hotelling model becomes a better predictor of human performance. Our results seem also to agree with our previous results[26] on model performance in x-ray coronary angiograms as a function of additive white noise. In that work we also found that all three models were good predictors of human performance.

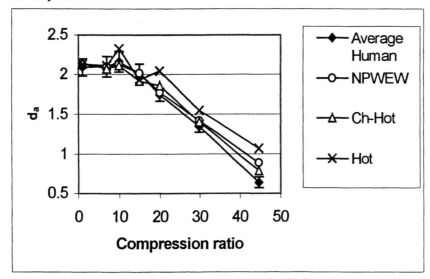

Figure 3. Human vs. model performance (NPWEW, Ch-Hot: channelized Hotelling; Hot: Hotelling) as a function of compression ratio. Model performance is degraded with internal noise to match human performance in the uncompressed conditions.

5. CONCLUSIONS

We have extended previous work by applying model observers to predict human visual detection of a simulated lesion embedded in real x-ray coronary angiograms as a function of different degrees of JPEG image compression. Overall, the non-prewhitening matched filter with an eye filter and the channelized Hotelling model (with internal noise proportional to the external noise) predicted the effect of JPEG image compression on human performance. These results suggest that model observers could potentially be used to evaluate image compression algorithms.

6. ACKNOWLEDGEMENTS

The authors would like to thank Cedric Heath and George Ruan for participation as observers in the study. This was work was supported by National Institute of Health (NIH) grant RO1-HL 53455.

7. REFERENCES

1. Eigler NL, Eckstein M P, Maher K, Honig D and Whiting JS, "Effect of a stenosis stabilized display on morphological feature detection," Circ., 89, 2700-2709 (1994).

2. Nissen SE et al., "Cardiac Aniography Without Cine Film: Erecting a Tower of Babel in the Cardiac Catheterization Laboratory," Journal of the American College of Cardiology, 24, 834-837 (1994)

3. Rigolin VH, Robiolio PA, Spero LA, Harrawood B.P., Morris KG, Fortin DF, Baker WA, Bashore TM, and Cusma JT, "Compression of Digital Coronary Angiograms Does Not Affect Visual or Quantitative Assessment of Coronary Artery Stenosis Severity." Am. J. of Card., 78, pp 131-135, (1996)

4. Baker WA et al., "Lossy (15:1) JPEG compression of digital coronary angiograms does not limit detection of subtle morphological features," Circ., 96, 1157-1164 (1997)

5. Whiting JS, Eckstein MP, Einav S, Eigler NL, Perceptual Evaluation of JPEG compression for medical image sequences, in OSA Annual Meeting Tech. Dig., Vol. 23, pp 161, (1992)

6. Bartroff J.L., Morioka CA, Whiting JS, Eckstein MP, Image compression and feature stabilization of dynamically displayed coronary angiograms, Proc. SPIE, Image Perception, Ed. E. Krupinski (1999)

7. Lo SC, Shen EL, Seong KM, An image splitting and remapping method for radiological image compression, Medical Imaging IV: Image Capture and Display, Proc. SPIE 1232, 312 – 321 (1990)

8. Chan KK, Lau CC, Lou SL, Hayrepatian, A, Ho BKT, Huang H.K., Three-dimensional Transform Compression of Image from Dynamic Studies, Medical Imaging IV: Image Capture and Display, Proc SPIE 1232, 322-326 (1990)

9. Goldberg M, Panchanathan S, Wang LA comparison of Lossy Techniques for Digitized Radiographic Images, Medical Imaging IV: Image Capture, Formatting and Display, Proc. SPIE 1987, 269-281, (1993)

10. Eckstein MP, Morioka CA, Whiting JS, Eigler N, Psychophysical evaluation of the effect of JPEG, Full-frame DCT and Wavelet image compression on signal detection in medical image noise, in Medical Imaging, Image Perception, Harold Kundel, Editor, Proc. SPIE 2436, 79-89 (1995)

11. Lubin J, The use of psychophysical data and models in the analysis of display system performance, in Digita images and human vision, Ed. A.B. Watson, MIT Press, 163-178, (1993)

12. Ahumada AJ, Jr., Watson AB, Rohally AM, "Models of human image discrimination predict object detection in natural backgrounds," in Human Vision, Visual Proc., and Digital Display VI, ed. B. Rogowitz and J. Allebach, 2411, 355-362, SPIE, (1995)

13. Watson AB, Gale AP, Solomon JA, Ahumada AJ, Visibility of DCT quantization noise: Effects of display resolution, Proceedings, Society for Information Display, San Jose, CA, Society for Information Display, pp. 697-700, (1995)

14. Barrett HH, Yao J, Rolland JP, Myers KJ. Model observers for assessment of image quality. Proc. Natl.Acad. Sci. USA, 90:9758- 9765, (1993).

15. Burgess AE, Wagner RB, Jennings RJ, and Barlow HB. Efficiency of human visual signal discrimination. Science, 214: 93-94, (1981)

16. Burgess AE, Ghandeharian H, Visual signal detection. II. Signal location identification. J. Opt. Soc. Am. A, 1: 900-905, (1984)

17. Burgess AE, Colborne B. Visual Signal Detection IV: Observer inconsistency. J. Opt. Soc. Am. A, 5:617-627, (1988)

18. Swesson RG, Judy PF, Detection of noisy visual targets: model for the effects of spatial uncertainty and signal to noise ratio. Percept. Psychophys, 29: 521-534, (1981)

19. Myers KJ, Barrett HH, Borgstrom MC, Patton, DD, Seeley GW. Effect of noise correlation on detectability of disk signals in medical imaging. J. Opt. Soc. Am.A , 2: 1752-1759, (1985)

20. Rolland JP, Barrett HH. Effect of random inhomogeneity on observer detection performance. J. Opt. Soc. Am. A, 9:649-658, (1992)

21. Abbey CK, Barrett HH, Linear iterative reconstruction algorithms: Study of observer performance, in Proc. 14th Int. Conf. On Information Processing in Medical Imaging (Yves Bizais, Christian Barillot, and Robert Di Paola, Eds.), Kluwer Academic, Dordrecht, 65-76, (1995)

22. Burgess AE, Li X., Abbey C.K., Visual signal detectability with two noise components: anomalous masking effects, J. Opt. Soc. Am. A 14(9):2420-2442, (1997)

23. Zhao B, Schwarz, LH, Kijewski, PK, Effect of lossy compression on lesion detection: Predictions of the nonprewhitening matched filter, Med. Phys., 25, 1621-1624, (1998)

24. Revesz G, Kundel HL, Graber MA. The influence of structured noise on the detection of radiologic abnormalities. Invest. Radiol., 9:479-486, (1974)

25. Eckstein MP, Whiting JS. Lesion detection in structured noise. Academic Radiology, 2:249-253, (1995)

26. Eckstein MP, Abbey CA, Whiting JS, Human vs model observers in anatomic backgrounds Proceedings SPIE Image Perception, 3340, 15-26, (1998)

27. Abbey CK, Barrett HH, Eckstein MP. Practical issues and methodology in assessment of image quality using model observers. in Medical Imaging Proc. SPIE, Ed. H. Roerhig The physics of medical imaging, 3032: 182-194, (1997)

28. Wagner RF, Weaver KE. An assortment of image quality indices for radiographic film-screen combinations- can they be resolved? In Application of Optical Instrumentation in Medicine I. P.L. Carson, WH Hendee, and WC Zarnstorff, eds, Proc. SPIE, 35, 83-94, (1972)

29. Ishida M, Doi K, Loo LN, Metz CE, Lehr JL, Digital image processing: effect of detectability of simulated low-contrast radiographic patterns, " Radiology 150, 569-575, (1984)

30. Burgess AE, Statistically defined backgrounds: Performance of a modified nonprewhitening matched filter model. J. Opt. Soc. Am. A, 11:1237-42, (1994)

31. Webster MA, Miyahara E, Contrast adaptation and the spatial structure of natural images, J. Opt. Soc. Am. A, 9, 2355-2366, (1997)

32. Barrett HH, Abbey CK, Gallas B, Eckstein MP, Stabilized estimates of Hotelling-observer detection performance in patient structured noise, Proc. SPIE 3340, (1998)

33. Myers K, Barrett HH, Addition of a channel mechanism to the ideal observer model, J Opt. Soc. Am. A, 4: 2447-2457, (1987)

34. Yao J, Barrett HH, Predicting human performance by a channelized Hotelling observer model, SPIE Math. Methods Med. Imaging, 1768:161-168, (1992)

35. Abbey CK, Barrett HH, Wilson DW, Observer signal to noise ratios for the ML-EM algorithm, Proc. SPIE 2712:47-58, (1996)

36. Marcelja S, Mathematical description of the responses of simple cortical cells, J. Opt. Soc. Am. A, 70, 1297-1300, (1980)

37. Watson AB, Detection and recognition of simple spatial forms, in Physical and Biological Processing of Images, OJ Bradick & AC Sleigh, Eds. New York: Springer-Verlag, (1983)

38. Eckstein MP, Abbey CK, Bochud FO, Visual signal detection in structured backgrounds III. Figures of merit for model observers with internal response correlations. J. Opt. Soc. Of Am., (submitted)

39. Green DM, Swets JA, Signal Detection Theory and Psychophysics (Wiley, NewYork, 1966)

40. Eckstein MP, Whiting JS, Visual signal detection in structured backgrounds I. Effect of number of possible locations and signal contrast, J Opt. Soc. Am. A, 13:1777-1787, (1996)

Visual Discrimination Model for Digital Mammography

Jeffrey P. Johnson[a], Jeffrey Lubin[a], Elizabeth A. Krupinski[b],
Heidi A. Peterson[a], Hans Roehrig[b], Andrew Baysinger[b]

[a] Sarnoff Corporation, Princeton, NJ 08543
[b] Department of Radiology, University of Arizona, Tucson, AZ 85724

ABSTRACT

Numerous studies have been conducted to determine experimentally the effects of image processing and display parameters on the diagnostic performance of radiologists. Comprehensive optimization of imaging systems for digital mammography based solely on measurements of reader performance is impractical, however, due to the large number of interdependent variables to be tested. A reliable, efficient alternative is needed to improve the evaluation and optimization of new imaging technologies. The Sarnoff JNDmetrix[TM] Visual Discrimination Model (VDM) is a computational, just-noticeable difference model of human vision that has been applied successfully to predict performance in various nonmedical detection and rating tasks. To test the applicability of the VDM to specific detection tasks in digital mammography, two observer performance studies were conducted. In the first study, effects of display tone scale and peak luminance on the detectability of microcalcifications were evaluated. The VDM successfully predicted improvements in reader performance for perceptually linearized tone scales and higher display luminances. In the second study, the detectability of JPEG and wavelet compression artifacts was evaluated, and performance ratings were again found to be highly correlated with VDM predictions. These results suggest that the VDM would be useful in the assessment and optimization of new imaging and compression technologies for digital mammography.

Keywords: image quality, observer performance, vision modeling, just-noticeable difference, digital mammography, image compression

1. INTRODUCTION

Digital mammography offers potential for significant improvements in diagnostic efficiency and accuracy[1-2], but as with any new imaging technology, a great deal of work is needed to optimize design and operating parameters in various components of the imaging system[3-4]. For example, there is still considerable disagreement about requirements for resolution, grayscale depth, signal dynamic range, and signal-to-noise ratio in both image capture and display. For image capture, signal-to-noise ratio is affected primarily by x-ray dose; for display, it is affected by various electronic noise sources and by image compression, often in unpredictable ways.

It is difficult to determine optimal settings of these and other imaging-system parameters, primarily because system performance depends on human performance in vision-based tasks. In mammography, the final arbiter of system performance must be the radiologist or other medical professional who is using the system to perform specific feature detection and classification tasks. But direct measurement of observer performance is a costly and time-consuming process that requires large numbers of radiologists and test images to achieve statistical reliability. The difficulty of this process is compounded by the fact that the various image capture and display parameters do not affect visual performance independently. For example, it is often possible to trade-off parameters such as spatial resolution and grayscale depth, while image compression parameters are known to interact in even more complex ways with various other parameters, such as signal-to-noise ratio of the image capture device. Comprehensive evaluation and optimization of a complete imaging system based on human performance measurements would require a prohibitively large number of parameter settings and combinations.

A reliable, efficient alternative to empirical performance studies is needed to more rapidly and effectively optimize imaging-system parameters for digital mammography. If, for example, there were a fast and accurate technique for predicting the performance of radiologists, this technique would ultimately improve screening and diagnosis, since it would ensure optimal performance from each component of the image capture, transmission, and display systems, and from the mammography system as a whole, thereby enabling the best possible visual performance by the radiologist using that system.

Part of the SPIE Conference on Image Perception and Performance
San Diego, California ● February 1999
SPIE Vol. 3663 ● 0277-786X/99/$10.00

The Sarnoff Corporation has developed a quantitative, computational model of human vision - the JNDmetrix[TM] Visual Discrimination Model (VDM) - which provides, via software, accurate estimates of human performance in visual detection, classification and rating tasks, as a function of imaging system parameters[5-6]. The VDM takes two images or image sequences as input, and returns accurate, robust, and rapid estimates of the perceptual discriminability between the two inputs. When the two inputs are similar signals with and without a feature of interest, such as a microcalcification cluster in a mammogram, the VDM can be applied to determine the range of imaging-system component specifications over which the feature of interest could be detected reliably.

The Sarnoff VDM has been rigorously tested in a wide range of image-analysis applications[7-9], but has not yet been applied, except in preliminary studies, to the domain of digital mammography. The purpose of the present study was to evaluate the applicability of the VDM for predicting effects of image display and processing parameters on reader performance in specific detection tasks in digital mammography. Successful demonstration of the accuracy and utility of the VDM will provide designers and integrators of softcopy mammography systems with a validated tool for optimizing and assessing the performance of their systems and components.

2. EXPERIMENTAL METHODS

2.1. Observer Performance Studies

2.1.1. Tone scale and luminance

The first observer performance study evaluated the effects of display tone scale and peak luminance on the detection of microcalcification clusters in digital mammograms. Test images were displayed on a DataRay DR110 monitor (DataRay Corp., Westminster, CO) using the three tone scales shown in Figure 1: the Default characteristic curve of the monitor, given approximately by a gamma power function with gamma=2.2, and two perceptually linearized curves derived by Barten[10] and Lubin-Pica[11], which were designed to produce equal increments in visual discriminability for each unit change in grayscale level. The three tone scales were applied initially with a peak display luminance of 140 fL. The peak luminance was then reduced by the application of neutral-density gelatin filters (Eastman Kodak, Rochester, NY) to the faceplate. Filters with an optical density of 0.2 or 0.5 were applied to reduce the peak luminance to 88 fL (63% transmission) or 45 fL (32% transmission), respectively. Only the Barten tone scale was used in tests of the reduced peak luminances.

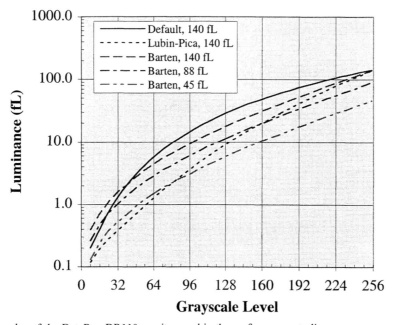

Figure 1. Tone scales of the DataRay DR110 monitor used in the performance studies.

Base images for the performance studies were selected from the Nijmegen[12] database of digital mammograms with identified microcalcification clusters. The raw images contained 2048x2048 pixels with 50-micron spatial resolution and 12-bit grayscale resolution. Fifty 256x256-pixel subimages containing identified regions of interest with at least one microcalcification cluster were cropped from the full images. These regions of interest varied in diameter from 22 to 192 pixels and were centered randomly within each subimage, which filled a 45x45 mm^2 area on the DataRay monitor.

For the first performance study, a set of 250 test images was generated by replicating each of the 50 base images at four reduced levels of contrast in the "target" microcalcification clusters. The 100% target contrast in the original, target-present images was reduced by processing the images with Adobe Photoshop software after linear rescaling of grayscale levels from 12 to 8 bits. Individual microcalcifications in the target-present images were first replaced with normal background texture to create target-absent (0% contrast) images. Additional test images with intermediate target contrasts of 25%, 50%, and 75% were generated by weighted linear superposition of the target-present and target-absent images. The five contrast levels for each base image were presented with different image orientations to inhibit recognition by the readers. The ordering of the test images for the test sessions was random with a constraint that no base image was repeated within 20 trials. Two consecutive series of the 250 test images were generated to create a total of 500 images for the test sessions.

Six radiologists from the University of Arizona Medical Center participated as readers. They viewed the 500 test images in each of the five tone scale (Default, Barten, and Lubin-Pica at 140 fL) and luminance (Barten at 88 and 45 fL) conditions. Images were displayed one at a time and the reader was asked to assign a numerical confidence rating for the presence of microcalcifications in the image on a six-point scale: 1=Absent, definite; 2=Absent, probable; 3=Absent, possible; 4=Present, possible; 5=Present, probable; 6=Present, definite. Images were viewed in a darkened room at a fixed viewing distance of 20±2 cm. Readers were not allowed to adjust display or window/level controls, but were given unlimited time to view each image. The readers participated in five one-hour sessions viewing images in only a single condition during a session. Each reader viewed each condition in a different randomized order. Each reading session was separated from the previous session by at least two weeks.

2.1.2. Image compression

A second performance study was conducted to evaluate the detectability of encoding artifacts in digital mammograms. Twenty of the base images from the first study were encoded by JPEG and wavelet techniques at five "quality" levels that produced a broad range of perceptible distortion in the decompressed images. Compression ratios ranged from 5 to 24 for the JPEG images and from 3 to 14 for the wavelet images. The test images were presented in a triangular "odd-man-out" configuration with the uncompressed reference image at the top and two versions of the same image presented side-by-side below it. In each trial, one of the side-by-side images was the decompressed (codec) image and the other was the uncompressed image, with random right/left assignment of image position. Readers were asked to identify which of the side-by-side images was the codec image and to rate their confidence in the selection using a six-point scale: 1=Right, definite; 2=Right, probable; 3=Right, guess; 4=Left, guess; 5=Left, probable; 6=Left, definite. Test images were displayed on the DataRay monitor with 140 fL peak luminance and a perceptually-linearized Barten tone scale. A total of 200 randomized trials (20 base images x 5 quality levels x 2 repetitions with different image orientation; no repetitions of any base image within 10 trials) were evaluated in each test session. Five readers from the first study evaluated the JPEG and wavelet images in two separate test sessions scheduled about two weeks apart. Three readers viewed the JPEG images in the first session; the other readers viewed the wavelet images in the first session.

2.2. Visual Discrimination Model

The Sarnoff Visual Discrimination Model (VDM) computes an image-fidelity metric called the just-noticeable-difference (JND) aggregate measure, or JAM, that quantifies the visually perceptible differences between a pair of reference and test images. Input images for the VDM were prepared by transforming the 256x256-pixel grayscale images used in the observer performance studies to luminance images using the tone scales shown in Figure 1. Reference images for the tone scale and luminance studies were the target-absent (0% target contrast) images. Each of these reference images was compared in VDM simulations to the four corresponding test images at 25%, 50%, 75%, and 100% target contrast. For the compression study, the reference images were the uncompressed base images, while the test images were the corresponding codec images for five levels of JPEG and wavelet compression.

Sarnoff's VDM software (version 7.3.C04) was used to compute a single JAM value for each pair of reference and test images. The JAM was computed over the full 256x256-pixel JND map for each pair of images. Mean JAM values were then computed over all trials of images at the same level of target contrast or compression. For comparison to an alternate image-fidelity metric, the mean luminance error between reference and test images was also computed.

3. RESULTS

3.1. Tone Scale and Luminance Study

Confidence ratings from the tone scale and luminance study were used to generate individual Receiver Operating Characteristic (ROC) curves and areas (Az) under the curve. Values for the six readers are given in Table 1 for the five combinations of tone scale and peak luminance and four levels of target contrast. Mean Az values from Table 1 are plotted in Figure 2. Analysis of Variance (ANOVA) revealed a significant main effect for target contrast (F = 838.43, df = 3, p < 0.0001), and a main effect that approached significance for tone scale (F = 3.46, df = 2, p = 0.07). Least-squares means post-hoc tests indicated that overall there was improvement in the detection of microcalcifications for both perceptually linearized tone scales, Lubin-Pica and Barten, relative to the Default scale, with the difference between the Barten and Default scales being significant (t = 2.58, df = 10, p = 0.03). With respect to target contrast, each 25% reduction in contrast significantly lowered the detectability of microcalcifications as measured by Az (all t-test comparisons p < 0.0001). Overall (F = 0.97, df = 6, p = 0.47) there was no significant interaction between target contrast and tone scale. Least-squares post-hoc results indicate that while the Barten curve outperformed (p < 0.04 for all comparisons) the Default at all target contrast levels, the Lubin-Pica scale yielded better detection rates than the Default scale at higher (> 50%) target contrast levels (p < 0.02), but not at lower (≥50%) target contrast levels (p > 0.05).

Table 1. Areas, Az, under the ROC curves for the first study involving five combinations of tone scale and peak luminance, five levels of microcalcification target contrast (0 to 100%), and six readers.

Target Contrast	Reader	Az for ROC Curves (Tone Scale / Peak Luminance)				
		Default 140 fL	Lubin-Pica 140 fL	Barten 140 fL	Barten 88 fL	Barten 45 fL
100%	1	0.864	0.983	0.984	0.979	0.925
	2	0.930	0.971	0.964	0.989	0.869
	3	0.980	0.986	0.988	0.938	0.945
	4	0.967	0.971	0.990	0.926	0.906
	5	0.975	0.987	0.989	0.910	0.899
	6	0.991	0.975	0.968	0.963	0.966
	Mean	0.951	0.979	0.981	0.951	0.918
75%	1	0.862	0.919	0.911	0.924	0.894
	2	0.857	0.928	0.918	0.908	0.882
	3	0.896	0.935	0.920	0.889	0.931
	4	0.901	0.906	0.919	0.887	0.861
	5	0.932	0.941	0.935	0.869	0.881
	6	0.931	0.913	0.926	0.934	0.887
	Mean	0.896	0.924	0.921	0.902	0.889
50%	1	0.643	0.762	0.755	0.781	0.745
	2	0.731	0.765	0.798	0.805	0.703
	3	0.778	0.774	0.762	0.798	0.727
	4	0.779	0.764	0.790	0.801	0.665
	5	0.798	0.781	0.753	0.778	0.732
	6	0.794	0.800	0.846	0.844	0.743
	Mean	0.754	0.774	0.784	0.801	0.719
25%	1	0.524	0.511	0.569	0.576	0.598
	2	0.519	0.509	0.555	0.565	0.502
	3	0.534	0.563	0.567	0.672	0.543
	4	0.535	0.544	0.539	0.620	0.486
	5	0.581	0.553	0.589	0.565	0.494
	6	0.609	0.610	0.632	0.556	0.586
	Mean	0.550	0.548	0.575	0.592	0.535

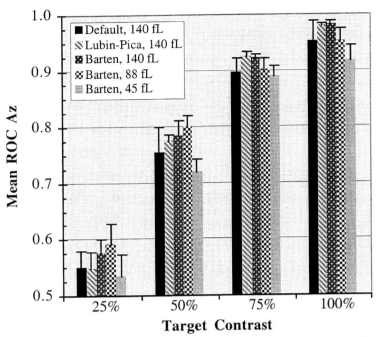

Figure 2. Mean area, Az, under the ROC curve for five combinations of tone scale and peak luminance and four levels of microcalcification target contrast. Vertical error bars show the 95% confidence intervals.

For the luminance conditions (Barten curve only), the ANOVA revealed significant main effects due to luminance (F = 16.04, df = 2, p = 0.008) and target contrast (F = 1340.87, df = 3, p = 0.001). Least-squares post-hoc tests indicated that the main effect of luminance was due primarily to a significant drop in performance at the lowest luminance (45 fL) compared to 140 fL (t = 5.08, df = 10, p = 0.0005) and 88 fL (t = 4.71, df = 10, p = 0.0008). Performance did not differ significantly for 140 fL versus 88 fL (t = 0.37, df = 10, p = 0.72). Values of Az declined monotonically with decreasing peak luminance for target contrasts > 50%, with the difference between 140 fL and 45 fL being significant (t = 3.62, df = 10, p = 0.001) at the 100% target contrast level. Az levels were somewhat higher at 88 fL than at 140 fL for lower (< 50%) contrast levels, with the differences between 140 fL and 88 fL compared to 45 fL being significant (p < 0.02) for both 50% and 25% target contrasts. Comparison of all five conditions at each target contrast revealed that the 45 fL Az performance was significantly lower (p < 0.05) for all target contrasts than any other condition.

Trends in the experimental dependence of mean Az values on tone scale and peak luminance were also evident in mean JAM values, shown in Figure 3a, computed by the Sarnoff VDM for the test images used in the observer performance study. The VDM successfully predicted the observed enhancement in microcalcification detection for the perceptually-linearized tone scales for target contrasts >25%, as well as the decline in reader performance at lower peak luminances. The VDM was somewhat too sensitive, however, to the effects of the Lubin-Pica scale, causing an overprediction of its impact relative to the Barten scale. The correlation between model JAM and experimental Az values was much greater than that obtained using an alternate image-fidelity metric, mean luminance error (MLE), shown in Figure 3b. Values of MLE for images simulated with the Lubin-Pica and Barten tone scales were significantly lower than those with the Default scale, suggesting that a *higher* target detection rate might be expected with the Default scale, contrary to both the experimental results and VDM predictions. Relative declines in MLE with decreasing peak luminance were much larger than the observed changes in mean Az, which were tracked more accurately by the VDM at target contrasts >50%.

The superior correlation of JAM values with experimental performance data is shown more explicitly in Figures 4a and 4b, which plot mean Az values as a function of mean JAM and MLE, respectively. The correlation was significantly higher for JAM (r=0.97) than for MLE (r=0.80) values for the same test images. Moreover, the relative variation in JAM for each datapoint was generally smaller than for MLE.

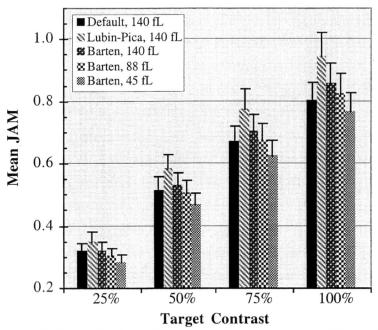

Figure 3a. Mean JAM values for five combinations of tone scale and peak luminance and four levels of microcalcification target contrast. Vertical error bars show the 95% confidence intervals.

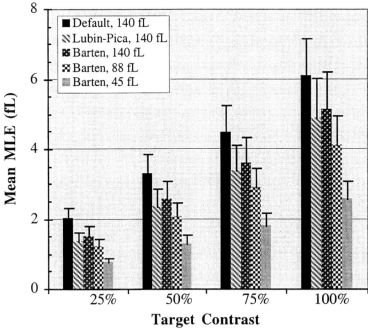

Figure 3b. Mean luminance error (MLE) for the same test images and conditions as in Figure 3a. Vertical error bars show the 95% confidence intervals.

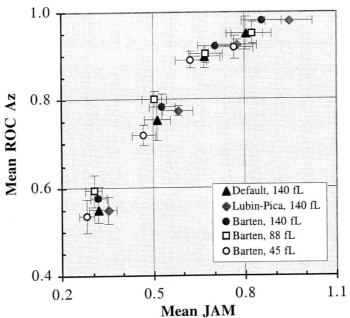

Figure 4a. Correlation of mean JAM values with area, Az, under the ROC curve for five combinations of tone scale and peak luminance. The correlation coefficient r = 0.97. Error bars represent the 95% confidence intervals.

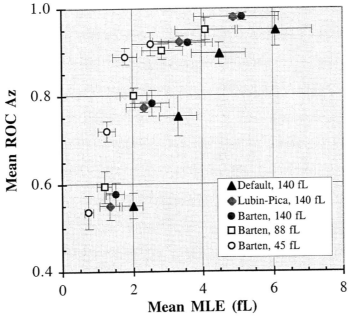

Figure 4b. Correlation of mean luminance error (MLE) with area, Az, under the ROC curve for the same test images and conditions as in Figure 4a. The correlation coefficient r = 0.80. Error bars represent the 95% confidence intervals.

3.2. Image Compression Study

The second performance study evaluated the ability of radiologists to detect JPEG and wavelet encoding artifacts in digital mammograms. The percentage of correct responses, averaged for five readers over all test images encoded with the same JPEG or wavelet compression parameter, are shown in Figure 5 as a function of the compression ratio for the test images. Mean confidence ratings (1=Low to 3=High) assigned to the same sets of images are shown in Figure 6. Distortions in the compressed images were highly visible (≥90% correct) for both encoding methods at compression ratios over 9. Reducing the mean detection rate to below 75% required compression ratios less than 5 for wavelet and 7 for JPEG encoding. It should be noted that these guidelines apply to the *mean* performances; individual variations among the readers in this study were large, and one reader was able to correctly identify the compressed images in more than 85% of the trials at all compression levels.

ANOVA results for the JPEG experiment showed significant differences due to compression level (F=8.57, df=4, p=0.0003), with post-hoc least-squares means analysis showing that each JPEG level differed significantly (p<0.03) from others two or more levels above or below it. For the wavelet experiment, ANOVA results showed a significant main effect (F=8.67, df=4, p=0.0003) for compression level. Least-squares means post-hoc analysis showed significant differences (p<0.02) between the following wavelet compression levels: level 1 to 3, 4 and 5; level 2 to 3,4 and 5; level 3 to 1 and 2; level 4 to 1 and 2; and level 5 to 1 and 2.

Reader performance in the compression study was correlated significantly with JAM values computed by the Sarnoff VDM for the same test images. The mean percentages of correct responses for JPEG and wavelet images are plotted in Figure 7a as a function of JAM values averaged over the 20 test images at each compression level. High correlation coefficients of r=0.97 were achieved when the JPEG and wavelet results were considered independently. Combining the two sets of results reduced the overall correlation coefficient to r=0.87 due to differences in vertical offset and slope of the trend lines for the two compression methods. The correlation of mean luminance error (MLE) with reader performance, shown in Figure 7b, was also high (r=0.97) when JPEG and wavelet results were considered separately. The combined correlation of both datasets, however, was significantly lower (r=0.71) than was demonstrated for the JAM values in Figure 7a.

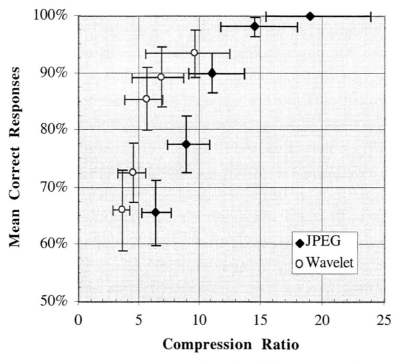

Figure 5. Mean percentages of correct responses for images encoded at five JPEG or wavelet quality levels, plotted as a function of the mean compression ratio for each level. Vertical bars represent 95% confidence intervals. Horizontal bars show the full range of compression for all images at each quality level.

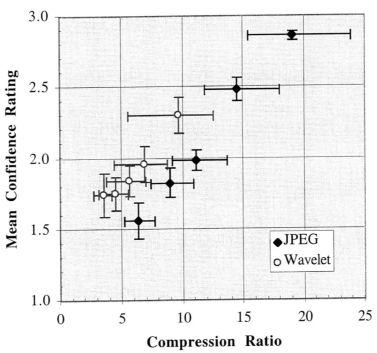

Figure 6. Mean confidence rating for images encoded at five JPEG or wavelet quality levels, plotted as a function of the mean compression ratio for each level. Vertical bars represent 95% confidence intervals. Horizontal bars show the full range of compression for all images at each quality level.

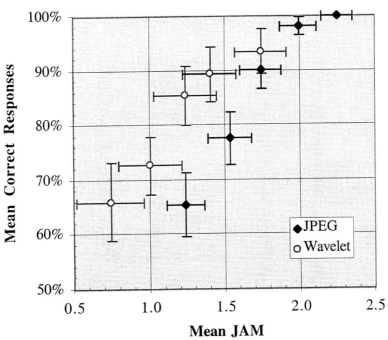

Figure 7a. Correlation of vision-model JAM with mean percentage of correct responses for images compressed to five JPEG or wavelet "quality" levels. The correlation coefficients for JPEG and wavelet datasets were 0.97 separately and 0.87 overall. Error bars represent 95% confidence intervals.

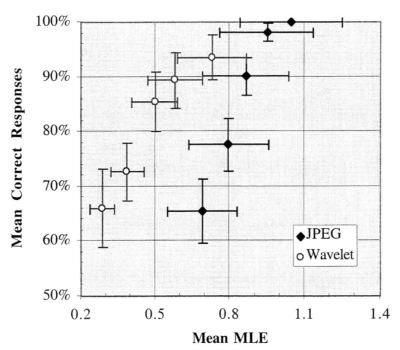

Figure 7b. Correlation of mean luminance error (MLE) with percentage of correct responses for images compressed to five JPEG or wavelet "quality" levels. The correlation coefficients for JPEG and wavelet datasets were 0.97 separately and 0.71 overall. Error bars represent 95% confidence intervals.

4. DISCUSSION

A high level of correlation was found between experimental reader performance and image-fidelity metrics computed by the Sarnoff VDM for two detection tasks in digital mammography. The VDM successfully predicted improvements in microcalcification detection using the perceptually linearized tone scales (Barten and Lubin-Pica) and higher peak luminances (88 and 140 fL). The correlation of VDM metrics with reader performance was significantly greater than that obtained using another objective image-fidelity metric, mean luminance error.

In the compression study, performance ratings for the perceptibility of JPEG and wavelet encoding artifacts were also better correlated with VDM predictions than with mean luminance error. The correlation between JPEG and wavelet results, however, was less than expected. One possible reason for this could be the difference in the perceptual ranges of compression artifacts in the wavelet and JPEG test images, which were viewed in separate test sessions. Another explanation could be the need for adjustments in the relative sensitivity of the VDM to JPEG and wavelet artifacts, since JPEG artifacts tend to be "blocky" with distinct edges, while wavelet artifacts tend to be more uniformly distributed and blurred in appearance. An improved experimental approach to resolving these issues would be to minimize the effects of different perceptual ranges of artifacts by first reducing the maximum JPEG compression to a level closer to the maximum wavelet level, and then combining the JPEG and wavelet images randomly in the same test session.

The correlation of VDM metrics with experimental reader performance confirmed earlier results in nonmedical imaging applications, and suggests that the VDM would be useful in the evaluation and optimization of new imaging and compression systems for digital mammography. Additional studies are warranted to extend the validation of the VDM to other tasks in digital radiology and medical imaging, and to demonstrate the practical value of the VDM in the development of improved technologies for medical image acquisition, processing, and display.

ACKNOWLEDGMENTS

This evaluation of the Sarnoff JNDmetrix™ VDM for applications in digital mammography was supported by the National Information Display Laboratory, Princeton, NJ and by DataRay Corporation, Westminster, CO.

REFERENCES

1. Cheung L, Bird R, Chitkara A, Rego A, Rodriguez C, Yuen J., "Initial operating and clinical results of a full field mammography system," In: Karssemeijer N, Thijssen M, Hendriks J, van Erning L, eds. Digital Mammography Nijmegen, 1998. Boston, MA: Kluwer Academic Publishing, 1998; 11-18.
2. Pisano ED. Initial clinical experience with full field digital mammography. In: Karssemeijer N, Thijssen M, Hendriks J, van Erning L, eds. Digital Mammography Nijmegen, 1998. Boston, MA: Kluwer Academic Publishing, 1998;391-394.
3. Mawdsley GE, Yaffe MJ, Maidment ADA, Niklason L, Williams M, Hemminger BM. Acceptance testing and quality control of digital mammography equipment. In: Karssemeijer N, Thijssen M, Hendriks J, van Erning L, eds. Digital Mammography Nijmegen, 1998. Boston, MA: Kluwer Academic Publishing, 1998;437-444.
4. Kimme-Smith C, Lewis C, Yang L, Bassett LW. An automated quality control program for whole breast digital image receptors. In: Karssemeijer N, Thijssen M, Hendriks J, van Erning L, eds. Digital Mammography Nijmegen, 1998. Boston, MA: Kluwer Academic Publishing, 1998;445-448.
5. Jackson WB, Beebee P, Jared DA, Biegelsen DK, Larimer JO, Lubin J, Gille JL. X-ray image system design using a human visual model. SPIE Medical Imaging 1996; 2708:29-40.
6. Jackson WB, Said MR, Jared DA, Larimer JO, Gille JL, Lubin J. Evaluation of human vision models for predicting human-observer performance. SPIE Medical Imaging 1997;3036:64-73.
7. Alphonse GA, Lubin J. Psychophysical requirements for seamless tiled large-screen displays. SID Digest 1992; 23:941-944.
8. Lubin J, Bergen JR. Pattern discrimination in the fovea and periphery. Invest Ophthalmology and Visual Science Supplement 1991; 32:1024.
9. Lubin J, Bergen JR. Cockpit display visibility modeling. NASA Contractor Report 177623, NASA/Ames Research Center, Moffet Field, CA, 1993.
10. Barten PGJ. Subjective image quality of high-definition television pictures. SID Sym Digest 1990; 31:239-243.
11. Lubin J, Pica A. A non-uniform quantizer matched to human visual performance. SID Sym Digest 1991; 32:619-622.
12. National Expert and Training Center for Breast Cancer Screening, Dept. of Radiology, Univ. of Nijmegen, the Netherlands.

Signal detection in a lumpy background: effects of providing more information to the human than just the raw data

B. D. Gallas[a][b] and H. H. Barrett[a][b][c]

[a]Dept. of Radiology, University of Arizona, Arizona Health Sciences Center, Tucson, AZ, 85724

[b]Program in Applied Mathematics, University of Arizona, Tucson, AZ, 85721

[c]Optical Sciences Center, University of Arizona, Tucson, AZ, 85721

ABSTRACT

In this paper we present a modification to the standard two-alternative forced-choice (2AFC) experiment in an attempt to help the human detect signals by providing redundant information. We call the old experiment 2AFC_RAW, and the new experiment, 2AFC_FILTER. In the 2AFC_FILTER experiment, we provide the observer with the pair of raw data images (as in 2AFC_RAW) *plus* filtered versions of the raw data. The thought behind this modification is that the human might benefit from generic pre-processing of the data into multiple images, each extracting different information.

We defined two different 2AFC_FILTER experiments, each using Laguerre-Gauss functions as the filters. The difference between the two was their defining Gaussian envelope. We tested human performance given a variety of image classes with the 2AFC_RAW and the two 2AFC_FILTER experiments. The same raw data were used in each.

We found that there was a significant human performance increase from the 2AFC_RAW to the 2AFC_FILTER experiment. It was also seen that the choice of the filters made a difference. Specifically, human performance was better when the Gaussian envelope of the Laguerre-Gauss functions matched the signal.

Keywords: signal detection, lumpy background, 2AFC, 2AFC_FILTER, channel observer, human performance, psychophysics, Laguerre-Gauss functions

1. INTRODUCTION

In attempts to better understand the human observer, we have been conducting two-alternative forced-choice (2AFC) experiments that measure the human's ability to detect signals in noisy radiographic images of random ("lumpy") backgrounds. In this paper we present results from 2AFC experiments where the images are the same, but the information we provide is different.

In our standard 2AFC experiment, which we will call 2AFC_RAW, the observer is provided pairs of images which are the raw data from an imaging system and a reference image of the signal. The imaging system is simulated as convolution (Gaussian blur) plus measurement noise. One image in each pair has the signal. The observer is then "forced" to choose which image has the signal.

Here, we are trying to help the human detect signals by providing redundant information. We call the new experiment the 2AFC_FILTER experiment. Using the 2AFC paradigm, we provide the observer with the pair of raw data images *plus* filtered versions of the raw data. The thought behind this modification is that the human will benefit from a generic pre-processing of the data. Each filtered image provides different information.

Gilland *et al.* have shown that filtering during tomographic reconstruction increases human performance in signal detection[4]. They also found that the optimal amount of smoothing is strongly dependent on the signal to be detected. Specifically for a Butterworth filter, they saw that a maximum increase in performance occurred when the Butterworth filter matched the signal. Similar results were seen by Abbey[1]. This dependence, though, is a little awkward because we don't know the signal in clinical images. In this paper we are investigating a hypothesis that by providing multiple versions of *generically* filtered images in addition to the raw data we can get a maximal increase in performance over filters.

Further author information for B. D. Gallas:
E-mail: gallas@math.arizona.edu, work: (520) 626-6963, fax: (520)626-2892

264

Part of the SPIE Conference on Image Perception and Performance
San Diego, California ● February 1999
SPIE Vol. 3663 ● 0277-786X/99/$10.00

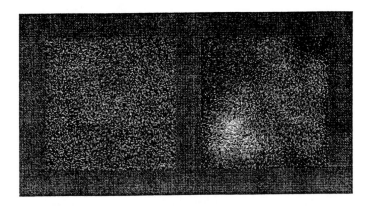

Figure 1. Example images generated with low-intensity (left) and high-intensity circ lumps (right).

This 2AFC_FILTER experiment was also inspired by work in our group with the channelized-Hotelling observer. Myers introduced this observer as a model of the human observer[5]. In this model, an ideal linear observer is restricted to a scalar output per information-selective channel. This usually reduces the data set. The channels, as mentioned above, can be chosen to model the human[1] or they can be defined in an attempt to estimate the ideal linear observer[2][3]. For the work here, instead of restricting the observer to scalar channel outputs, we provide the observer with an entire image per channel.

This paper begins by describing the images that will be used throughout this paper. Then we will motivate and introduce the 2AFC_FILTER experiment. We will discuss the filters we chose, and outline the psychophysical experiments. Then we will present and compare the results of the human experiments. For the most part, these results are telling us to look further. Therefore, we will outline current and upcoming experiments that will investigate the effect of *multiple* channels of information in signal-detection tasks.

2. IMAGES

The images used here come from a simple model for imaging a 2D random object. The distribution on each pixel is modeled as the continuous-to-discrete mapping of an object f by an operator $\mathcal{H}$ plus measurement noise. This is written

$$\mathbf{g} : [\mathbf{g}]_i = [\mathcal{H}f]_i + n_i, \tag{1}$$

The operator $\mathcal{H}$ is modeled here as convolution with a Gaussian followed by sampling on a pixel grid. The noise n_i is modeled as Gaussian noise with mean equal to zero and variance equal to $[\mathcal{H}f]_i$. As a result, the $\mathbf{g}_i$ are approximately Poisson distributed, which is a good model for radiographic images.

In addition to the randomness coming from the measurement noise, we define the objects randomly too[6]. Each object is made up of a constant background B to which we add some number of lumps K dispersed randomly throughout the scene. Finally, a signal, Gaussian for the work here, may or may not be added to get

$$f(\mathbf{r}) = B + \sum_{k=0}^{K} b(\mathbf{r} - \mathbf{r}_k) \quad (+s(\mathbf{r})). \tag{2}$$

In the definition 2, the number of blobs K is a taken to be a Poisson random variable with mean $\overline{K}$ and the location of each lump $\mathbf{r}_k$ is taken to be a uniform random variable on the domain.

The lumps for our experiments are either Gaussian, circ or besinc (see Fig. 2). The circ function is defined as one within a circle and zero outside. Hence, the circ is spatially compact and has long tails in the frequency domain. The besinc is the two-dimensional Fourier transform of the circ. As such, it is compact in the frequency domain with long tails in the spatial domain.

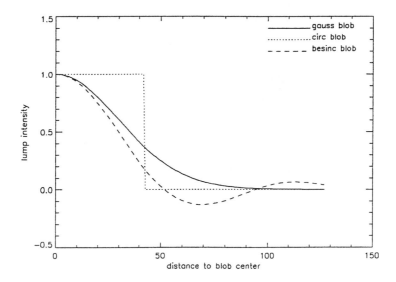

Figure 2. Radial profiles of the lump shapes.

The shapes were chosen because they are quite different from one another; they vary from completely spatially compact and monotonic to very non-compact and oscillating. We vary the intensity of the lumps, affecting the relative contributions of measurement noise and background inhomogeneity. Qualitatively, the higher the lump intensity, the more obvious the lumps become (see 1). We vary the lump intensity because we know the performance of the Hotelling observer is quite different for each background shape as we vary the intensity of the lumps. Therefore, by varying the lump shape and intensity, we attempt to test the robustness of our conclusions.

We found it necessary to rescale the signal as we varied lump intensity. We decided to keep human performance approximately the same as we increased the lump intensity of the Gaussian lumps. The same rescaling of the signal was done for each lump shape.

3. EXPERIMENT

3.1. Channel Observer

A model observer that we have found to be useful in our analyses is the channelized-Hotelling observer, or channel observer for short. This observer has as its inputs u_d where $d = 1, 2...D$. Each u_d is the raw-data image passed through a corresponding filter $\mathbf{t}_d$. This can be expressed as

$$\mathbf{u} = T^t \mathbf{g}, \quad \text{where } T = [\mathbf{t}_1, \mathbf{t}_2, ... \mathbf{t}_D], \tag{3}$$

where $\mathbf{u}$ is a $D \times 1$ vector (D equals the number of channels), $\mathbf{g}$ and $\mathbf{t}_i$ are $M \times 1$ vectors (M equals the number of measurements) and T is an $M \times D$ matrix. The channel observer is defined to be the signal image (as seen by a set of channels) operated on by the inverse covariance matrix of the channel outputs like

$$\mathbf{v}_{\text{ch}} = K_{\text{ch}}^{-1} \mathbf{s}_{\text{ch}}. \tag{4}$$

So, $\mathbf{v}_{\text{ch}}$ and $\mathbf{s}_{\text{ch}}$ are $D \times 1$ vectors and K_{ch}^{-1} is a $D \times D$ matrix. Note that the channel observer can also be defined in the image space,

$$\mathbf{w}_{\text{ch}} = \sum_{d=1}^{D} v_d \mathbf{t}_d, \tag{5}$$

which is just a weighted sum of the channels.

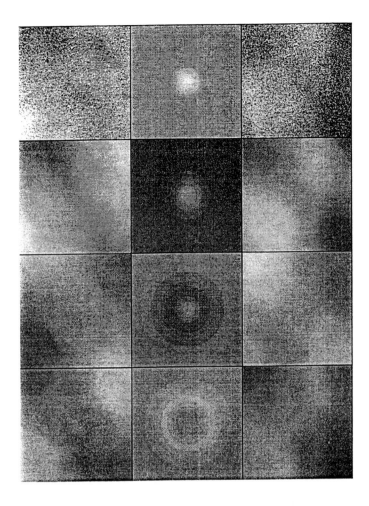

Figure 3. The top row in this image is a sample image pair plus the reference image of the signal for the 2AFC_RAW experiment. In the 2AFC_FILTER experiments, the observer gets the raw data column plus 6 additional rows (only 3 shown). Each row is the raw data image passed through a different filter. The middle column shows what the signal looks like when passed through each filter. Contour effects can perhaps be seen in printed versions of this document. However, they were not seen on the monitor in the experiments.

The channel observer was originally designed to incorporate the physiology of the visual system. As such, the channels were defined according to psychophysical and electrophysiological measurements. Using this type of channel observer attempts to decrease the performance of the Hotelling observer for the purpose of modeling the human.

A different purpose of the channel model is to estimate or approximate the Hotelling observer or, equivalently, its template. This methodology was presented by Barrett at last year's SPIE conference[2] . This method was shown to be successful for images like the ones we are using here with Laguerre-Gauss functions as the channels. We presented this work at the 1999 conference of the Optical Society of America which was held in Baltimore[3] . Laguerre-Gauss channels were chosen because the Hotelling template is rotationally symmetric and thus has a Laguerre-Gauss representation. The template is rotationally symmetric, because the signal and background correlation structure are both rotationally symmetric (by construction).

The benefit of this type of channel observer is that the channels may be chosen so that the channel observer can perform as well as the Hotelling observer while reducing the dimensionality of the data. In other words, the smaller channel data contains as much information about the detection task as the raw data. Therefore, filtering the images with channels that can estimate the Hotelling observer should not, by themselves, result in any loss in detectability. The 2AFC_FILTER experiment is an attempt to marry ideas about the channel observer and the 2AFC experiment

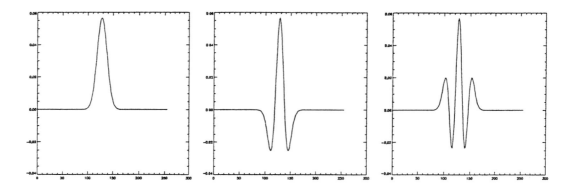

Figure 4. Examples of the first three Laguerre-Gauss functions.

with the hoped-for result of increasing human performance given the same raw data.

3.2. 2AFC_FILTER

In the 2AFC_RAW experiment, the observer is given pairs of raw data images and a reference image of the signal. For example, the observer is presented the first row in Fig. 3. In each pair of raw-data images, one image contains the signal and the other does not. The task is to choose which image in each pair has the signal. The performance of the observer for this task is measured as the percent correct.

In the 2AFC_FILTER experiment, we give the observer filtered versions of each image to make a decision *in addition to* the pair of raw data images. An example of what the observer is given can be seen in Fig. 3. Each row below the raw data is the raw data passed through a different filter. Percent correct is again the measure of performance.

The motivation for this modification to the experiment is to improve signal detection. We shouldn't decrease the human's performance by providing the extra information unless we overwhelm or confuse him or her. However, by pre-processing the raw data, we do some noise averaging and extract different information for each filter. This could prove useful to the human.

3.3. Laguerre-Gauss Functions

As mentioned, the Laguerre-Gauss functions were used in previous analyses that had success in estimating the Hotelling observer with channel observers. Therefore, we chose them to be the filters used in the 2AFC-FILTER experiment. The main rationale, again, is that the filtered images contain much of the detectability information by themselves.

The radial dependence of each Laguerre-Gauss function is the product of a polynomial and a Gaussian. Examples of the first three Laguerre-Gauss functions are presented in Fig. 4. This set of functions is parameterized by the spread of the Gaussian envelope. This Gaussian defines the domain of interest of the functions. In other words, finite combinations of these functions give approximations that are more accurate within the defining Gaussian envelope than outside. Regardless of the spread, the Laguerre-Gauss functions are a complete set of orthonormal functions on the set of functions that are rotationally symmetric.

3.4. Summary of Psychophysical Experiments

The human data were collected for 5 observers, one of which was the first author. There were three experiments, beginning with the 2AFC_RAW experiment. The two other experiments were 2AFC_FILTER experiments using Laguerre-Gauss functions for the filters. In the first of these, the defining Gaussian envelope of the Laguerre-Gauss functions had a spread of 15 pixels and in the other it was 25 pixels. A Gaussian with a spread of 15 pixels approximately matches the Gaussian signal to be detected, and a spread of 25 pixels was used to see the impact that the filter spread has on detectability. We give these two experiments the abbreviated notation 2AFC_FILTER (lgg15) and 2AFC_FILTER (lgg25), respectively.

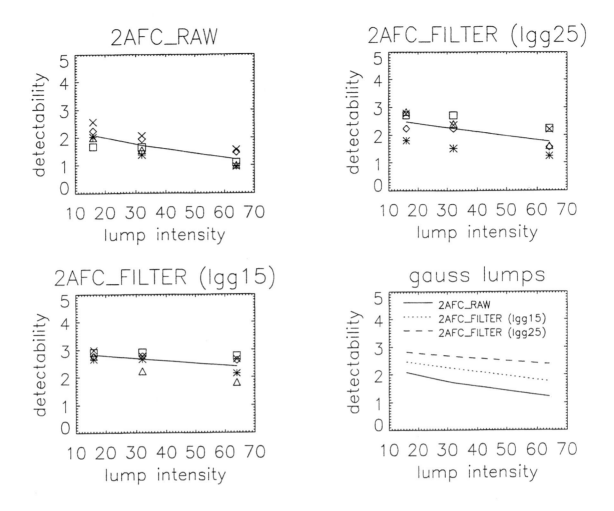

Figure 5. Human detectability for the images with Gaussian lumps. Symbols track individual observers and lines track observer-averaged performance. Top-left: experiment with just the raw data. Top-right: experiment with raw data plus the raw data passed through 6 Laguerre-Gauss filters with a spread of 25 pixels. Bottom-left: experiment with raw data plus the raw data passed through 6 Laguerre-Gauss filters with a spread of 15 pixels. Bottom-right: observer-averaged detectabilities from all three experiments.

Within each experiment, we realized images from Gaussian, circ and besinc lumps at three lump intensities for a total of 9 modalities. For each modality there were 500 raw data images, 100 of which were training images. The total number of images created, then, was 4500 raw data images. The same 4500 raw data images were used in each of the 2AFC_RAW, 2AFC_FILTER (lgg15) and 2AFC_FILTER (lgg25) experiments to remove the variability possible from introducing different images.

To begin each experiment, the observers ran through all the training images to acquaint themselves with the experiment. Then for each modality, the observers began with the modality-specific training set of 100 images in order to develop their signal detection strategy for that image class. Finally, the observers ran through the other 400 images broken up into four separate trials for the estimate of their performance.

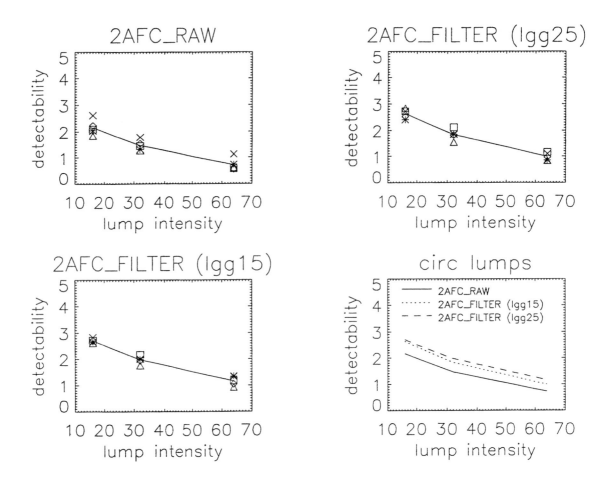

Figure 6. Human detectability for the images with Gaussian lumps. Symbols track individual observers and lines track observer-averaged performance. Top-left: experiment with just the raw data. Top-right: experiment with raw data plus the raw data passed through 6 Laguerre-Gauss filters with a spread of 25 pixels. Bottom-left: experiment with raw data plus the raw data passed through 6 Laguerre-Gauss filters with a spread of 15 pixels. Bottom-right: observer-averaged detectabilities from all three experiments.

4. PSYCHOPHYSICAL RESULTS

In Fig. 5 we present the human results for the experiment with Gaussian lumps. In all the plots, we present the percent correct mapped to detectability. This is just a monotonic transformation of the data. Specifically,

$$\text{detectability} = \sqrt{2}\Phi^{-1}(\text{proportion correct}) \tag{6}$$
$$\text{where } \Phi(x) = \int_{-\infty}^{x} \exp(-x^2)\, dx.$$

This measure is often used in order to compare human results with model observers.

The top-left plot in Fig. 5 tracks the detectability of the human observers vs. lump intensity for the 2AFC_RAW experiment with images defined with Gaussian lumps. Each symbol indicates the detectability of one observer and the line is the observer-averaged detectability. The top-right and bottom-left plots show the human observer results for the 2AFC_FILTER (lgg25) and 2AFC_FILTER (lgg15) experiments. The bottom-right plot summarizes the data showing the observer averaged detectabilities for each experiment. Specifically, observer-averaged performance increased when we added filtered information to the experiment. Also, there was more of an increase when we used

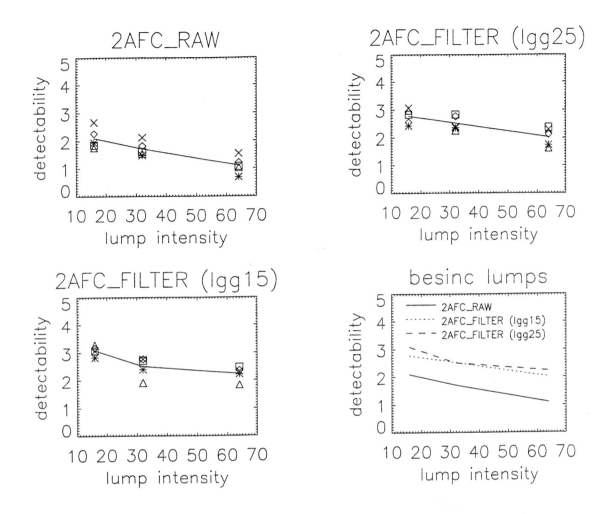

Figure 7. Human detectability for the images with besinc lumps. Symbols track individual observers and lines track observer-averaged performance. Top-left: experiment with just the raw data. Top-right: experiment with raw data plus the raw data passed through 6 Laguerre-Gauss filters with a spread of 25 pixels. Bottom-left: experiment with raw data plus the raw data passed through 6 Laguerre-Gauss filters with a spread of 15 pixels. Bottom-right: observer-averaged detectabilities from all three experiments.

the filters defined with the Gaussian envelope that matched the signal. This trend is seen when the images were defined with circ and besinc lumps too (Figs. 6 and 7). However, the differences between results from the two 2AFC_FILTER experiments are not as obvious.

We tested the significance of the observed differences using the paired t-test on the detectability differences. First, we compared the detectabilities from the 2AFC_RAW and the 2AFC_FILTER (lgg15) experiments. So, for each modality and observer, we subtracted the 2AFC_RAW detectability from the 2AFC_FILTER (lgg15) detectability. Thus, there are 45 sample differences (9 modalities and 5 observers) for this t-test. The null hypothesis is that the mean difference is zero. The results are that we can reject this hypothesis at a p-value less than .001. We can also reject the null hypothesis when we compare the detectabilities from the 2AFC_RAW and 2AFC_FILTER (lgg25) experiments. Finally, we can even reject the null hypothesis when we compare the detectabilities from the two 2AFC_FILTER experiments.

We took this analysis a step further. We also tested the significance on a modality-by-modality basis using the Wilcoxon signed-rank test on paired observations (a total of 9 tests each with 5 samples). When we compared the detectabilities from the 2AFC_RAW and 2AFC_FILTER (lgg15) experiments, we were able to reject the null hypothesis that the differences are zero at a p-value of .01 for *all* modalities. Qualitatively, with 5 observers, this was a result of the fact that each observer performed better in the 2AFC_FILTER (lgg15) experiment than in the 2AFC_RAW experiment. When we compared detectabilities from the 2AFC_RAW and 2AFC_FILTER (lgg 25) experiments, we were able to reject the null hypothesis for all modalities *except* Gaussian lumps with lump intensity 16 and circ lumps with lump intensity 64. For these two modalities, one observer performed better in the 2AFC_RAW experiment than in the 2AFC_FILTER (lgg 25) experiment. Finally, when we compared detectabilities from the 2AFC_FILTER experiments, we were able to reject the null hypothesis for all images with lump intensities equal to 64 and circ lumps with lump intensity equal to 32.

5. CONCLUSIONS

In summary, providing redundant information in the form of filtered versions of the raw data improves human signal detection performance across a variety of image classes. However, it is not clear yet whether the performance improvement is a result of one filter, or whether the human is using the multiple channels of visual input to make a decision.

We also note that for lumpy images with large lump intensities (more difficult experiments), the actual filter spread affected the human performance. Specifically, it seems that the human observers were able to use the filtered images better when the defining Gaussian envelope of the filters matched the signal.

In order to resolve whether human observers can utilize multiple channels of information, we are continuing experiments. Specifically, we are repeating the 2AFC_FILTER experiments, but we are providing 3 channels of filtered images (instead of 6) and no raw data to the observer. Finally, we plan to repeat the experiments one last time, providing the image passed through only one filter. This will give us a baseline (performance from pure smoothing) from which we can check if there is any additional improvement when more information is provided to the observer.

REFERENCES

1. Abbey C. K. "Assessment of reconstructed images," *PhD. Dissertation, Graduate Interdisciplinary Program in Applied Mathematics, University of Arizona, 1998.*
2. H. H. Barrett, Craig K. Abbey, B. Gallas and Miguel Eckstein. "Stabilized Estimates of Hotelling-Observer Detection Performance in Patient Structured Noise", Proc. SPIE Medical Imaging, 1998, 3340:27-43.
3. B. D. Gallas and H. H. Barrett. "Approximating Optimal Templates for Signal Detection in Stochastically Defined Images", Optical Society of America Annual Meeting, Baltimore, MD, October, 1998. (www.math.arizona.edu/~gallas/radiology/rad_home.html)
4. Gilland D. R., Tsui B. M. W., McCartney W. H., Perry J. R. and Berg J. "Determination of the optimum filter function for SPECT imaging," *The Journal of Nuclear Medicine, May 199,* **29-5**, 643-650.
5. K. J. Myers "Visual Perception in correlated noise," *PhD. Dissertation, Optical Sciences Center, University of Arizona, 1985.*
6. J. P. Rolland and H. H. Barrett "Effect of Random Background Inhomogeneity on Observer Detection Performance," *J. Opt. Soc. Am. A., May 1992,* **9-5,** 649-658.

Further investigation of the effect of phase spectrum on visual detection in structured backgrounds

François O. Bochud[*], Craig K. Abbey and Miguel P. Eckstein

Dept. of Medical Physics and Imaging, Cedars Sinai Medical Center, Los Angeles, CA 90048

ABSTRACT

Medical images can be described by their power and phase spectra. Therefore, it is of interest to know how these components influence human observers in detection tasks. Whereas the power spectrum appears to correctly describe the useful statistical properties of computer generated noise images (like white noise, filtered white noise or lumpy backgrounds), this might not be the case for patient structured images. The present study investigates the role of stationarity, power and phase spectra of two types of medical images (mammography and angiography). We consider different categories of images that all have the same mean, and power spectrum. Two-alternative forced-choice experiments are performed on patient structured images, random phase, filtered white noise, and clustered lumpy background. This latter has the property to contain visible structures similar to the ones observed on real mammograms, and (unlike real patient structure) to be stationary by construction. It is shown that model observers can take non-stationarity into account of real images in two different ways. The safest and easiest way consists of applying the model template directly on the images. The other way consists of correcting the performance computed from global quantities with a factor that takes into account local statistical values in the area of interest. Finally, patient structured backgrounds are not fully described by their power spectrum and we show that human observers are able to use some information contained in the phase spectrum.

Keywords: Image noise, power spectrum, phase spectrum, stationarity, detection experiment, mammography, angiography.

1. INTRODUCTION

The detection of a signal superimposed on computer generated image noise has been successfully predicted by a number of computer model observers (e.g. Hotelling, non-prewhitening matched filter with an eye filter and channelized Hotelling observers). Performance predictions of these model observers are often obtained from evaluation of closed form expressions that include information about the signal profile and the covariance or the Wiener spectrum of the image[1-3]. The statistics used in these calculations do not take into account any phase spectrum present in the image, and therefore, the derived model observer performance is phase-invariant. In particular, patient structured images are not stationary and have a phase spectrum that may influence task performance.

In a previous work[4] we showed that human detection performance on patient structured backgrounds were higher than on computer generated images that have the same mean, variance, and power spectrum (random phase noise). This human behavior contrasts with the model performance computed using the power spectrum. Since both types of backgrounds had the same mean, variance and power spectrum, the model performance was the same. The conclusion drawn from that experiment was that the power spectrum was not adequate to describe patient structured images in relation to human performance given that human observers were somehow able to use information contained in the phase spectrum (e.g. in the actual background structure).

However, two possibilities that could explain the previously observed results, but were not investigated, are image non-stationarity, or a difference in higher order statistics. The goal of this study is to investigate these possibilities. In order to isolate human observers' ability to use information in the phase spectrum from effects of background non-stationarity, we first obtain model performance by direct application of the model templates to the images, a method that can take into account some of the local properties of the image. Second, we introduce a computer-generated background (clustered lumpy background[5]) that has local structures but, unlike real patient background, is stationary. Therefore, if human performance degrades from the clustered lumpy background to the random phase it cannot be due to background non-stationarity and must be due to the observers' ability to use information in the phase spectrum.

---

[*] Correspondence: Email: francois@medphysics.csmc.edu; Web: http://www.csmc.edu/medphysics; Phone: +1-310-855-7770; Fax: +1-310-652-8338

Part of the SPIE Conference on Image Perception and Performance
San Diego, California • February 1999
SPIE Vol. 3663 • 0277-786X/99/$10.00

We conduct two-alternative forced-choice (2-AFC) experiments on images that have the same statistical properties (mean, variance, and power spectrum). The considered backgrounds are patient structured images (mammograms and coronary angiograms), clustered lumpy backgrounds (matching the mammographic power spectra), random phase and filtered noise.

2. METHOD AND MATERIAL

2.1. Phase and power spectra

The Fourier transform of an image can be decomposed into an amplitude spectrum and phase spectrum. If we consider a stationary ensemble of images, and compute their Fourier transforms, the ensemble average of the square of the amplitude spectra is the power spectrum (also called Wiener spectrum)[6]. The power spectrum describes the amount of variations present in the images at a given spatial frequency. The phase spectra of an ensemble of images are unlikely to average to any particular pattern because the phase of a given image describes the spatial distribution of the frequency contained in the image. If the images are stationary, then the probability density of the phase of each frequency computed across samples is uniform between 0 and 2π.

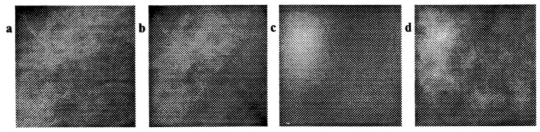

Fig. 1: Example of the role of power and phase spectra on a mammographic image (128x128 pixels, pixel size: 0.3mm). (a) Original image. (b) Image with the same phase spectrum as image-a but with a power spectrum equal to mean value of the entire set. (c) Image with the same power spectrum as image-a but with a random phase spectrum. (d) Image with power spectrum equal to mean value of the entire set and a random phase spectrum.

As an example, Fig. 1 shows the meaning of phase and power spectrum in the case of a mammographic image. Image (a) is a sample mammographic image. In image (b) the power spectrum is replaced by the mean power spectrum computed from an ensemble of images. The phase spectrum remains identical to (a). In image (c), the amplitude spectrum is unchanged and the phase spectrum is random. Finally, image (d) has a random phase spectrum (the same as image (c)) and the mean power spectrum computed from the entire image set.

Comparison of images (a) and (b) (or (c) and (d)) shows that the phase spectrum contains the information about the localization of the structures within the image. Comparison of images (a) and (c) (or (b) and (d)) shows that the power spectrum contains the information about the amount of fluctuations throughout the image without any concern about the location. This is especially visible when comparing images (a) and (c) where the amount of fluctuations (power spectra) is the same but the localizations of these fluctuations (phase spectra) are different. In one case, the phase spectrum is such that some structures can be easily recognized, whereas in the other case the randomness of the phase spectrum makes the appearance of such structures very unlikely.

2.2. Image backgrounds

We investigated two types of patient structured backgrounds and three categories of computer generated images.

2.2.1. Patient structured backgrounds

The patient structured backgrounds are square samples taken from digital mammograms and digital coronary angiograms at monitor screen resolution. Because patient structured images contain low frequency structures, the computation of their power spectra with a discrete Fourier transform method requires caution with regard to edge discontinuities. This problem can be solved by applying a window on the images prior computing to their Fourier transform[7]. For a complete description of the method used in this study, the reader is referred to reference[5]. The measured power spectra for the two backgrounds of interest are displayed in Fig. 2. It can be seen that both these spectra have a power law shape at low frequency (with a slope of -3.7 for mammography and -3.4 for angiography) that begin to plateau at high frequency.

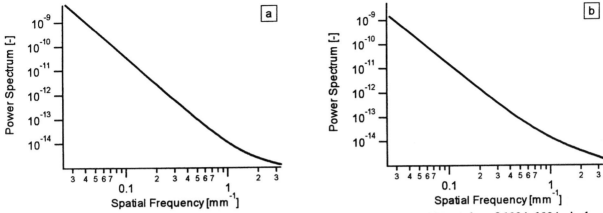

Fig. 2: Radially averaged power spectra measured on (a) mammograms (85 samples of 1024x1024-pixel images, pixel size=0.04mm), and (b) angiograms (212 samples of 256x256-pixels images, pixel size=0.3mm)

2.2.2. Random phase noise

Most of the time, images are assumed stationary and fully described by their mean, variance, and power spectrum. This motivated us to generate stationary backgrounds that have a power spectrum equal to the one measured on patient structured images[4]. These backgrounds are generated in the Fourier domain. Their amplitude is equal to the square root of the power spectrum, and their phase spectrum is random and independent in each frequency with a uniform probability density between 0 and 2π. In order to obtain real images, the symmetry of the phase spectrum (ϕ) is odd:

$$g_r(\mathbf{r}) = \mathfrak{I}^{-1}\left\{\sqrt{W(\mathbf{u})}e^{i\phi(\mathbf{u})}\right\} \quad , \tag{1}$$

where "$\mathfrak{I}$" is the Fourier transform operator, $\mathbf{r}$ is the spatial coordinate and $\mathbf{u}$ is the frequency coordinate. If the power spectrum is set equal to the one of the patient structured images, and if we have a pseudo-random number generator for the phase spectrum, we can get an infinite number of realizations of images having the same power spectrum as the real images.

2.2.3. Filtered white noise

As a verification of the random phase noise, we also performed the experiment on filtered white noise with a power spectrum W. A realization of this kind of noise is obtained by filtering a white noise image ($n(\mathbf{r})$) with the square root of the power spectrum:

$$g_f(\mathbf{r}) = \mathfrak{I}^{-1}\left\{\sqrt{W(\mathbf{u})}\,\mathfrak{I}\{n(\mathbf{r})\}\right\} \quad . \tag{2}$$

This type of background is very similar the random phase noise and is not expected to induce any detectability difference.

2.2.4. Clustered lumpy background

Random phase and filtered white noise backgrounds are very unlikely to contain recognizable structures similar to those found in patient structured images. This is the reason why we developed a third category of simulated backgrounds that can be adjusted to have the same statistics (mean, and power spectrum) as the real images. This type of background, called "clustered lumpy background"[5] is a generalization of the type I lumpy background described by Rolland and Barrett[8]. It can be shown to be stationary and to contain structures that look like the real mammograms. Moreover, its statistical properties are analytically tractable

The clustered lumpy background is generated by first producing a random uniform distribution of K delta functions as in the type I lumpy background method. This serves as a "cluster map". Each of these positions ($\mathbf{r}_k$) is used as an origin for a second process whereby a random number (N_k) of delta functions are randomly positioned. The number N_k in the kth cluster is a Poisson random variable and the positions $\mathbf{r}_{kn}$ are selected using a probability density function f($\mathbf{r}$). The K delta functions are then removed from the image and replaced by K clusters of delta functions. Finally each delta function serves as the origin for a blob defined using a function b($\mathbf{r}/a, \mathbf{R}_\theta$), where a is a random scaling factor, $\mathbf{R}_\theta$ is the rotation matrix that rotates the whole blob, and the angle θ is a random variable. A different angle and scale can be used for each of the

$M = \sum_{k=1}^{K} N_k$ delta function locations. The blobs are then summed to create the image. Formally, the value of an image g at position **r** is then:

$$g(\mathbf{r}) = \sum_{k=1}^{K} \sum_{n=1}^{N_k} b\left(\frac{1}{a_{kn}}(\mathbf{r} - \mathbf{r}_k - \mathbf{r}_{kn}), \mathbf{R}_{\theta_{kn}}\right) \quad . \tag{3}$$

For a given condition (mammography or angiography) and for all the categories of backgrounds (original, random phase, filtered white noise, and clustered lumpy) the first order statistics are controlled by the background mean and variance. All mammographic images have a mean value of 114.5 gray levels and a standard deviation of 40 gray levels. For the angiographic images, the average mean value measured over the whole set of real images is 100.0 gray levels and the average standard deviation is 20.5 gray levels. For the random phase and filtered white noise with angiographic power spectrum, each image mean is 100.0 gray levels and each image standard deviation is 20.5 gray levels.

2.3. Generation of signals

The imaging systems investigated in this study have gray levels proportional to the radiation exposure. Therefore, an image containing the signal (g_s) is simulated by multiplication of the background (**b**) and the signal shape pixel by pixel:

$$\mathbf{g}_s = (\mathbf{s} + 1) \otimes \mathbf{b} \tag{4}$$

where "$\otimes$" means pixel by pixel multiplication, and where $s+1 = \exp(-\mu t)$. The attenuation coefficient μ defines the signal contrast and **t** is the simulated object thickness. In this study, the signal is a 2D-projected sphere (1cm diameter) filtered by the modulation transfer function of the image system.

We considered 128x128 pixel images at a pixel size equal to the monitor pixel (0.3mm). This means that the angiogram were displayed without modification, whereas the real mammograms have been averaged in order to have a pixel size close to 0.3mm. For each condition, we used 300 different image realizations. Fig. 3 shows an example of each background condition.

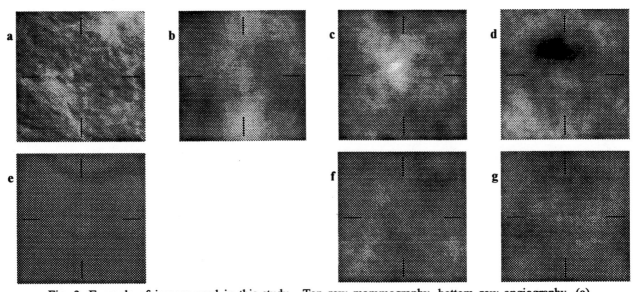

Fig. 3: Example of images used in this study. Top row mammography, bottom row angiography. (a) original, (b) clustered lumpy, (c) random phase, (d) filtered white noise, (e) original, (f) random phase, (g) filtered white noise.

2.4. Psychophysical studies

We performed a two-alternative forced-choice experiment (2-AFC) in which the observer had to detect a 2D projected sphere (1cm diameter) superimposed on a noisy background (either patient structured or computed generated noise). Each image is divided in two parts of 128x128 pixels. Possible target locations are at the center of each image part, and are indicated by cues in order to minimize location uncertainty. The backgrounds of the two locations are independent in order to avoid correlation of the responses from one location to another.

Four human observers were involved in this study. All are well trained to this kind of experiment and were using their usual sight correction (glasses or lenses). The viewing distance was free, but observers tended to a mean distance of about 50cm.

2.5. Data analysis

Once trained for the detection task, the observers performed five sessions of 100 trials for each condition of interest. The measured performance is the percent of correct answers (PC) transformed into a detectability index (d_a):

$$d_a = \sqrt{2}\, \Phi^{-1}(PC) \quad , \tag{5}$$

where Φ is the cumulative Gaussian function. The detectability index d_a is equivalent to the standard d' under the assumption of Gaussian observer responses[9]. The index of detectability is approximately linear with signal contrast and independent of number of locations[10].

2.6. Material

The digital mammograms were obtained by a digital 510(K)-Bennett mammographic unit (Trex Medical Corporation, Waltham, MA-USA) (courtesy of University of California Los Angeles Medical Center). They have a pixel size of 0.04mm and are coded as 14 bits per pixel. The coronary angiograms were obtained on an 8-bit 512x512 pixels digital unit. They have a pixel size of 0.3mm. Both imaging systems have gray levels proportional to the x-ray exposure.

Images were presented on an Image systems M17L 0.3mm pixel size monochrome gray-scale monitor operated by a Md2/PCI video board (Dome Imaging System, inc., Waltham, MA-USA). This board uses a 10-bit digital-to-analog converter and gives the opportunity to truly adjust the relationship between digital value (e.g. gray level) and monitor output (e.g. luminance). The experiments were performed with a perceptually linearized gray level output[11].

2.7. Model observers

We also consider two simple linear observers: the non-prewhitening matched-filter observer (NPW), and the non-prewhitening matched-filter observer with an eye filter (NPWE). The NPW observer is equivalent to the ideal observer in white noise[1]. The NPWE observer has a behavior similar to human observers in low-pass noise[12]. By definition, a linear observer computes its response by performing the scalar product of a quantity called "template" with the same dimensionality as the image.

The strategy of the NPW observer consists of performing the scalar product of the mean signal (s) and the image (g). The response of this observer is a scalar given by:

$$\lambda_{NPW}(g) = s^t g \quad , \tag{6}$$

If we assume that the image noise is stationary and Gaussian distributed, it can be shown that the detectability (d') of this observer is expressed as a ratio of integrals in the Fourier domain.

$$d'^2_{NPW} = \frac{2\bar{b}^2 \left(\int |\tilde{s}(u)|^2 du \right)^2}{\int |\tilde{s}(u)|^2 W(u) du + \int |\tilde{s}_1(u)|^2 W(u) du} \tag{7}$$

where $\tilde{s}(u) = \Im\{s(r)\}$, $\tilde{s}_1(u) = \Im\{s(r)(s(r)+1)\}$, and $\bar{b}$ is the mean background level.

The NPWE observer applies a similar strategy except that the signal by which the image is multiplied is filtered by the square of the visual response function (v).

$$\lambda_{NPWE}(g) = \left(DFT^{-1}\left\{ DFT\{s\}|v|^2 \right\} \right)^t g \quad , \tag{8}$$

where "DFT" is the discrete Fourier transform operator. The used visual response function is the one proposed by Burgess[12]. It is a 2D isotropic band-pass filter that peaks at 4 cycles/degree. The detectability of this observer can also be expressed as a ratio of integrals in the Fourier domain:

$$d'^2_{NPWE} = \frac{2\bar{b}^2 \ \left(\int |\tilde{s}(\mathbf{u})|^2 |\tilde{v}(\mathbf{u})|^2 \, d\mathbf{u}\right)^2}{\int |\tilde{s}(\mathbf{u})|^2 \, W(\mathbf{u}) |\tilde{v}(\mathbf{u})|^4 \, d\mathbf{u} + \int |\tilde{s}_2(\mathbf{u})|^2 \, W(\mathbf{u}) \, d\mathbf{u}} \quad , \tag{9}$$

where $\tilde{s}_2(\mathbf{u}) = \Im\left\{\Im^{-1}\left\{\tilde{s}(\mathbf{u})|\tilde{v}(\mathbf{u})|^2\right\}(s(\mathbf{r})+1)\right\}$.

There are two differences between the two expressions of d' (Eq. 7 and 9) and their additive signal equivalent[12]. First, the numerator is multiplied by $2\bar{b}^2$, which comes from the fact that the signal amplitude is proportional to the background level. Second, the denominator contains an additive term that takes into account the fact that the noise has a slightly different spectrum when the signal is present.

3. RESULTS

3.1. Human observers

Fig. 4 shows the performance of the four human observers for the different categories of image tested. Each point is d_a computed from the mean value of PC across five experiment sessions (Eq. 5), and the error bars are standard errors computed on PC across the five sessions and transformed into d_a. It can be seen that for either mammographic or angiographic backgrounds, random phase noise and filtered white noise do not result in different performance levels. It is also seen that the performance with original medical images is higher than the performance with random phase. Finally, the clustered lumpy background induces a performance significantly higher than random phase and original images.

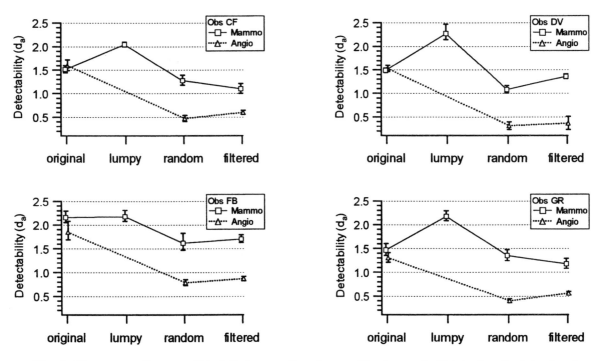

Fig. 4: Observers performance (d_a) plotted versus the category of background. Original: patient structured image; lumpy: clustered lumpy background (mammography only); random: random phase noise; filtered: filtered white noise. Error bars are standard errors computed from performance variability across 5 sessions.

3.2. Model observers

The performance of the two model observers (NPW and NPWE) are computed in two different ways. . First, d' is directly computed from the image statistics (power spectrum) according to Eq. 7 and 9. Fig. 5 shows the results of the two models. Second, the model performance is measured by applying the template on each image used by the human observers according to Eq. 6 and 8. This method (unlike the former) takes into account background non-stationarity. Model templates are applied to the images in three sessions of 100 trials each randomly chosen without replacement out the whole set of 300 different images. It can be seen that the frequency formulas and the application of the template on the images give the same results for all stationary backgrounds (clustered lumpy, random phase, and filtered white noise). This equivalence also holds for original angiographic background but not for the original mammographic background. This shows that mammographic background is non-stationary and that computation of d' from the power spectra (which assumes stationarity) can lead to error in the predicted performance.

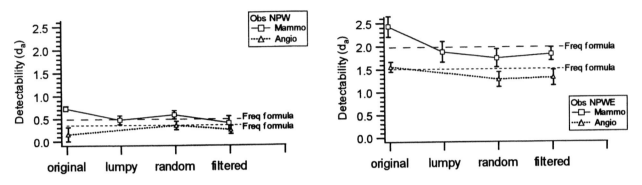

Fig. 5: Model observer performance plotted versus the categories of background. The points correspond to the results of the applied templates on the images (d$_a$) and the horizontal dashed lines are the results of computation in the Fourier domain (d').

4. DISCUSSION

4.1. Image non-stationarity and computation of model performance

For the original mammographic background, the fact that the model performance computed by direct application of the template is higher suggests that some local image properties might be different in the area around the signal (non-stationarity). This is actually the case and Fig. 6 shows a contour plot of the mean and standard deviation of each pixel measured across all image samples. These plots demonstrate that the mammographic backgrounds are clearly not stationary: the left part of the image has a higher mean level and the center part of the image has less fluctuation than the borders. We surmise that this kind of non-stationarity comes from the low frequencies present in the real images that define the global shape of the breast. Our results therefore show that model performance for the mammographic backgrounds should be computed by direct application of the model on the image and that the frequency domain integration (assuming stationarity) might introduce errors in performance predictions.

An interesting possibility is to correct the value of d' computed from the Fourier domain integration by the local values of mean level and standard deviation that are in the center of the image (where the signal actually appears). By taking a mean value of 120 and a standard deviation of 32 rather than 114.5 and 40 as originally assumed, the value of d' obtained from the frequency calculation has to be corrected by a factor of 1.31 ($= \frac{120}{114.5} \frac{40}{32}$). This gives us a value of d'$_{NPWE}$ equal to 2.59 which is no longer significantly different than the value obtained by direct application of the model on the images. Therefore, a computation of the model performance by Fourier integration with a correction, that takes into account some of the local properties of the image around the signal location, is equivalent to the performance obtained by application of the template on the images[13-15]. This implies that local stationarity in the area of the signal appears to be a reasonable assumption.

4.2. Human observer ability to use information in the phase spectrum

Human and model performances (by direct application of the templates) are degraded from the mammographic and angiographic background to the random phase noise. Our results suggest that the degradation in human performance in these and past experiments can at least be partly explained by image non-stationarity. However, the magnitude of the degradation for the human observer (especially in the angiographic background) seems to be larger than the model degradation suggesting that perhaps image non-stationarity might not account for all the human degradation.

In order to experimentally isolate effects of non-stationarity from human observers' ability to use phase information, we introduced a computer generated background with local structures that is nevertheless stationary, isotropic, and has the same mean, variance, and power spectrum as the random phase backgrounds. Our results show that human observers perform significantly better in clustered lumpy backgrounds than in random phase noise, whereas model observers are insensitive. Since we controlled for image non-stationarity, this experiment shows conclusively (unlike the experiments with real patient backgrounds) that human observers are not simply cross-correlating the image like the NPW or the NPWE observers. The human observer strategy might be either another type of cross-correlation or might be non-linear. In both cases, the human observer has to be influenced by the phase spectrum; otherwise, there would not be detectability difference between clustered lumpy backgrounds and random phase backgrounds.

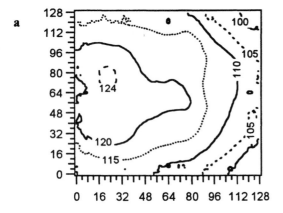 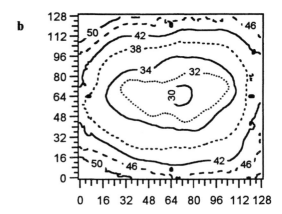

Fig. 6: Contour plot of the mean (a) and standard-deviation (b) of each pixel of the original mammograms measured across the whole set of images (the units are in gray levels). Each individual image has an image mean of 114.5 and a standard-deviation of 40 gray levels.

5. CONCLUSION

The goal of this study was to evaluate the role of the power and phase spectra, and the applicability of model observer to describe detection performance in patient structured images. It is shown that due to non-stationarity in the real patient structured backgrounds model observer should be computed by direct application of the template and use of the Fourier integration might lead to errors in the predicted performance. However, a correction that takes into account the non-stationarity effect (which is basically a low-frequency effect) in the Fourier integration formula can correctly predict model performance.

Like in past experiments we found that human performance degraded from original patient structured backgrounds to random phase. Unlike our previous work, our present results suggest that this degradation is in part or all due to image non-stationarity. However a final experiment that controlled for image non-stationarity (clustered lumpy backgrounds) still showed human performance degradation from the original to the random phase condition. This result allows us to conclude that human observers use information in the phase spectrum. This might imply that human observers apply a more complex linear or non-linear strategy.

ACKNOWLEDGMENTS

We are very grateful to Dr Carolyn Kimme-Smith from University of California Los Angeles who made the digital mammograms available for this study. We would also like to acknowledge Darko Vodopich, George Ruan and Christie Follett who spent long sessions observing images. This work has been funded by the Swiss National Fund for Scientific Research and the National Institute of Health (NIH) ROI HL 53455.

REFERENCES

1. Wagner RF, Brown DG, "Unified SNR analysis of medical imaging systems", Physics in Medicine and Biology **30**, 489-518, 1985.

2. Barrett HH, Yao J, Rolland JP, Myers KJ, "Model observers for assessment of image quality", Proceeding of the National Academy of Science, USA **90**, 9758-9765, 1993.
3. Burgess AE, Li X, Abbey C, "Visual signal detectability with two noise components: anomalous masking effects", Journal of Optical Society of America A **14**, 2420-2442, 1997.
4. Bochud FO, Verdun FR, Hessler C, Valley JF, "Detectability on radiological images: The effect of the anatomical noise", proceedings SPIE **2436**, 156-164, 1995.
5. Bochud FO, Abbey CK, Eckstein MP, "Statistical texture synthesis of mammographic images with clustered lumpy backgrounds", Optics Express **4**, 33-43 (1999). [http://epubs.osa.org/oearchive/source/7241.htm]
6. Dainty JC, Shaw R, *Image Science*, Academic, London, 1974.
7. Papoulis A, *Probability, random variables, and stochastic processes*, McGraw-Hill, Inc., New-York, 1991.
8. Rolland JP, Barrett HH, "Effect of random background inhomogeneity on observer detection performance", Journal of Optical Society of America A **9**, 649-658, 1992.
9. Green DM, Swets JA, *Signal detection and psychophysics*, R.E Krieger Publishing Company, New York, 1966.
10. Eckstein MP, Whiting JS, "Visual signal detection in structured backgrounds. I. Effect of number of possible spatial locations and signal contrast", Journal of Optical Society of America A **13**, 1777-1787, 1996.
11. Krupinski E, Roehrig H, Furukawa T, Tang C, "Influence of monitor luminance and tone scale on observer detection performance", proceedings SPIE **3340**, 99-104, 1998.
12. Burgess AE, "Statistically defined backgrounds: Performance of a modified non-prewhitening observer model", Journal of Optical Society of America A **11**, 1237-1242, 1994.
13. Eckstein, M.P., Whiting, J.S., Lesion detection in structured noise, Academic Radiology **3**, 249-253 (1995)
14. Eckstein MP, Abbey CK, Whiting JS, "Human versus model observers in anatomic backgrounds", proceedings SPIE **3340**, 16-26, 1998.
15. Eckstein MP, Bartroff J, Abbey CK, Bochud FO, Whiting JS, "Effect of image compression in model and human observers", proceedings SPIE **3663**, -, 1999.

SESSION 8

Modeling Visual Signal Detection II

Estimation of human-observer templates in two-alternative forced-choice experiments.

Craig K. Abbey,* Miguel P. Eckstein, and François O. Bochud

Dept. of Medical Physics and Imaging, Cedars-Sinai Medical Center, Los Angeles, CA

ABSTRACT

A method is presented for directly estimating the weights, or "linear template" used by an observer performing a signal-known-exactly detection task in a two-alternative forced-choice (2-AFC) experiment. The approach generalizes prior work by Ahumada, and Beard and Ahumada, to 2-AFC experiments and correlated image noise, and yields an unbiased estimate of the observer template. The estimation procedure is checked against a known linear detection strategy, and human-observer templates estimated from some preliminary psychophysical experiments are shown.

Keywords: Visual signal detection, observer template, model observer, two-alternative forced-choice detection.

1 INTRODUCTION

Modeling human visual detection has become an important focus of research in medical imaging because accurate models would allow for efficient optimization of imaging modalities in terms of task performance[1-.8] To this end, a number of linear detection strategies (often referred to as model observers) have been proposed for predicting human performance in noise-limited signal-known-exactly detection tasks. These model observers are typically validated by comparing their performance to the performance of trained human observers in psychophysical studies. However, performance does not uniquely determine the detection strategy since two different strategies can yield identical performance indices over a range of conditions. Hence it is unclear that an observer that predicts performance effects of human observers in one circumstance will generalize to other situations.

The purpose of this work is to describe an alternative to comparisons of performance. We propose to estimate a human-observer template - the array of pixel weights used by the observer - directly from the images and the corresponding observer responses in a two-alternative forced-choice (2-AFC) experiment. The derived observer template can then be compared for similarity to a number of proposed model observers. The derivation of the observer template presented here is an extension of previous work by Ahumada,[9] and Beard and Ahumada[10] for yes-no detection experiments. The basic idea of the method presented here is to take the average difference between the image chosen in a 2-AFC trial (whether its correct or not) and the image that is not chosen. When the images in the 2-AFC experiment are drawn from a multivariate Gaussian distribution, the expected value of this average can be computed analytically. A transformation of the resulting expected value is directly related to the observer template. The technique accommodates correlated noise in the images and internal noise in the observer.

---

*Correspondence: Email: abbey@medphysics.csmc.edu; Telephone: 310 965 8413; Fax: 310 652 8338

Part of the SPIE Conference on Image Perception and Performance
San Diego, California • February 1999
SPIE Vol. 3663 • 0277-786X/99/$10.00

In this paper, we derive the relationship between a linear observer template and the expected difference between the chosen and not-chosen images in a 2-AFC experiment under Gaussian assumptions on the images that are described in detail below (Section 2.3). We have tested this relationship using linear model observers in Gaussian noise (where all the assumptions built into the derivation are satisfied). We also report some preliminary findings with human observers in white noise.

We believe this approach may be a helpful tool for understanding how human observers perform noise limited detection tasks, and therefore, for predicting human performance in detection tasks relevant to medical imaging. The computational requirements for obtaining the necessary average images can be made relatively modest by a judicious choice of image correlation structure, and hence the method can be implemented into existing 2-AFC experimental protocols fairly easily.

2 THEORY

The main intuition behind our approach is that somehow the difference between the image that was chosen as containing the signal and the one that was not chosen yields some information about the observer template used to make the decision. In this section we derive an explicit relationship between the observer template and the expected difference in the chosen and not-chosen images.

Three key assumptions are used to obtain the main result of this paper. Therefore, before proceeding with the derivation, we list and describe each assumption in general terms.

Assumptions:

1. A human observer uses a **linear** detection strategy to perform the detection task. This assumption means that the observer applies a weight to each pixel in the image and then sums the result (along with some internal noise) to create an internal response variable. The weights are fixed (nonadaptive) from trial to trial.

   Human observers are clearly able to use image intensities in a nonlinear fashion in many circumstances or else they would be totally incapable of performing many kinds of texture discrimination tasks. Nonlinear processes (i.e. nonlinear transducers or contrast-gain control) have long been used to analyze human detection performance in noise-free detection tasks with stimuli that are often presented for short durations by medical standards[11,12].

   Linear detection strategies have been successful models of human observers in noise limited detection of a fixed (nonrandom), spatially compact signal profile with long presentation times[13-17] (greater than 200ms). Furthermore, when the image intensities obey a Gaussian distribution with the same covariance matrix in both the signal-present and signal-absent images, there is no intrinsic advantage to a nonlinear detection strategy. In this case, the ideal observer can be shown to use a linear detection strategy.[14] Nevertheless, the presumption of a linear observer is a strong assumption that limits the applicability of this approach to tasks in which it applies.

2. Internal noise in the human observer response obeys a Gaussian distribution and is statistically independent of the images. Since the internal noise component is inherently unobservable for humans, we are free to model it with any distribution that provides reasonable fits to observed data. Evidence supporting a Gaussian internal noise component in noisy detection tasks can be found in work be Burgess et al[13,18], Pelli,[19] and more recently by Eckstein et al.[20]

3. The distribution of image intensities obeys a multivariate Gaussian distribution with a specified mean image and covariance matrix. It is often the case that the "two" images in a 2-AFC experiment are in fact two separate subregions of a single image. In this case the two subregions must be spatially separated enough

that they are effectively uncorrelated. This step is not so much an assumption as a requirement since it can be implemented by the investigator using images generated with pseudo-random numbers.

The derivation of the method we propose is somewhat involved. In particular, it requires a complete model of how a 2-AFC task is performed for a linear detection strategy, and how the generation of 2-AFC decisions obtained from Gaussian-distributed images are related to figures of merit for the detection task. Sections 2.1 through 2.4 describe this process in some detail. In section 2.5, the main theoretical result of the paper is presented linking the observer template to a expectation involving the images used in the 2-AFC experiment and the decisions derived from these images. In section 2.6 this relationship is used to obtain an unbiased estimate of the observer template by replacing expectations with sample averages.

2.1   Formation of internal response variables

An observer can be presumed to perform a 2-AFC detection task by formulating scalar responses to the two images in each trial of the experiment. The image that elicits the larger response is the one chosen by the observer as containing the signal. This approach does not involve any assumptions (yet) since any strategy for performing a 2-AFC task can be described by the comparison of scalar response variables.

We will represent the two images in a trial of a 2-AFC experiment as the vectors $\mathbf{g}^+$ and $\mathbf{g}^-$. The number of elements in each vector is equal to the number pixels in each image. The superscript "+" or "−" refers to the presence or absence of the signal. If necessary, a particular trial is indicated by a subscript. Hence, $\mathbf{g}_i^+$ is the vector of pixel intensities for the signal-present image in the ith trial and $\mathbf{g}_i^-$ is the corresponding signal-absent image vector.

The formation of a response variable from an image is mathematically modelled by a scalar-valued function of the pixel intensities. As described above in assumption 1, we follow much of the work on noise-limited detection of spatially compact signals and assume that this function is a linear combination of the pixel intensities. Hence the observer response can be implemented through an inner product of the image ($\mathbf{g}^+$ or $\mathbf{g}^-$) with an observer template $\mathbf{w}$. Each element of $\mathbf{w}$ is a weight associated with corresponding pixel in the image. Hence $\mathbf{w}$ itself can be displayed as an image. Since human observers are subject to internal noise in the response variables (this is why it is possible to obtain different decisions from the same pair of images in repeated trials), we add a scalar random variable to the output of the inner product in forming the response. The resulting formula defining the response to the signal-present image is given by

$$r^+ = \mathbf{w}^t \mathbf{g}^+ + \varepsilon^+, \tag{1}$$

and the response to the signal-absent image is given by

$$r^- = \mathbf{w}^t \mathbf{g}^- + \varepsilon^-, \tag{2}$$

where ε^+ and ε^- represent the internal noise in each response.

Although it is an explicit component of both (1) and (2), $\mathbf{w}$ is not presumed to be known in this work. The goal is to estimate $\mathbf{w}$ from the results of a 2-AFC experiment.

2.2   2-AFC decisions

From the images $\mathbf{g}^+$ and $\mathbf{g}^-$, the observer identifies one of the two images as containing the signal by comparing r^+ to r^-. If the response to the signal present image is larger than the signal absent image, then a correct decision is made, if not, an incorrect decision is made. This step is written

$$r^+ \overset{\text{incorrect}}{\underset{\text{correct}}{\lessgtr}} r^-.$$

An equivalent expression for this comparison utilizing (1) and (2) is

$$\mathbf{w}^t\left(\mathbf{g}^+ - \mathbf{g}^-\right) + \left(\varepsilon^+ - \varepsilon^-\right) \overset{\text{incorrect}}{\underset{\text{correct}}{\lessgtr}} 0.$$

For convenience we will define $\Delta\mathbf{g} = \mathbf{g}^+ - \mathbf{g}^-$ and $\Delta\varepsilon = \varepsilon^+ - \varepsilon^-$. With this change in notation we can write

$$\mathbf{w}^t\Delta\mathbf{g} + \Delta\varepsilon \overset{\text{incorrect}}{\underset{\text{correct}}{\lessgtr}} 0. \tag{3}$$

The result of (3) tells us whether a correct decision was made, but does not clearly specify which image was chosen. We can specify the difference between the image that was chosen and the image not chosen for a given trial in terms of $\mathbf{w}$, $\Delta\mathbf{g}$, and $\Delta\varepsilon$. Let $\mathbf{g}^{\text{chosen}}$ be the image chosen by an observer in a trial and let $\mathbf{g}^{\text{not chosen}}$ be the image not chosen in the trial. We can express the difference between $\mathbf{g}^{\text{chosen}}$ and $\mathbf{g}^{\text{not chosen}}$ by

$$
\begin{aligned}
\mathbf{g}^{\text{chosen}} - \mathbf{g}^{\text{not chosen}} &= \Delta\mathbf{g}\, \text{sgn}\left(r^+ - r^-\right) \\
&= \Delta\mathbf{g}\, \text{sgn}\left(\mathbf{w}^t\Delta\mathbf{g} + \Delta\varepsilon\right).
\end{aligned} \tag{4}
$$

where sgn is the scalar-valued "signum" function[21] defined by

$$\text{sgn}\left(x\right) = \left\{ \begin{array}{ll} 1, & \text{if } x > 0 \\ 0, & \text{if } x = 0 \\ -1, & \text{if } x < 0 \end{array} \right. . \tag{5}$$

Equation (4) tells us that if the observer chooses the correct image $(r^+ - r^- > 0)$, then $\mathbf{g}^{\text{chosen}} - \mathbf{g}^{\text{not chosen}} = \Delta\mathbf{g}$. If the observer has chosen incorrectly $(r^+ - r^- < 0)$, then $\mathbf{g}^{\text{chosen}} - \mathbf{g}^{\text{not chosen}} = -\Delta\mathbf{g}$. We will assume continuous densities on the observer responses and hence the probability of an equivocal decision $(r^+ - r^- = 0)$ is zero. The second line in (4) recasts the argument of the signum function in terms of $\mathbf{w}$, $\Delta\mathbf{g}$, and $\Delta\varepsilon$.

2.3 Distribution of images and internal noise

We will now appeal to assumptions 2 and 3 above, and impose distributions on the images and internal noise components. Multivariate-normal (Gaussian) distributions are specified for $\mathbf{g}^+$ and $\mathbf{g}^-$. We denote these distributions by

$$\mathbf{g}^+ \sim \text{MVN}\left(\mathbf{s} + \mathbf{b}, \mathbf{K}\right) \qquad \mathbf{g}^- \sim \text{MVN}\left(\mathbf{b}, \mathbf{K}\right), \tag{6}$$

where MVN is meant to indicate the multivariate normal distribution with a given mean and covariance matrix. The image vector $\mathbf{s}$ is the profile of the signal to be detected. In assumption 1 we outlined our rationale for restricting attention to signals with a fixed profile at a fixed location. Hence, $\mathbf{s}$ is considered nonrandom here. The vector $\mathbf{b}$ is the background on which the signal rests. Typically, $\mathbf{b}$ is a uniform (nonrandom) constant in all elements that serves mainly to keep the mean value of the image in the middle of the display range of the monitor on which the 2-AFC experiment is conducted. However, recently some researchers have begun to use random variations in the background as a way to investigate observer internal noise in what are called "twin" background studies[22],[8] In these studies, the background is random from trial to trial but identical in the signal-absent and signal-present images within any given trial. For the purposes of this work, either the fixed background or the twin background may be investigated. For twin background studies, the distributions given in (6) must be interpreted as conditional distributions of the signal-present and signal-absent images given the common background component $\mathbf{b}$.

The covariance $\mathbf{K}$ governs the noise correlation structure in each of the two images. As stated in assumption 3, the noise fluctuations in the signal-present image are presumed to be independent of the noise in the signal-absent image. If "white" noise is used in the experiment, then $\mathbf{K} = \sigma^2 \mathbf{I}$ where σ^2 is the pixel variance and $\mathbf{I}$ is the identity matrix.

From the image distributions in (6), the distribution of $\Delta \mathbf{g}$ is given by

$$\Delta \mathbf{g} = \mathbf{g}^+ - \mathbf{g}^- \sim \text{MVN} \left(\mathbf{s}, 2\mathbf{K} \right). \tag{7}$$

Because the background is the same in both $\mathbf{g}^+$ and $\mathbf{g}^-$, $\mathbf{b}$ disappears from the mean difference leaving only the signal profile $\mathbf{s}$. The uncorrelated noise in the two images leads to addition of the image covariance matrices in their difference.

We note in passing that the method we derive is general enough to accommodate different covariance matrices for $\mathbf{g}^+$ and $\mathbf{g}^-$. This generalization only modifies the covariance of (7) from $2\mathbf{K}$ to $\mathbf{K}_{\mathbf{g}^+} + \mathbf{K}_{\mathbf{g}^-}$, where $\mathbf{K}_{\mathbf{g}^+}$ is the covariance matrix of the signal-present images and $\mathbf{K}_{\mathbf{g}^-}$ is the covariance matrix of the signal-absent images. In this case, the different noise correlation structures, which can be thought of as a different image texture when the signal is present, provide useful information for performing the task. However, a linear detection strategy is incapable of using these second-order, or textural, differences. Hence, we will not pursue this generalization here since it seems highly unlikely that an observer would adopt a linear detection strategy in these circumstances.

Univariate normal distributions are specified for the internal noise components ε^+ and ε^- in (1) and (2). Both components are presumed to be zero-mean with equal variance and to be independent of each other, and hence,

$$\varepsilon^+, \varepsilon^- \sim \text{N} \left(0, \sigma_\varepsilon^2 \right),$$

where σ_ε^2 is the common internal noise variance. With this choice of a distribution on ε^+ and ε^-, the internal noise difference, $\Delta \varepsilon$, is distributed according to

$$\Delta \varepsilon \sim \text{N} \left(0, 2\sigma_\varepsilon^2 \right). \tag{8}$$

As was the case with the image covariance matrices described above, the proposed method can be modified to handle correlations between ε^+ and ε^- or unequal variances. Since models of internal noise do not typically incorporate these extensions, we will not pursue them here.

2.4 Measures of performance

The most general measure of performance in a 2-AFC experiment is the proportion of correct responses, P_C. In terms of decisions made according to (3), the proportion correct is defined by an expectation over both $\Delta \mathbf{g}$ and $\Delta \varepsilon$ as

$$P_C = \left\langle \text{step} \left(\mathbf{w}^t \Delta \mathbf{g} + \Delta \varepsilon \right) \right\rangle_{\Delta \mathbf{g}, \Delta \varepsilon}, \tag{9}$$

where the step function is defined to be 0 for arguments less than 0 and 1 for arguments greater than 0 (note that $\text{step}(x) = \frac{1}{2} + \frac{1}{2} \text{sgn}(x)$). When $\Delta \mathbf{g}$ and $\Delta \varepsilon$ obey the distributions given in (7) and (8), the proportion correct is directly related to another figure of merit, the detectability index d'. For the notation defined above, the observer detectability index is defined by

$$d'_{\mathbf{w}} = \frac{\mathbf{w}^t \mathbf{s}}{\sqrt{\sigma_\varepsilon^2 + \mathbf{w}^t \mathbf{K} \mathbf{w}}}. \tag{10}$$

Note that the detectability index has a subscript to indicate the dependence of the index on the detection strategy incorporated through the observer template $\mathbf{w}$. The relationship between proportion correct and the observer detectability under the normality assumptions used here is given by

$$P_C = \Phi \left(\frac{d'_{\mathbf{w}}}{\sqrt{2}} \right), \tag{11}$$

where Φ is the cumulative normal distribution function.

In a 2-AFC experiment, the proportion correct is typically estimated by

$$\hat{P}_C = \frac{N_C}{N_T}, \tag{12}$$

where N_C is the number of correct decision trials in an experiment, and N_T is the total number of trials in the experiment.

2.5   The expected difference image

The basis of the proposed method is to take the expectation of both sides of (4), and hence we will consider the quantity

$$\langle \mathbf{g}^{\text{chosen}} - \mathbf{g}^{\text{not chosen}} \rangle = \langle \Delta \mathbf{g} \, \text{sgn} \left(\mathbf{w}^t \Delta \mathbf{g} + \Delta \varepsilon \right) \rangle_{\Delta \mathbf{g}, \Delta \varepsilon}. \tag{13}$$

The expectations encompass both the external noise (from the images) in $\Delta \mathbf{g}$ and the internal noise (from the observer) in $\Delta \varepsilon$. Since (4) is a vector equation, the expectation in (13) is interpreted as an expected value in each vector element. If we use the fact that $\Delta \varepsilon$ is statistically independent of $\Delta \mathbf{g}$ (as per assumption 2), equation (13) simplifies to

$$\langle \mathbf{g}^{\text{chosen}} - \mathbf{g}^{\text{not chosen}} \rangle = \langle \Delta \mathbf{g} \, \langle \text{sgn} \left(\mathbf{w}^t \Delta \mathbf{g} + \Delta \varepsilon \right) \rangle_{\Delta \varepsilon} \rangle_{\Delta \mathbf{g}}, \tag{14}$$

where the expected value with respect to the internal noise component has been reduced to a scalar-valued expectation involving the signum function.

The expectation with respect to $\Delta \varepsilon$ in (14) can be computed analytically as[23]

$$\langle \text{sgn} \left(\mathbf{w}^t \Delta \mathbf{g} + \Delta \varepsilon \right) \rangle_{\Delta \varepsilon} = 2\Phi \left(\frac{\mathbf{w}^t \Delta \mathbf{g}}{\sqrt{2} \sigma_\varepsilon} \right) - 1. \tag{15}$$

Utilizing (15) in (14) yields

$$\begin{aligned}
\langle \mathbf{g}^{\text{chosen}} - \mathbf{g}^{\text{not chosen}} \rangle &= \left\langle \Delta \mathbf{g} \left(2\Phi \left(\frac{\mathbf{w}^t \Delta \mathbf{g}}{\sqrt{2} \sigma_\varepsilon} \right) - 1 \right) \right\rangle_{\Delta \mathbf{g}} \\
&= 2 \left\langle \Delta \mathbf{g} \Phi \left(\frac{\mathbf{w}^t \Delta \mathbf{g}}{\sqrt{2} \sigma_\varepsilon} \right) \right\rangle_{\Delta \mathbf{g}} - \langle \Delta \mathbf{g} \rangle_{\Delta \mathbf{g}}. \tag{16}
\end{aligned}$$

From the distribution of $\Delta \mathbf{g}$ given in (7), the expectation in Equation (16) can be computed analytically. The second term on the right side of (16) is given directly from the distribution of $\Delta \mathbf{g}$ by

$$\langle \Delta \mathbf{g} \rangle_{\Delta \mathbf{g}} = \mathbf{s}. \tag{17}$$

The first term of (16) can also be computed analytically but involves a somewhat lengthy derivation. We state the result here as[23]

$$\left\langle \Delta \mathbf{g} \Phi \left(\frac{\mathbf{w}^t \Delta \mathbf{g}}{\sqrt{2} \sigma_\varepsilon} \right) \right\rangle_{\Delta \mathbf{g}} = \Phi \left(\frac{\mathbf{w}^t \mathbf{s}}{\sqrt{2 \left(\sigma_\varepsilon^2 + \mathbf{w}^t \mathbf{K} \mathbf{w} \right)}} \right) \mathbf{s} + \frac{1}{\sqrt{\pi \left(\sigma_\varepsilon^2 + \mathbf{w}^t \mathbf{K} \mathbf{w} \right)}} \exp \left(-\frac{\left(\mathbf{w}^t \mathbf{s} \right)^2}{4 \left(\sigma_\varepsilon^2 + \mathbf{w}^t \mathbf{K} \mathbf{w} \right)} \right) \mathbf{K} \mathbf{w}. \tag{18}$$

This equation can be simplified somewhat using the definition of $d'_\mathbf{w}$ given in (10), and the relation between $d'_\mathbf{w}$ and P_C in (11). With these substitutions, equation (18) simplifies to

$$\left\langle \Delta \mathbf{g} \Phi \left(\frac{\mathbf{w}^t \Delta \mathbf{g}}{\sqrt{2} \sigma_\varepsilon} \right) \right\rangle_{\Delta \mathbf{g}} = P_C \mathbf{s} + \frac{1}{\sqrt{\pi \left(\sigma_\varepsilon^2 + \mathbf{w}^t \mathbf{K} \mathbf{w} \right)}} \exp \left(-\left(\frac{d'_\mathbf{w}}{2} \right)^2 \right) \mathbf{K} \mathbf{w}. \tag{19}$$

Substituting (17) and (19) into (16) yields a final form for the expected difference of

$$\left\langle \mathbf{g}^{\text{chosen}} - \mathbf{g}^{\text{not chosen}} \right\rangle = (2P_C - 1)\,\mathbf{s} + \frac{2}{\sqrt{\pi\left(\sigma_\varepsilon^2 + \mathbf{w}^t\mathbf{K}\mathbf{w}\right)}}\exp\left(-\left(\frac{d'_{\mathbf{w}}}{2}\right)^2\right)\mathbf{K}\mathbf{w}. \tag{20}$$

Equation (20) is the main theoretical result of this paper. Note that the observer template appears explicitly as a vector in the second term of the right-hand side. This fact is the motivation for the estimation procedure described next.

2.6 Estimation of the observer template

The basis of the estimation method is to replace the expectation on the left side of (20) by a sample average. For simplicity, let us denote the expected difference by the variable $\mathbf{z} \equiv \left\langle \mathbf{g}^{\text{chosen}} - \mathbf{g}^{\text{not chosen}} \right\rangle$. We can manipulate the terms of (20) to get

$$\mathbf{K}^{-1}\left(\mathbf{z} - (2P_C - 1)\,\mathbf{s}\right) = \frac{2}{\sqrt{\pi\left(\sigma_\varepsilon^2 + \mathbf{w}^t\mathbf{K}\mathbf{w}\right)}}\exp\left(-\left(\frac{d'_{\mathbf{w}}}{2}\right)^2\right)\mathbf{w}. \tag{21}$$

The right side of this equation is the vector of interest, $\mathbf{w}$, multiplied by a nonnegative scalar also dependent on $\mathbf{w}$. In terms of decisions made using (3) (and both the figures of merit P_C and $d'_{\mathbf{w}}$), the magnitude of $\mathbf{w}$ is arbitrary as long as the variance of the internal noise component remains proportional to $\|\mathbf{w}\|^2$. In other words, a linear observer specified by an observer template $\mathbf{w}$ and internal noise variance σ_ε^2 is identical to the linear observer described by the template $c\mathbf{w}$ and internal noise variance $c^2\sigma_\varepsilon^2$ for any $c > 0$. We can therefore define the quantity on the right side of (21) as the quantity of interest without loss of generality.

An estimate of $\mathbf{w}$ is formed by replacing $\mathbf{z}$ and P_C in (21) by their sample estimates. In a 2-AFC experiments with N_T trials, $\mathbf{z}$ can be estimated from the sample average

$$\widehat{\mathbf{z}} = \frac{1}{N_T}\sum_{i=1}^{N_T}\left(\mathbf{g}_i^{\text{chosen}} - \mathbf{g}_i^{\text{not chosen}}\right).$$

The sample estimate of proportion correct, $\hat{P}_C$, is given in (12). The resulting estimate of $\mathbf{w}$ is given by

$$\widehat{\mathbf{w}} = \mathbf{K}^{-1}\left(\widehat{\mathbf{z}} - \left(2\hat{P}_C - 1\right)\mathbf{s}\right). \tag{22}$$

Since $\widehat{\mathbf{z}}$ is an unbiased estimate of $\mathbf{z}$ (under general conditions a sample average is an unbiased estimate of its mean value[24]) and $\hat{P}_C$ is well known to be an unbiased estimate of P_C, $\widehat{\mathbf{w}}$ is therefore an unbiased estimate of $\mathbf{K}^{-1}\left(\mathbf{z} - (2P_C - 1)\,\mathbf{s}\right)$.

3 EXPERIMENTAL RESULTS

Two sets of experimental results are presented. The first is a validation experiments in which a linear observer template is used to generate data. The goal of the experiments is to see how well the estimation method reproduces this known template, In the second set of experiments some preliminary human data are used to obtain a human-observer template in white noise.

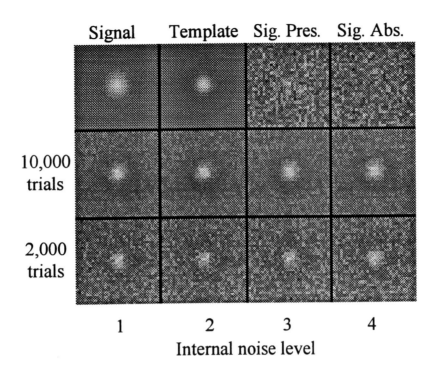

Figure 1: Sample images from Validation experiments. The images in the top row are the mean signal image, the NPWE template, and noisy sample signal-present and signal-absent images. The next two rows of images are estimated templates from 10,000 and 2,000 trials respectively assuming the NPWE strategy. The different columns in each row correspond to difference levels of internal noise.

3.1 Validation experiments

As a check of the estimation procedure, 2-AFC experiments have been conducted using a known template for the detection of a Gaussian "bump" in white noise. The images were 32×32 pixels with a mean intensity of 128 grey-levels (GL). The noise in the images was white (independent from pixel to pixel) with a common variance of 25.0 GL. The signal-present images were generated by adding a Gaussian profile with a standard deviation of 3.0 pixels and an amplitude of 10.0 GL in the center of each image. These images closely resemble the stimuli used by Burgess[13] to investigate human-observers in noise-limited detection tasks.

The observer template used to generate responses is a discrete version of the Modified Nonprewhitening Matched Filter used by Burgess.[17] We will follow Burgess' notational convention and denote this observer by the acronym NPWE (for **Nonprewhitening** observer with **Eye** filter). The observer template is defined as the expected signal filtered by a model of the contrast sensitivity function of the human visual system. Operationally, the template is defined by

$$\mathbf{w}_{\text{NPWE}} = \text{DFT}_{2\text{D}}^{-1} \left(\mathbf{E} * \text{DFT}_{2\text{D}} \left(\mathbf{s} \right) \right),$$

where $\text{DFT}_{2\text{D}}$ is the two-dimensional Discrete Fourier Transform, and $\mathbf{E}$ is the eye-filter. The eye-filter is defined by the function $E\left(\rho\right) = \rho^\alpha \exp\left(-\beta\rho\right)$. The elements of $\mathbf{E}$ are obtained by evaluating $\left|E\left(\rho\right)\right|^2$ at the frequencies of the DFT. Following Burgess, the parameter α was set to 1.3, and β was set so that the maximum point of the eye filter occurred at 4 cycles per degree visual angle. For these experiments, β was set to 5.08 corresponding to an assumed viewing distance of approximately 50.0 cm and a pixel size of 0.60mm. With this value of β, the filter

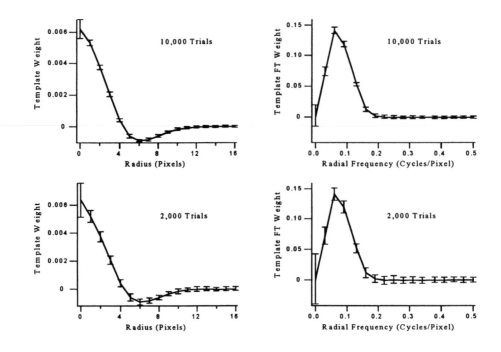

Figure 2: Plots of Radial Averages and errors for 100 templates estimated from 10,000 and 2,000 trials per template. Each plot contains two graphs: the true template weights and the average of the estimated templates with sample error bars computed from the 100 estimated templates. The agreement between the true and average templates is generally below the resolution of the plot.

peak occurs at 0.26 cycles per pixel in the image spectrum. Images of the signal and NPWE-observer template, as well as an example signal-present and signal-absent image are given in the top row of Figure 1. In the observer template, note the darker "surround" that circles a brighter center. The surround is due to the low-frequency suppression implemented by the eye filter.

Four levels of internal noise were checked to see if internal noise in the observer strongly affected the estimation procedure. In each case, the variance of the internal noise was set to be proportional to $\mathbf{w}_{\mathrm{NPWE}}^{t}\mathbf{K}\mathbf{w}_{\mathrm{NPWE}}$, the variance of the observer response due to the (external) image noise. The constants of proportionality used were 0.0 (no internal noise), 0.3, 0.6, and 0.9.

In the first set of experiments, the observer template was estimated 100 times using 10,000 independent trials per estimate at each level of internal noise. Example estimates at each level of internal noise are given in the second row of Figure 1. While the estimates have some visible noise, the center-surround profile of the observer template is clearly visible at all internal noise levels. There does not appear to be any evidence of degradation in the estimates with the internal noise levels tested.

In the second set of experiments, the estimates of the observer template are derived from 2,000 trials per estimate. The purpose of these experiments was to see if the features of the observer template are present in estimates from a more realistic number of trials. Example estimates at each level of internal noise are given in the second row of Figure 1. While the estimates are clearly noisier at 2,000 trials per estimate, the general center-surround character of the observer template still appears to be visible in the estimates.

A more quantitative assessment of the of the quality of the template estimates is given in Figure 2. The template estimates are displayed in terms of radial averages and radial frequency averages. In each plot, the

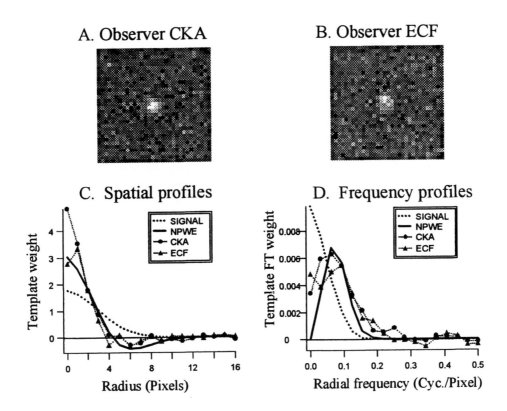

A. Observer CKA

B. Observer ECF

C. Spatial profiles

D. Frequency profiles

Figure 3: Results of psychophysical studies. The images in A and B are the estimated templates for the two observers (CKA and ECF) that participated in the experiments. The plots in C and D compare radial averages of the estimated templates to the signal profile and NPWE observer.

average radial profile and standard deviation – derived from the 100 sample estimates – are plotted along with that of the true template (weighted according to Equation (21)). In most cases, the difference between the true template value and the sample average is less than the resolution of the plot, and hence, the plots only appear to have a single line. The larger error bars near the origin of all the plots is due to the relatively small number of points included in the radial average at these positions. In all cases, the true template is well bracketed by the error bars of the samples. At 2,000 trials per estimate, the template errors are still relatively small compared to the magnitude of the template features.

3.2 Preliminary human-observer study

As an example of how the proposed method can be used to study human observers, we present estimated templates derived from human observer studies on white-noise images. Two observers performed 2,000 2-AFC trials – in 20 sessions of 100 trials – of the white noise detection task described in the previous section. One of the observers (CKA) is an author of this paper and (hopefully) fully aware of research goals of this work. The other observer (ECF) is naive to the goals of the study and compensated for performing the experiments. Both observers have participated in numerous detection tasks of this sort previously. Specific training for this task was conducted in 4 training sessions totalling 210 2-AFC trials.

All experimental data were collected on a high performance monitor (Model M21LMAX, Image Systems Inc., Hopkins, Minnesota), using a display program that was written in the IDL programming environment by the authors. The monitor lookup table was calibrated to a linear scale with a mean luminance setting of 16.0 cd/m^2. The images were displayed against a dark background. Because of the small size of the images (32×32 pixels) the images were upsampled by a factor of 2 for display yielding an effective pixel size of 0.60mm. Furthermore, the two images in each 2-AFC trial were separated by a gap of 32 pixels (19.2mm) on the display.

The results of the psychophysical studies are summarized in Figure 3. The images in Figures 3-A and 3-B are the estimated templates for the two observers. The plots in Figures 3-C and 3-D are radial averages of the two estimated templates, the signal profile, and the NPWE observer in both the spatial domain and the Fourier domain. Note that because of the white noise in the images, the signal profile is in fact the observer template used by the ideal observer. Hence the signal profile represents the optimal weights for performing the task. The plots of the signal and NPWE templates have been scaled by a constant that minimizes the least-squares error with the average of the two human-observer templates. Generally good agreement between the two human observers is seen throughout the figure. When compared to the signal profile in Figure 1, the estimated templates in Figures 3-A and 3-B appear to be noticeably narrower in the their spatial extent. This observation is borne out in the radial plots of Figure 3-C. Both estimated templates appear to be falling off substantially faster than the signal profile, and possibly faster than the NPWE observer template. In Figure 3-D, some low frequency suppression appears to be present in the human-observer templates which does not match the signal profile near the origin of the plot. However, the human observers do not appear to have quite the same level of low frequency suppression found in the NPWE observer template. The data in Figure 3-D indicate a weak "surround" (low-frequency suppression) in the human observers. Also of interest in Figure 3-D is relatively slow falloff of the human observer template at higher frequencies (0.15 to 0.25 cycles/pixel). The human observers appear to be incorporating some spatial frequencies with little or no signal content into their observer templates.

4 CONCLUSIONS

The purpose of this paper has been to present an extension of the observer template estimation method used by Ahumada et al to the 2-AFC experimental paradigm and to accommodate the effects of correlated Gaussian noise in the images. Derivation of an unbiased estimator for a linear observer template is the main theoretical result of the paper. The estimator was validated by repeatedly computing estimates at $10,000$ and $2,000$ trials per estimate. The method was observed to be unbiased (as predicted by the theory) with a reasonable degree of errors in radial averages.

The method was also tested on preliminary psychophysical data from two human observers performing a detection task in white noise. The resulting templates exhibit apparent low frequency suppression that falls somewhere between the full suppression found in the NPWE observer and the total lack of low frequency suppression found in the ideal observer. The human observer templates also appear to extend somewhat further into the frequency domain than either the ideal observer or the NPWE observer. These features of the human-observer templates bear further investigation.

5 REFERENCES

[1] R.F. Wagner and D.G. Brown, "Unified SNR analysis of medical imaging systems," *Phys. Med. Biol.*, Vol. 30, No. 6, 489-518, 1984.

[2] H.H. Barrett, K.J. Myers, and R.F. Wagner, "Beyond signal-detection theory," *Proc. SPIE* 626:231-239, 1986.

[3] K.M. Hanson, "Method of evaluating image-recovery algorithms based on task performance," *J Opt Soc Am A*, 7:1294-1304, 1990.

[4] H.H. Barrett, "Objective assessment of image quality: Effects of quantum noise and object variability," *J Opt Soc Am A*, 7:1266-1278, 1990.

[5] H.H. Barrett, T Gooley, K Girodias, J Rolland, T White, and J Yao, "Linear discriminants and image quality," *Image Vision Comput.* 10, 451-460, 1992.

[6] H.H. Barrett, J. Yao, J. Rolland, and K.J. Myers, "Model observers for assessment of image quality," *Proc. Natl. Acad. Sci.* USA 90, 9758-9765, 1993.

[7] M.P. Eckstein, and J.S. Whiting, "Lesion detection in structured noise," *Acad. Radiol.* 2:249-253, 1995.

[8] A.E. Burgess, X. Li, and C.K. Abbey, "Visual signal detectability with two noise components: anomalous masking effects," *J Opt Soc Am A*, 14:2420-2442, 1997.

[9] A.J. Ahumada, "Perceptual classification images from vernier acuity masked by noise," *Perception* 26, pp. 18, 1996.

[10] B.L. Beard and A.J. Ahumada, Jr., "Relevant image features for vernier acuity," *Perception* 26, pp. 38, 1997.

[11] G.E. Legge, and J.M. Foley, "Contrast masking in human vision," *J Opt Soc Am*, 70, 1458-1471, 1980.

[12] J.M. Foley, "Human luminance pattern-vision mechanisms: masking experiments require a new model," *J Opt Soc Am A*, 11, 1710-1719, 1994.

[13] A.E. Burgess, and H. Ghandeharian, "Visual signal detection. II. Signal-location identification," *J Opt Soc Am A*, 1:900-905, 1984.

[14] K.J. Myers, *Visual perception in correlated noise*, Ph.D. Dissertation, University of Arizona, Tucson, 1985.

[15] J. Rolland, and H.H. Barrett, "Effect of random background inhomogeneity on observer detection performance," *J. Opt. Soc. Am. A*, 9:649-658, 1992.

[16] J. Yao, *Model observers for predicting human performance on signal-detection tasks*, Ph.D. Dissertation, University of Arizona, Tucson, 1994.

[17] A.E. Burgess, "Statistically defined backgrounds: performance of a modified nonprewhitening matched filter model," *J Opt Soc Am A*, 11:1237-1242, 1994.

[18] A.E. Burgess, and B. Colborne, "Visual signal detection. IV. Observer inconsistency," *J Opt Soc Am A*, 5:617-627, 1988.

[19] D. Pelli, *Effects of visual noise*, Ph.D. Dissertation, Cambridge University, Cambridge, 1981.

[20] M.P. Eckstein, and J.S. Whiting, "Visual signal detection in structured backgrounds I. Effect of number of possible locations and signal contrast," *J Opt Soc Am A*, 14:2406-2419, 1996.

[21] G. Dahlquist, Å. Björck, and N. Anderson, *Numerical Methods.* Prentice-Hall, New Jersey. pp. 64, 1974.

[22] M.P. Eckstein, A.J. Ahumada, and A.B. Watson, "Visual signal detection in structured backgrounds. II. Effects of contrast gain control, background variations, and white noise," *J Opt Soc Am A*, 13:1777-1787, 1997.

[23] Detailed derivations of Equations (15) and (18) are available from the authors.

[24] K.V. Mardia, J.T. Kent, and J.M. Bibby, *Multivariate Analysis.* Academic press, San Diego. pp. 51-2, 1979.

Quantitative image quality of spatially filtered x-ray fluoroscopy

Kadri N. Jabri[a] and David L. Wilson[a,b]

[a]Department of Biomedical Engineering
Case Western Reserve University
Cleveland, OH 44106

[b]Department of Radiology
University Hospitals of Cleveland &
Case Western Reserve University
2074 Abington Road
Cleveland, OH 44106

ABSTRACT

One potential method to lower x-ray fluoroscopy dose without compromising image quality is to acquire images at a decreased exposure rate and digitally filter to reduce noise. In both single image frames and image sequences, we investigated the effect of noise-reduction spatial filtering on the detection of stationary cylinders that mimicked arteries, catheters, and guide wires in x-ray imaging. We simulated ideal edge-preserving spatial filters by filtering the noise only and then adding targets for detection. Filters used were three different center-weighted averagers that reduce pixel noise variance by factors of 0.75, 0.5, and 0.25. Detection performance in unfiltered and spatially filtered noisy image sequences and single frames was measured using a reference/test, 9-alternative, adaptive forced-choice method. Performance level was fixed and results were obtained in the form of signal contrast sensitivity. In single images, the effect of filtering on detection was insignificant at all filtering levels. On the other hand, filtering in image sequences improved detectability by as much as 23%, yielding a potential x-ray dose savings of 34%. Comparing results with the prewhitening matched filter model indicated that human observers have improved detection efficiency in spatially filtered image sequences, as compared to white-noise sequences. We conclude that edge-preserving spatial filtering is more effective in sequences than in single frames. Such filtering can potentially improve image quality in noisy image sequences such as x-ray fluoroscopy.

Keywords: x-ray fluoroscopy, medical imaging, image perception, quantitative image quality, detection, spatial filtering

1. INTRODUCTION

X-ray fluoroscopy results in a high radiation dose to patients undergoing long-duration interventional procedures. Cases of severe skin injury following fluoroscopic imaging are documented.[1] One potential method to reduce dose without degrading image quality is to acquire images at a decreased exposure rate and digitally filter to reduce noise.[2-4] To quantitatively assess the effect of different filters on image quality, we measure human observers' ability to detect low-contrast objects in noisy image sequences. As part of ongoing research to better understand and optimize the processing and acquisition of x-ray fluoroscopy,[5-11] we used such studies to investigate temporal filtering of image sequences.[12] In this paper, we investigate simulated edge-preserving, noise-reduction spatial filtering.

Linear low-pass image filters blur edges. To avoid this, a multitude of nonlinear filtering algorithms have been developed to reduce noise without introducing any significant blur.[13] In our experiments, we filter the noise by a low-pass linear filter and then add the signal for detection. This simulates an ideal edge-preserving filter since signal edges and signal energy are perfectly preserved. This simulation method allows for easy modification of the transfer function, thereby allowing different levels of noise reduction and different characteristics of the noise power spectrum.

Further author information: (Send correspondence to D.L.W.)
K.N.J.: Email: knj2@po.cwru.edu
D.L.W.: Email: dlw@po.cwru.edu; Telephone: 216-368-4099; Fax: 216-368-4969

296

Part of the SPIE Conference on Image Perception and Performance
San Diego, California • February 1999
SPIE Vol. 3663 • 0277-786X/99/$10.00

A number of advanced edge-preserving filters are available,[14-16] and our noise-only filtering technique is a reasonable simulation.

In addition to noise reduction and edge blurring, another effect of low-pass filtering is spatial noise correlation. Several reports investigate the effects of spatially correlated noise,[17-19] and structured backgrounds[20-22] on detection in single, or static, images. These studies show that human detection performance is generally degraded by the presence of noise correlation. Recent experiments by Burgess *et al.*[21] indicate that human observers in some situations can partially compensate for spatial noise correlation, but still perform worse than an observer model that can fully prewhiten, or decorrelate, image noise.

In the case of a spatially filtered image sequence, where filtering is applied independently to each frame, noise is spatially correlated but temporally uncorrelated. We anticipate that digital spatial filtering of image sequences might be more advantageous than that of single images since it combines spatial noise reduction with the human observer's ability to filter and reduce the effective noise across time. Moreover, we hypothesize that the adverse effect of spatial noise correlation on detection will be diminished when viewing a sequence where noise correlation in each frame is independent of that in the next. With and without spatial filtering, we measure detection performance in terms of signal contrast sensitivity in single frames and in image sequences.

For convenience, image sequence filters are often evaluated by comparing pixel noise variance before and after filtering.[2,3,23] Based on perception studies on single images, this is probably a naive evaluation. Therefore, in addition to comparing measurements to two observer models, we examine the error associated with using pixel noise reduction as an image quality predictor after filtering.

2. THEORY

2.1. Observer Models

We have extended to the temporal domain two popular signal detection models. The first is the prewhitening matched filter (PWMF), which is also the ideal Bayesian observer for the case of additive noise.[24] The second is a non-prewhitening matched filter model (NPW-HVS) which is modified to incorporate a psychophysically-measured spatiotemporal human visual system (HVS) response. PWMF can fully compensate for spatial noise correlation while NPW-HVS cannot.

2.1.1. PWMF

The PWMF model is a signal detector with exact knowledge of signal and noise characteristics, and it is useful for comparing human observer performance with the best-possible performance. The spatiotemporal signal-to-noise ratio (SNR) of the PWMF model is given by

$$SNR^2_{PWMF} = \iiint \frac{|S(u,v,f)|^2}{N(u,v,f)} \, du \, dv \, df \tag{1}$$

where $S(u,v,f)$ is the signal spectrum, $N(u,v,f)$ is the noise power spectrum, u and v are the spatial frequency coordinates, and f is the temporal frequency coordinate. In our experiments, noise is either white or spatially filtered by the transfer function $H(u,v)$. For a stationary target, the signal spectrum is separable, $S(u,v,f) = S_s(u,v)S_t(f)$. For an image sequence, SNR is given by

$$SNR^2_{PWMF} = \int |S_t(f)|^2 \, df \iint \frac{|S_s(u,v)|^2}{|H(u,v)|^2 \, N_o} \, du \, dv \tag{2}$$

where N_o is the constant power spectrum of the white noise before filtering, and $H(u,v) = 1$ for unfiltered images. To calculate the SNR in single images, the temporal factor, $\int |S_t(f)|^2 \, df$, is simply removed.

2.1.2. NPW-HVS

The modified non-prewhitening matched filter was developed by others to model detection in single images,[25,26] and we have extended it to the time domain.[9,10] In its general form, the SNR of NPW-HVS is given by

$$SNR^2_{NPW-HVS} = \frac{\left[\iiint |S(u,v,f)|^2 |V(u,v,f)|^2 \, du \, dv \, df\right]^2}{\iiint |S(u,v,f)|^2 |V(u,v,f)|^4 N(u,v,f) \, du \, dv \, df + \iiint N_i(u,v,f) \, du \, dv \, df} \tag{3}$$

where $V(u,v,f)$ is the spatiotemporal frequency response of the HVS, and $N_i(u,v,f)$ is the observer internal noise spectrum. We consider a special case where the HVS response is separable, $V(u,v,f) = V_s(u,v)V_t(f)$, and internal noise is zero, $N_i = 0$. SNR is given by

$$SNR^2_{NPW-HVS} = A \, \frac{\left[\iint |S_s(u,v)|^2 |V_s(u,v)|^2 \, du \, dv\right]^2}{\iint |S_s(u,v)|^2 |V_s(u,v)|^4 |H(u,v)|^2 N_o \, du \, dv} \tag{4}$$

where

$$A = \frac{\left[\int |S_t(f)|^2 |V_t(f)|^2 \, df\right]^2}{\int |S_t(f)|^2 |V_t(f)|^4 \, df}. \tag{5}$$

The spatial contrast sensitivity response, $V_s(u,v)$, is based on measurements from traveling sinewave stimuli with a stabilized visual field.[27] It has no DC (zero-frequency) response, and it is similar in form to "eye filter" models used by Burgess.[25] To calculate SNR in single images, the temporal dimension is removed by setting $A = 1$.

2.2. Spatial Filters Applied to Image Frames

We investigate three different spatial 3×3 center-weighted averagers, with three different weight assignments, that are applied independently to each frame in an image sequence. The output of the center-weighted averager, $y(m,n)$, is given below where m and n are discrete spatial coordinates in image space, and K is the center-weight.

$$y(m,n) = \frac{\sum_{i=-1}^{+1} \sum_{j=-1}^{+1} a_{ij} \, x(m+i, n+j)}{K+8}, \quad where \;\; a_{ij} = \left\{ \begin{array}{ll} K & \text{if } i = j = 0 \\ 1 & \text{otherwise} \end{array} \right. \tag{6}$$

We use three levels of filtering that reduce pixel noise variance by factors of 0.75, 0.50, and 0.25, corresponding to K values of 51.13, 18.58, and 6.883, respectively.

In experiments, we simulate ideal edge-preserving spatial filters by first filtering the background noise and then adding the signal for detection. As a result, no edge blurring is introduced and we isolate the effect of edge blurring from those of noise reduction and spatial correlation.

3. METHODS

3.1. Experimental Sessions and Data Collection

We used a variation on an adaptive, interspersed 9-alternative forced-choice technique.[7] For each trial, a low-contrast stationary cylinder was randomly placed in the center of one of 9 fields on the display (Fig. 1). Observers had unlimited viewing time and they indicated where they thought the cylinder resided by using a mouse. Feedback was provided in the form of an audible beep when the response was correct.

Four types of presentation were used: white noise (no filtering) and three levels of spatial filtering. Different types of presentation were randomly interspersed within a single session to reduce the effect of subject effort and attention level on the comparison of results. Observers underwent at least two training sessions before data collection. There were 200 trials for each presentation type.

For each presentation type, contrast was adapted during the course of an experiment to maintain an 80% probability of correct detection, corresponding to a detectability index $d'_{80\%} = 2.405$.[7] Performance level was therefore fixed, and results were gathered in the form of signal contrast sensitivity (inverse of the cylinder contrast, C, as determined below) at the 200th trial. A higher contrast sensitivity measurement indicated an improved ability to detect the target.

Three graduate students, with normal or corrected-to-normal vision, participated as observers. One was an author (KJ), and the two others were naive to the hypotheses. Viewing was binocular at a fixed distance of one meter in a darkened room.

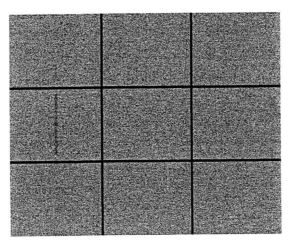

Figure 1. A sample frame from the 9-alternative forced-choice display. A stationary vertical cylinder is randomly placed in the center of one of 9 fields. Noise in this figure is unfiltered and contrast is increased for clarity.

3.2. Image Generation and Display

Image sequences were created by first constructing noise-only frame sequences from unfiltered or spatially filtered zero-mean noise, and then adding uniform background and signal. Unfiltered noise-only sequences were created on-the-fly immediately before each presentation using white, zero-mean Poisson noise with a standard deviation of 30. Filtering proved too slow for real-time implementation, so filtered noise-only sequences were created and stored beforehand and were read from disk before each trial. There were 100 noise sequences for each filtered presentation type, and over the 200 trials in a measurement each sequence was used twice.

Image sequences were constructed in real-time during an experimental session using the noise-only frames. A constant gray level of 128 was added to each frame, which was then divided into 9 fields. A 5-pixel-diameter vertical cylinder with the appropriate contrast was then projected in the center of one of the 9 image fields. Contrast without normalization, C, was defined as

$$C = g_b - g_c \tag{7}$$

where g_b is the background gray level, and g_c is the minimum noise-free cylinder gray level. X-ray system blur was introduced in each frame by convolving the cylinder profile with a one-dimensional kernel representing the line spread function (LSF).

The display system consisted of software running on a PowerMac 9500/200 personal computer (Apple Computer, Inc., Cupertino, CA) with an 8-bit linearized display monitor. The display refresh rate was 66Hz (non-interlaced), and images were repeated once to simulate 33 acquisitions/s x-ray fluoroscopy. For image sequence experiments, 64 frames were displayed in a repeating loop. For single image experiments, only the first frame was displayed. Images were 480 × 384 pixels in size and subtended a visual angle of 13.75 × 11.0 degrees at the 1 m viewing distance.

4. RESULTS

In Fig. 2, signal contrast sensitivity is plotted as a function of filtering level for both single images and image sequences. A higher contrast sensitivity value indicates improved detection. Each sensitivity value was estimated over 200 trials and the estimated coefficient of variation is $\approx 5\%$. For image sequences, a paired t-test (that does not take into account the standard error estimates of each data point) shows a significant effect of filtering at all levels as compared to no filtering ($p < 0.05$). However, the effect of filtering on single images is not significant ($p > 0.05$).

In Fig. 3, we examine the ratio of sensitivity measurements in order to compare the effect of spatial filtering on sequences with that on single images. The average ratio is 2.9 for the unfiltered case, and it significantly increases ($p < 0.05$) to 3.2, 3.2, and 3.4 at successive filtering levels. This direct comparison clearly shows that spatial filtering is more advantageous in sequences as compared to single images.

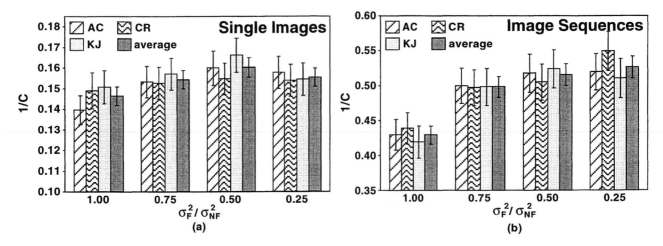

Figure 2. Signal contrast sensitivity as a function of spatial filtering for single images (a) and image sequences (b). A variance ratio of 1.0 indicates no filtering, and more filtering is achieved as one goes from left to right along the x-axis. Measurements from three observers, as well as an average across observers are shown.

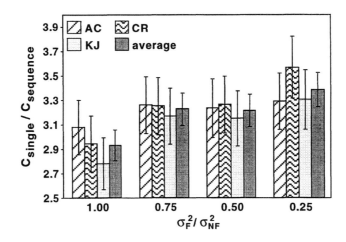

Figure 3. The ratio of signal contrast sensitivity in an image sequence to that in a single image as a function of spatial filtering.

In Fig. 4, we compare the change in measured contrast sensitivity to observer models and to predictions from pixel noise variance. For the purpose of comparison, all predictions are normalized by the human observer measurement for the unfiltered case. For single images (Fig. 4a), the improvement of sensitivity with filtering is not significantly different than either NPW-HVS or PWMF, and it is much less than predicted by pixel noise reduction. For image sequences (Fig. 4b), PWMF and NPW-HVS considerably underestimate the effect of filtering on detection. At higher levels of filtering, the detection improvement is far below the pixel noise prediction.

5. DISCUSSION

Image processing textbooks generally recommend low-pass spatial filtering to enhance images corrupted by Gaussian noise.[28-30] However, the advantages of such filtering are not always apparent in noise-limited detection tasks. Others have studied spatial processing of single images and report varying effects on detection performance.[17,18] In the case of a simple low-pass spatial filter, processing reduces pixel variance and creates noise spatial correlation. It also blurs edges and potentially reduces signal energy. Our experiments remove the latter effects on the signal by filtering the

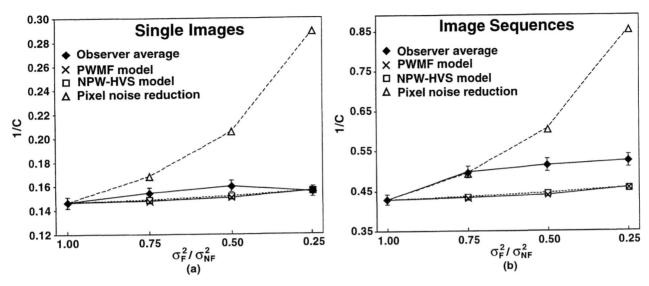

Figure 4. Predictions (normalized) from two observer models and from pixel noise variance reduction are compared to sensitivity improvement as a function of spatial filtering for single images (a) and image sequences (b). Contrast sensitivity for the models is the inverse of the signal contrast needed to achieve an SNR equal to $d'_{80\%}$. To obtain predictions from pixel variance, we scale sensitivity in the unfiltered case by the square root of the variance ratio.

noise only. Even in this idealized case, there is no significant improvement in detection after filtering of single images. However, an improvement is evident in the case of image sequences.

5.1. Applicability to X-ray Fluoroscopy

Although we refer to our image sequences as simulated x-ray fluoroscopy, this is a simplification. We do not consider factors in conventional fluoroscopy such as image intensifier spatial blurring, camera-lag temporal blurring, and anatomical backgrounds. We choose to selectively study the effect of spatial filtering which is optimally done in a simplified, controlled setting.

The present human observer detection results indicate that spatial processing can be an effective noise-reduction method in x-ray fluoroscopy. Potential dose savings are of particular interest. Detection results predict an x-ray dose savings of 26% to 34% with spatial filtering, a clinically substantial effect.

In Fig. 4, measurements are compared to predictions from pixel noise reduction, a measure commonly used to assess filters in x-ray fluoroscopy.[3,4,23] Several studies have shown that this is a misleading measure of image quality for single images,[18,21] and our results lead to the same conclusion for spatially filtered image sequences. The prediction error can be large. For example, at a pixel variance ratio of 0.25, noise reduction predicts a 100% improvement in contrast sensitivity while we measure only 23%.

With the introduction of recently developed semiconductor-based flat-panel x-ray detectors into fluoroscopy, spatial and temporal blurring that exist in conventional systems will virtually be eliminated. As a result, there is a rejuvenated interest in digital spatiotemporal processing. Quantitative image quality studies like the one presented here should lead to filtering strategies that are optimized for the human observer.

5.2. Measurements and Observer Models

Many of our previous experiments demonstrated that visual temporal processing reduces the effective noise.[5,6,11,12] The ratio of detection performance in a sequence to that in a single image measures the effect of human temporal processing. This ratio increases with increased spatial filtering (Fig. 3) indicating that humans are more effective at combining data across time as spatial processing increases. This effect is not predicted by either the PWMF or the NPW-HVS model. In general, results cannot be described by any model with independent linear processing across time.

One possible explanation for this effect is the following scenario. Spatial filtering creates clusters of locally correlated pixels that degrade detection. In image sequences, these noise clusters are temporally uncorrelated and move in a manner inconsistent with the stationary target. This situation improves detection by reducing the probability of false-positive detection as compared to single, static images. Alternatively, mathematical observer models, like those incorporating spatiotemporal channels[31,32] or internal noise sources that are functions of external noise correlation,[21] might decribe the effect.

6. CONCLUSION

We conclude that edge preserving, spatial filtering has applicability for effective noise reduction in x-ray fluoroscopy sequences. The negative effect of spatial noise correlation that is found in single frames is reduced whenever images are viewed in a sequence. Only through careful quantitative testing of image quality can one uncover such important interactions between image processing and human visual perception.

ACKNOWLEDGMENTS

This work is supported by NIH grant R01-HL48918.

REFERENCES

1. T. B. Shope, "Radiation-induced skin injuries from fluoroscopy," *Radiology* **197(P)**, p. 209, 1995. abstract.
2. D. T. Kuan, A. A. Sawchuk, T. C. Strand, and P. Chavel, "Adaptive noise smoothing filter for images with signal-dependent noise," *IEEE Trans. Pattern Anal. Mach. Intell.* **PAMI-7**, pp. 165–177, 1985.
3. C. L. Chan, A. K. Katsaggelos, and A. V. Sahakian, "Image sequences filtering in quantum-limited noise with applications to low-dose fluoroscopy," *IEEE Trans. Med. Imag.* **12**, pp. 610–621, 1993.
4. R. Aufrichtig and D. L. Wilson, "X-ray fluoroscopy spatio-temporal filtering with object detection," *IEEE Trans. Med. Imag.* **14**, pp. 733–746, 1995.
5. R. Aufrichtig, P. Xue, C. W. Thomas, G. C. Gilmore, and D. L. Wilson, "Perceptual comparison of pulsed and continuous fluoroscopy," *Med. Phys.* **21**, pp. 245–256, 1994.
6. P. Xue and D. L. Wilson, "Pulsed fluoroscopy detectability from interspersed adaptive forced choice measurements," *Med. Phys.* **23**, pp. 1833–1843, 1996.
7. P. Xue, C. W. Thomas, G. C. Gilmore, and D. L. Wilson, "An adaptive reference/test paradigm: Application to pulsed fluoroscopy perception," *Behavior Research Methods, Instruments, & Computers* **30**, pp. 332–348, 1998.
8. R. Aufrichtig, C. Thomas, P. Xue, and D. L. Wilson, "A model for perception of pulsed fluoroscopy image sequences," *J. Opt. Soc. Am., A* **11**, pp. 3167–3176, 1994.
9. P. Xue and D. L. Wilson, "Effects of motion blurring in x-ray fluoroscopy," *Med. Phys.* **25**, pp. 587–599, 1998.
10. P. Xue and D. L. Wilson, "Detection of moving objects in pulsed x-ray fluoroscopy," *J. Opt. Soc. Am., A* **15**, pp. 375–388, 1998.
11. D. L. Wilson, P. Xue, and R. Aufrichtig, "Perception of fluoroscopy last-image-hold," *Med. Phys.* **21**, pp. 1875–1883, 1994.
12. D. L. Wilson, K. N. Jabri, P. Xue, and R. Aufrichtig, "Perceived noise versus display noise in temporally filtered image sequences," *Journal of Electronic Imaging* **5**, pp. 490–495, 1996.
13. J. Astola and P. Kuosmanen, *Fundamentals of Nonlinear Digital Filtering*, CRC Press, Boca Raton, FL, 1997.
14. L. Alvarez, P.-L. Lions, and J.-M. Morel, "Image selective smoothing and edge detection by nonlinear diffusion. II," *SIAM Journal on Numerical Analysis* **29**, pp. 845–866, 1992.
15. N. H. C. Yung and A. H. S. Lai, "Performance evaluation of a feature-preserving filtering algorithm for removing additive random noise in digital images," *Optical Engineering* **35**, pp. 1871–1885, 1996.
16. G. Z. Yang, P. Burger, D. N. Firmin, and S. R. Underwood, "Structure adaptive anisotropic image filtering," *Image and Vision Computing* **14**, pp. 135–145, 1996.
17. P. A. Guignard, "A comparative method based on ROC analysis for the quantitation of observer performance in scintigraphy," *J. Opt. Soc. Am. A* **4**, pp. 945–953, 1987.
18. K. J. Myers, H. H. Barrett, M. C. Borgstrom, D. D. Patton, and G. W. Seeley, "Effect of noise correlation on detectability of disk signals in medical imaging," *J. Opt. Soc. Am. A* **2**, pp. 1752–1759, 1985.
19. K. T. Blackwell, "The effect of white and filtered noise on contrast detection thresholds," *Vision Research* **38**, pp. 267–280, 1998.
20. J. P. Rolland and H. H. Barrett, "Effect of random background inhomogeneity on observer detection performance," *J. Opt. Soc. Am. A* **9**, pp. 649–658, 1992.
21. A. E. Burgess, X. Li, and C. K. Abbey, "Visual signal detectability with two noise components: Anomalous masking effects," *J. Opt. Soc. Am. A* **14**, pp. 2420–2442, 1997.

22. M. P. Eckstein, A. J. A. Jr., and A. B. Watson, "Visual signal detection in structured backgrounds. II. Effects of contrast gain control, background variations, and white noise," *J. Opt. Soc. Am. A* **14**, pp. 2406–2419, 1997.

23. J. C. Brailean, R. P. Kleihorst, S. N. Efstratiadis, A. K. Katsaggelos, and R. L. Lagendijk, "Noise reduction filters for dynamic image sequences: A review," *Proc. IEEE* **83**, pp. 1272–1292, 1995.

24. R. N. McDonough and A. D. Whalen, *Detection of Signals in Noise. 2nd Ed.*, Academic Press, San Diego, CA, 1995.

25. A. E. Burgess, "Statistically defined backgrounds: Performance of a modified nonprewhitening observer model," *J. Opt. Soc. Am. A* **11**, pp. 1237–1242, 1994.

26. M. Ishida, K. Doi, L.-N. Loo, C. E. Metz, and J. L. Lehr, "Digital image processing: Effect on detectability of simulated low-contrast radiographic patterns," *Radiology* **150**, pp. 569–575, 1984.

27. D. H. Kelly, "Motion and vision, II: Stabilized spatio-temporal threshold surface," *J. Opt. Soc. Am.* **69**, pp. 1340–1349, 1979.

28. A. K. Jain, *Fundamentals of Digital Image Processing*, Prentice-Hall, Englewood Cliffs, NJ, 1989.

29. R. C. Gonzalez and R. E. Woods, *Digital Image Processing*, Addison-Wesley, Reading, MA, 1992.

30. W. K. Pratt, *Digital Image Processing. 2nd Ed.*, John Wiley and Sons, Inc., New York, 1991.

31. C. van den Branden Lambrecht and M. Kunt, "Characterization of human visual sensitivity for video imaging applications," *Signal Processing* **67**, pp. 255–269, 1998.

32. T. Matsui, "Theoretical analysis of perceptual responses to flashed sinusoidal waves using a multichannel spatiotemporal human vision model," *Electronics and Communications in Japan, Part 3* **81**, pp. 51–62, 1998.

On the detection of lesions in mammographic structure

Arthur E. Burgess, Francine L. Jacobson, and Philip F. Judy

Radiology Dept., Brigham & Women's Hospital,

Harvard Medical School, 75 Francis St., Boston, MA 02115

ABSTRACT

This paper is a report on very surprising results from recent work on detection of real lesions in digitized mammograms. The experiments were done using a novel experimental procedure with hybrid images. The lesions (signals) were real tumour masses extracted from breast tissue specimen radiographs. In the detection experiments, the tumours were added to digitized normal mammographic backgrounds. The results of this new work have been both novel and very surprising. Contrast thresholds increased with increasing lesion size for lesions larger than approximately 1 mm in diameter. Earlier work with white noise, radiographic image noise, computed tomography (CT) noise and some types of patient structure have accustomed us to a particular relationship between lesion size and contrast for constant detectability. All previous contrast/detail (CD) diagrams have been similar, the contrast threshold decreases as lesion size increases and flattens at large lesion sizes. The CD diagram for lesion detection in mammographic structure is completely different. It will be shown that this is a consequence of the power-law dependence of the projected breast tissue structure spectral density on spatial frequency. Mammographic tissue structure power spectra have the form $P(f) = B/f^\beta$, with an average exponent of approximately 3 (range from 2 to 4), and are approximately isotropic (small angular dependence). Results for two-alternative forced-choice (2AFC) signal detection experiments using 4 tumour lesions and one mathematically generated signal will be presented. These results are for an unbiased selection of mammographic backgrounds. It is possible that an additional understanding of the effects of breast structure on lesion detectability can be obtained by investigating detectability in various classes of mammographic backgrounds. This will be the subject of future research.

Keywords: Mammograms, tumour detection, signal detection, observer performance, CD diagrams, image structure, masking, structured noise.

1. INTRODUCTION

It has been frequently demonstrated that the signal amplitude (contrast) required to maintain a constant level of detection accuracy increases as signal size decreases. This has been the case for noiseless images[1], white noise[2], fluoroscopic and radiographic noise[3], computed tomography noise[4] and for detection in patient structure using skull radiographs[5], and liver CT images[6]. Surprisingly, lesion detection in mammographic structure shows the opposite effect – lesion amplitude in mammograms must be increased as size *increases* to maintain a constant detection accuracy. This unusual effect is due to the fact that the power spectrum of normal tissue structure in mammograms has a power-law frequency dependence of the form, $P(f) \approx B/f^\beta$. The average exponent β is about 3 for an collection of 64 mammographic measurement regions, with exponents for individual regions in the range from 2 to 4. The following is a simplistic explanation of the threshold amplitude versus size effect. As signal size increases, with amplitude held constant, its energy spectrum is increasingly concentrated at low spatial frequencies. The spectral density of patient structure is also increasing rapidly as frequency decreases. If the power-law exponent is large enough (greater than 2), then as lesion size increases, the ratio of signal energy and structure spectrum power will actually *decrease*. So lesion amplitude must be *increased* to maintain constant detectability. This effect will be demonstrated for model observers in the following theoretical section. The results for 2AFC experiments will also be presented, demonstrating that the effect also occurs for human observers.

304

Part of the SPIE Conference on Image Perception and Performance
San Diego, California • February 1999
SPIE Vol. 3663 • 0277-786X/99/$10.00

2. THEORY

Ideal (Prewhitening) observer model: Recent studies[7,8,9,10,28] have indicated that human signal detection in low-pass filtered noise and statistically defined backgrounds can be reasonably well described by a suboptimal Bayesian observer model which includes partial prewhitening. This implies that humans can partially compensate for positive spatial correlations in noise. The lowpass noise in those studies included cases with both well defined correlation distance (using Gaussian low-pass filters) and undefined correlation distance (using power-law filters). Consider detection of a 2D isotropic signal with radial dependence, s(r), and Fourier transform, S(f), in noise with a power spectrum P(f) that depends only on radial spatial frequency, f. The ideal observer (prewhitening matched filter) detectability index for this signal is given[11,12] by the integral

$$(d')^2 = 2\pi \int_0^\infty \frac{|S(f)|^2 f df}{P(f)} . \tag{1}$$

Non-prewhitening observer model: Another popular observer model is the non-prewhitening matched filter. There is now considerable evidence[7,10,13] suggesting that this model (in its unmodified form) is not very useful for describing human visual signal detection performance. However, a particular version of this model (NPWE), which includes an eye filter, has been shown to be useful[10] under carefully selected conditions (when noise bandwidth is large compared to signal bandwidth). The model also has the advantage of allowing closed-form performance calculations and convenient Monte Carlo simulations - again with careful attention to its restricted range of validity. So it will be described and evaluated for the sake of completeness. Its detectability index is given by[13]

$$(d'_{NPWE})^2 = \frac{\left| 2\pi \int_0^\infty |S(f)|^2 |E(f)|^2 f df \right|^2}{2\pi \int_0^\infty \left\{ |E(f)|^2 (1+\beta) P(f) + N_i \right\} |E(f)|^2 |S(f)|^2 f df} \tag{2}$$

where the eye filter has the form $E(f) = f \exp(-bf)$ with the constant, b, selected to give a peak at 4 cycles per degree. The $(1+\beta)$ multiplier of P(f) represents the effect of observer induced internal noise[14] and N_i is the spectral density of observer internal noise.

One point on terminology should be noted. In this work, signals are described by amplitude profiles rather than contrast. Signal contrast is usually calculated by normalizing amplitude by the local image mean value, L_0, in the vicinity of the signal. So the signal contrast profile is defined by $c(r) = s(r)/L_0$. If the contrast representation is used for the signal, then it must also be used to normalized the noise fluctuations. It is straightforward to demonstrate the contrast representation leads to the term $(L_0)^2$ in both the numerator and denominator of equations (1) and (2). The L_0 normalizations cancel. So there is no benefit obtained from using the contrast representation in signal detectability calculations.

Detectability and signal size: The variation of detectability with signal size will first be described for the two observer models using the case of detection of a 2D Gaussian signal with two-component noise that had been used in previous investigations[10]. One component, N_1, had a broad band (white) spectrum designed to simulate image noise. The other (background) component was filtered to simulate power-law noise of the form $N_2(f) = N_2 \cos(\pi f)/\{f_0^3 + f^3\}$ with f_0 equal to 1/128 cycles per pixel. The cut-off frequency was selected to equal one cycle per image width with the goal of preventing the noise power spectrum from approaching infinity as frequency decreased to zero. More recent experience with the statistics of mammographic spectra suggests that use of an arbitrary cut-off frequency in earlier work was misguided, since there is no evidence of flattening of breast structure spectral at low frequencies. However, it will be used here for demonstration purposes. Equations (1) and (2) were solved numerically for a range of signal sizes. Model performance was also investigated by Monte Carlo simulation of 2AFC detection. The results are shown in figure 1. There is good agreement between the numerical and Monte Carlo results for large signals. The slight disagreement at small sizes is probably due to quantization effects in the Monte Carlo experiment. Note that the PW model results are fitted by a slope of +0.5, this point will be addressed in more detail below. The numerical integration results for the two models reach a maximum at a Gaussian signal standard deviation of about 20, log(std. dev.) = 1.3, and decrease at larger sizes. This effect is due to the fact that the background component power spectrum had a low-frequency cut-off. Below that frequency the spectrum becomes flat. When the noise power spectrum becomes flat within the signal energy bandwidth (i.e. for large signal size), the CD diagram slope for large signal size tends toward the Rose model slope of -1. One would expect a similar transition for small signal sizes since the combined two component noise spectrum will be dominated by the uncorrelated image noise component at high spatial frequencies. This is not seen in figure 1 because it would have occurred for Gaussian signal standard deviations below one pixel in the Monte Carlo simulation, but will be seen in the human observer results in figure 5.

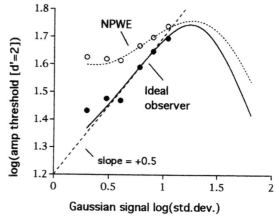

Figure 1. Amplitude threshold (d'=2) as a function of size for detection of a 2D Gaussian signal in two-component noise, $N(f)=N_1+ N_2\cos(\pi f)/\{(f_0)^3 + f^3\}$. The results are for two observer models, the Bayesian ideal and a non-prewhitening matched filter (NPWE) model with an eye filter, see equations (1) and (2). Curves are for numerical integration results. Circles are for Monte Carlo simulation.

CD diagram slopes: The above results demonstrated a very surprising positive CD diagram slope of 0.5 for the ideal observer model for detection in power-law noise with exponent equal to 3. Now consider changes in signal detectability as signal size and amplitude are both varied for a range of power-law exponents. This problem can be treated in a general way using a scalable signal described by, $s_W(r) =As(r/W)$, where W is a positive real-valued size scaling factor and A is an amplitude (contrast) scaling factor. The Hankel transform of this scalable signal is[15]

$$S_W(f) = AW^2 S(Wf). \qquad (3)$$

Assume, for the moment, that the combination of image noise and breast structure can be described by a second-order (weakly) stationary stochastic process, with a power spectrum $P(f) = N(f) + K/f^\beta$, where $N(f)$ is the spectral density of the image noise and K/f^β is an idealized model of the spectral density of projected breast tissue structure. In order to simplify the mathematics the image noise will be neglected and a high frequency cut-off, f_2, for the detectability index integral (equation 4) will be used instead. It can be argued that it is not physically reasonable for breast tissue to have a power-law spectrum to arbitrarily low spatial frequency. Spectral analysis results given in related papers in this conference[16,17] do not provide evidence of a flattening of the spectrum at low frequencies. However, this finding may say more about the problems related to digital spectral analysis than about the nature of the spectra themselves. The possibility of low-frequency flattening of $P(f)$ will accounted for by including a low frequency cut-off, f_1, in the following detectability index integral. Substituting in equation (1), the signal detectability index for the

Bayesian ideal observer in polar form (equation 1) becomes

$$(d')^2 = 2\pi \int_{f_1}^{f_2} \frac{|S_W(f)|^2 f df}{P(f)} = \frac{2\pi A^2 W^4}{K} \int_{f_1}^{f_2} |S_W(Wf)|^2 f^{1+\beta} df. \tag{4}$$

This equation can be transformed to a new coordinate system with radial frequency $v = Wf$ to give

$$(d')^2 = \frac{2\pi A^2 W^{2-\beta} I_v}{K} \quad ; \text{where} \quad I_v = \int_{f_1}^{f_2} |S(v)|^2 v^{1+\beta} dv \cdot \tag{5}$$

Note that this coordinate transformation is valid since only the signal size is scaled. The image noise is not scaled. The value of the integral I_v does not depend on either the spatial or amplitude scaling factors. One can define a detection threshold amplitude, A_t, using the criterion of d' equal to some arbitrarily selected constant, δ. Then the signal amplitude required to reach this amplitude as a function of signal scale factor W is given by

$$A_t = \delta \sqrt{K / 2\pi I_v} \; W^{(\beta-2)/2} \tag{6}$$

For comparison purposes, the conventional log-log representation is more convenient. The relationship between log(amplitude threshold, A_t) and log(signal size scale factor , W) then becomes

$$\log(A_t) = C + m[\log(W)], \quad \text{where} \quad C = \log\left(\delta \sqrt{K / 2\pi I_v}\right) \quad \text{and} \quad 2m = \beta - 2 \tag{7}$$

Since C is a constant for a given signal and noise, the slope of the constant threshold line on a log-log CD plot is $m = (\beta - 2)/2$. The relationship between the CD diagram slope and the noise power spectrum exponent for this idealized prewhitening observer model is shown in figure 2.

Figure 2. Plot of CD diagram slope versus the exponent of power-law noise, $1/f^\beta$, for the (ideal) pre-whitening matched filter observer model. White noise has a CD diagram slope of -1 and an exponent of zero. CT noise has a CD diagram slope of -1.5 an exponent of -1 (in this β exponent notation, which is of course unusual for describing CT noise) An average mammogram has a power-law spectrum with exponent of about 3 and ideal observer CD diagram slope of +0.5. The range of exponents for all mammograms evaluated was from 2 to 4.

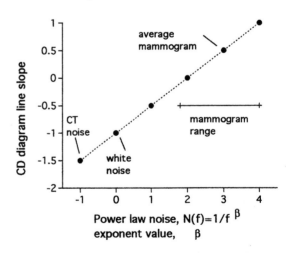

For the case of white noise, β equals zero and one obtains the well known Rose model[2] result that threshold amplitude decreases in inverse proportion to signal size (CD diagram slope = -1). Another well known case is for 2D image reconstruction from projections (such as x-ray computed tomography[4]) which has P(f) proportional to frequency for low frequencies, so contrast thresholds are proportional to $W^{-3/2}$ (CD diagram slope m = - 1.5). For the average mammogram, the power spectrum exponent, β, is about 3, so the model predicts that threshold amplitude (contrast) increases as the square root of signal size (m = +

0.5). The distribution of mammographic power spectrum exponent values found in this work ranges from 2 to 4. The consequences of this range of exponents for lesion detection will be discussed below and in figure 6.

3. EXPERIMENTAL METHODS

The human observer experiments were done using the 2AFC method by adding realistic tumour signals (extracted from digitized breast tissue specimen radiographs) to digital mammographic structure background images. An overview of methods will be given first, then details. Four tumour images (3 malignant and one fibroadenoma) were selected from 25 examples. The mammographic backgrounds were selected from a digitized mammogram database. All observer experiments were done using 512x512 background image regions with 120 micron sampling and a log-exposure amplitude scale (more on this point below). The regions were selected so that added lesion could be placed completely within that part of the mammogram where breast thickness was estimated to be constant. During each observer trial, two randomly selected regions were displayed side-by-side with one side containing the lesion to be detected. Observers selected the most probable side. The experiments were done using the signal-known-exactly (SKE)) paradigm, so the same lesion was used for all 128 decision trials in a given block and the two potential lesion locations were identified using a circle cue. An example display is shown in figure 3.

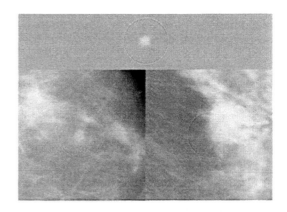

Figure 3. Example 2AFC experiment display for detection of a real breast lesion added to one of two 512x512 pixel (61x61 mm) background regions from different mammograms. A reference high amplitude version of the lesion (a ductal carcinoma in this example) is placed above the regions. Both backgrounds have circle cues[25] added in order to indicate the two alternative lesion locations.

The mammographic backgrounds were selected from a digitized mammogram database of 105 normal cases provided by Dr. Larry Clarke of the Univ. of South Florida. Details about the database are given in another conference paper[17]. The images were reduced to 120 micron sampling for observer experiments. The choice of 120 microns was based on two considerations. First, power spectrum analysis indicated that mammogram image noise rather than patient structure was the dominant factor for spatial frequencies greater than 1 cycle per mm, so 120 micron was considered to be adequate. Second, a smaller sampling distance would have required an expensive 2Kx2.5K format CRT display system. The acquisition of such a system is planned in the future but was not really required for the present study.

The images were first converted to optical density scale using the calibration curve of the digitizer and then converted to the log-exposure scale using calibration data supplied by Sterling Diagnostic Imaging[18]. There is considerable variation of apparent film speed and less marked variation in the shape of the H&D curve over time because of changes in processing conditions. So a fixed transformation from optical density to log-exposure must be regarded as an approximation. Using the simplifying assumption of a monoenergetic x-ray beam, the logarithm of x-ray exposure value at image location (x,y) is given by the product, $logE(x,y) = \mu_z(x,y)t(x,y)$, of patient part thickness, $t(x,y)$, and average linear attenuation variation, $\mu_z(x,y)$, along the x-ray projection ray path from the image position to the x-ray focus. This simple model ignores a number of complicating factors such anode heel effect, beam hardening, spatial varying secondary radiation, random variation in film sensitivity and processor chemical concentration. The amplitude transformations do have the effect of correcting the measured data values (to first order) for the major aspects of nonlinear film response as well the physics of the digitizer and x-ray imaging system.

One more step was necessary - elimination of tissue thickness variation. During mammography, the breast is compressed between two plastic plates to reduce thickness, increase x-ray transmission and reduce secondary radiation. The plates are approximately parallel. So there is a region within the mammogram where tissue thickness is approximately constant and a surrounding transition region where thickness systematically decreases. As is described in another paper[17], several methods were developed to estimate the boundary between these two regions to confine subsequent analyses and experiments to constant thickness regions. In this constant thickness region, $\log E(x,y) \approx \mu_z(x,y)T$, where T is the tissue thickness. Unfortunately, breast thicknesses were not recorded during the mammogram acquisitions so one can proceed no further with correction for geometry.

Only craniocaudal (CC) views were used because image segmentation methods are more straight forward then for mediolateral oblique (MLO) views. First, the approximately parabolic boundary of the constant thickness region of each mammogram was estimated. Then all visible chest wall muscle boundaries present in images were identified and localized by interactive visual inspection. For images with no visual evidence of chest wall muscle, an arbitrary boundary was identified 7.7 mm from the chest side of the mammogram. Next, a large number of possible lesion locations were identified on a square lattice within the constant thickness region with centers 7.7 mm apart. This spacing is half the largest lesion size (15.6 mm) used in the experiments. As an added precaution, the centers of possible lesion locations were limited to a subregion so that no center position was closer than 23 mm from the nearest estimated boundary. This gave 10,750 possible lesion locations. A total of 2048 possible lesion locations were then randomly selected for the detection experiments.

It was necessary to select a particular background region size for 2AFC experiment display. The purpose of displaying tissue outside the possible lesion location was to allow observers to get a 'feel' for the local statistics of the mammogram structure. From the author's previous experience with human observer experiments using statistically varying backgrounds and that of others[19], it was estimated that a background region about 3 times larger than the largest lesion was adequate. To be on the safe side a multiplier of 4 was selected. Since the largest lesion size was selected to be 128x128 (0.12 mm sampling), each background region was 512x512 pixels (61x61 mm). Whenever possible the lesion location was centered in the region. In some cases this centering was not possible because the selected location was too close to the edge of the source mammogram. The mean and variance of log-exposure was measured within a 23 mm (192 pixel) diameter circular region centered on the potential lesion location for selection of a linear transformation (window and level) of image amplitudes for display. Each 512x512 background was extracted from the source image, the mean value was subtracted, and region images were stored as records in the background database file.

Five signals were used in the observer experiments. Four were real breast tumours and one was a mathematically generated nodule signal. The tumour images that were extracted from digitized breast tissue specimens radiographs (50 micron pixels) by methods described in a companion paper in these proceedings[20]. The tumour images are also shown in that paper. All tumours (original size range 8 to 18 mm) were first rescaled to fit within a square array (256x256) and then minified during experiments on detectability as a function of size. The lesion size range was selected to be from 0.5 to 15.6 mm (4 to 128 pixels) with size steps of a factor of two, plus one additional size category of 96 pixels. At the smallest size (0.5 mm), the lesions did not resemble tumours and can be regarded as simulations of compact calcifications. The lesions began to visually resemble tumours when the 4 mm (32 pixel) scale was reached. The designer nodule had the equation $a(\rho)=A(1-\rho^2)^{1.5}$, where ρ is a normalized radius. This equation provides a good fit to lung nodules[8]. The designer nodule is, of course, not designed to mimic breast tumours. It was used in preliminary experiments for two reasons: (1) theoretical and experimental convenience and (2) to allow comparisons with previous observer experiments done using two-component simulated power-law noise[8].

The image display system included a Macintosh 9600 computer and an Image Systems model M24L 24 inch diagonal high-resolution grey-scale monitor[21] with a maximum luminance of 75 cd/m[2] and a 1200(V) by 1600(H) pixel format. The control software was written in IDL[22]. Two background regions were included in each 2AFC image, randomly selected from the database of 2048 possible lesion locations. If the two regions came from the same breast image, then one was replaced by another randomly selected from a different breast. Given the highly variable mammogram structure[17], both within and between images, and the limited dynamic range of CRT display, we used a novel adaptive window and level grey scale transformation method to prevent contrast-limited presentation of any image. Before loading each 61 mm square background segment into the 2AFC image, the zero mean (as defined above) data values were amplified by a gain dependent on the measured local variance about the potential lesion location. Local variance was used rather than the full 512x512 region variance because both the variance measurement and the variability of that measurement in a region increase as the region size increases. This point is discussed in two related papers[17,16]. A different transformation was used for each the two alternative image segments and the lesion amplitude was scaled by the gain of the side to which it was assigned. Finally, the complete 2AFC image (which included the two unrelated breast regions) was scaled by a fixed linear transformation to fit within the 8-bit dynamic range of the display memory. The variable gain range covered a factor of 3.5. The satellite lesion reference images (see below) gave the observer information about the pair of gains used for each trial. It is possible that observers cannot effectively use this information so detectability of one selected lesion was measured with the same gain in both fields. The results of this separate experiment are presented below.

Several steps were taken to ensure that the usual assumption of signal-known-exactly (SKE) conditions were valid in the experiment. Only one selected tumour lesion with fixed size was used for each block of 128 trials. Three reference copies of the lesion was placed above the two image fields (see figure 3). The central reference copy was displayed at high amplitude so the observer could see all lesion details (these details would, of course, rarely be seen at the signal amplitudes corresponding to 92% correct, d'=2). The satellite copies were at shown at the amplitude and gain that would have been used if the lesion were present on that side. Lesion amplitude was adjusted during the 2AFC trials using a modified staircase procedure[23] to maintain a value close to that giving 92% correct responses. After each incorrect decision the lesion amplitude was increased by one step. After six successive correct responses the amplitude was decreased by one step. The staircase amplitude steps were one-quarter octave (1.091 ratio). Because of the highly variable tissue structure there was a marked variation is lesion visibility from trial to trial so the staircase procedure was modified to include a lower limit, 2 steps below the estimated amplitude for 92 percent correct based on previous observer results. The goal was to ensure that decision trials were done with lesion amplitudes near that required to give the lowest coefficient of variation due to sampling statistics (d'=2)[24]. To assist observers in using lesion location information, unobtrusive circle cues[25] were placed around the two possible lesion locations. The cues were bipolar, consisting of contiguous bright and dark rings with diameter dependent on lesion size. An algorithm relating cue diameter and lesion size was developed, based on subjective evaluation. If the circle was too close to the lesion it interfered with detection. If was too far away then the lesion location became more difficult to determine. For the smallest lesion size (4 pixels, 0.5 mm), the selected cue diameter was 32 pixels. The following list gives the other paired lesion and cue sizes in pixels: (8,46), (16,64), (32,90), (64,128), (96,156), (128,182). Since observers were not constrained to a particular viewing distance, they tended to use a short distance for small lesions and longer distances for larger lesions. This caused the visibility of the circle cue to vary. To compensate for this effect, two cue ring thicknesses were used. The dark and bright rings were one pixel thick for small lesions (circle diameters less than 100 pixels). The rings were 2 pixels thick for larger lesions. The contrast of the bipolar rings was also subjectively selected to maximize the benefit of the cue. The same contrast was used for all cue sizes.

Three very experienced observers (the authors) took part in the experiment, two physicists and a board certified radiologist. Viewing time was not limited and feedback as to correctness of response was used. A block of 128 decision trials took between 6 and 12 minutes. Observers were encouraged to vary viewing distance as desired. Both a magnifying and minifying lens were available for use. The estimate of amplitude required for d' equal to 2 was obtained by pooling all observer response trials for a given lesion and size. This gave estimates of percentage correct as a function of lesion amplitude. The corresponding d' values were calculated. The threshold amplitude estimate (for d'=2) was then determined by linear regression of d' versus amplitude. Since the range of amplitudes was small and bracketed d' of 2, we used prior knowledge for mathematical stability. The regression line was forced to pass through the value of d' = -0.3 and zero lesion amplitude. This offset agreed with many previous complete psychometric function measurements (d' versus signal amplitude) for forced choice experiments by the author[26,27] and others[28].

4. EXPERIMENTAL RESULTS

Designer nodule signal: The first human observer 2AFC detection experiment was done using the 2D designer nodule signal added to digital mammogram backgrounds. The results of this preliminary experiment are shown in figure 4 and demonstrate that the predicted positive CD diagram slope also holds for human observers. The data are for one very experienced observer (the author) with 512 decision trials per datum. The best fit slope is 0.4 for the log-log relationship between amplitude threshold (d' =2) and signal size. This is slightly lower than the value of 0.45 predicted for the ideal observer (see figure 1) for the current best estimate of the average exponent for the mammographic structure power spectrum. The difference is consistent with previous findings suggesting that humans cannot completely compensate for positive noise correlations[8,9,10,13]. The discrepancy may also arise from the difficulty in accurately estimating the power spectrum of mammographic structure. This point is discussed in another paper in the conference[17].

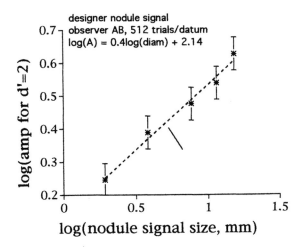

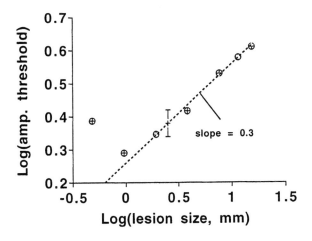

Figure 4. Amplitude threshold (relative units) versus signal size for a designer nodule signal added to mammogram backgrounds. One observer (AB) and 512 trials per datum. Best fit (log-log) slope is +0.4.

Figure 5. Amplitude threshold (relative units) versus size for four real lesions[20] added to mammographic backgrounds. Results are pooled for three observers (two experienced physicists and one board-certified radiologist) who are also authors of this paper. The best fit slope is +0.3 for sizes greater than 1 mm

Extracted tumour signals: The results of the 2AFC tumour detection experiments with hybrid digital mammograms and four lesions (a fibroadenoma and three ductal carcinomas) are shown in figure 5. The data are pooled results for three observers. Once again, the CD diagram slope is positive for lesion sizes greater than 1 mm. Since the 2D tumour profiles are highly variable, there is a problem with normalizing the data to a common (amplitude, size) equivalence scale. A number of 'equivalent size' definitions have been proposed for mathematically defined signals in simulated noise and backgrounds. Normalization based on detectability by the ideal observer model has been a good choice for filtered noise[10]. It is probable that this will also be true for mammographic lesions and backgrounds but that hypothesis remains to be tested. In the interim, the results for each lesion were scaled vertically to yield the same average threshold across the entire lesion size range.

Same gain experiment: As was mentioned in the methods section, different gains were used for the two mammographic backgrounds in the experiments to ensure that detection was always limited by either breast structure or image noise, and that detection was never limited solely by human contrast sensitivity. This conceivably could have had an unexpected effect on experimental results. So, a separate measurement was made of the detectability of the fibroadenoma with identical gains for the two sides in each 2AFC trial. The procedure, in this subsidiary experiment, was to calculate the gain for each side using the previous variance-based algorithm and then to use the lower of the two gains for both sides. This would give reduced contrast gain for about half the backgrounds. Three sizes of lesion were used: 1 mm, 4 mm and 15.6 mm (8, 32, and 128 pixels). Two very experienced observers (AB and PJ) took part in this experiment. The ratios of measured detectabilities for the two observers and 3 lesion sizes had an average of 1.00 and individual values of 1.03, 0.91, and 1.14 for AB and 0.95, 0.93, and 1.03 for PJ for the three sizes respectively. These variations are consistent with sampling statistics for 256 trials per condition. So it appears that using different gains for the two alternative regions does not affect performance. It also suggests that lower gains could have used for the experiments without approaching human contrast sensitivity limitations.

5. DISCUSSION

Summary: The numerical integration results for signal detection by model observers with power-law noise (figure 1) gave the surprising suggestion that CD diagram slopes would be positive for exponents, β, greater than 2. When the author first encountered that result, he was convinced that it was due to a computer coding problem. However, subsequent investigation by Monte Carlo simulation confirmed the theoretical predictions. These results were reported in an oral presentation at the October 1998 annual meeting of the Optical Society of America. The human observer results with mammographic background structure (figures 4 and 5) are in good agreement with the theoretical predictions. So we conclude that a CD diagram with positive slope is likely to apply in general for tumour detection in mammograms. This is a consequence of the power-law spectrum of mammogram structure. These experimental results suggest that, for the purposes of predicting tumour detectability, breast tissue can be considered to be approximately equivalent to random noise with the same power spectrum. This conclusion about random noise equivalence is supported by phase spectrum measurements reported in a related conference paper[16]. The human results for small lesion sizes (smaller than 1 mm) suggests that detection limits for objects such as microcalcifications and microcalcification clusters are mainly due to the standard effects of image noise and resolution. These surprising findings for detection of objects larger than 1 mm raise a number of questions and implications.

Breast structure as noise: Visual inspection of mammograms shows a large variety of tissue structure and textures. Some examples include linear structures such as ducts and blood vessels of a variety of sizes and orientations, filaments of connective tissue (Cooper's ligaments), lobular clumps of glandular tissue as well as a variety of fat distributions. The important point is that these 3D structures occur at a variety of scales with random orientation and position. The mammogram, of course, is a 2D projection with these structures randomly superimposed. The structural variations are readily apparent in mammograms and it is obvious that breast tissue structure is visually very different from simulated power-law noise created by isotropically filtering white noise. By contrast to visual inspection, statistical analyses and detection experiments must, by their very nature, involve averaging over a number of selected image regions from a variety of patients. Since the present experiments were a first step into this new territory, care was taken to use a large and unbiased selection of normal breast tissue regions. Averaging will inevitably destroy all evidence of any spatial phase coherence that may be present in the individual images. The signal known exactly (SKE) detection process, for model observers, involves template matching (with the signal as a template) and 2D integration. Since breast tumours, to a first approximation, are circular objects, the 2D integration process destroys any angular dependence of the breast tissue structure. There is considerable evidence[26,27,28] that human observers also use a Bayesian template matching strategy for SKE detection experiments. The above considerations suggest that, to a first approximation, the breast tissue can be considered to have the same effect on detection as random noise with the same power spectrum. Results on breast structure phase spectrum measurements reported in another paper in this conference[16] are consistent with this point of view.

Detectability by tissue classification: Statistical and spectral analysis[16,17] of all the collection mammograms in the database has made it clear that breast tissue is considerably more variable than a ensemble of filtered power-law noise images with an fixed exponent. Note use of the word 'collection' was used for the mammograms, rather than the term 'ensemble' that is usually associated with a set of sample functions from a random process. First, we do not know definitely whether mammogram structure can be characterized as a random process. Also, there is the question of second-order stationarity - does it apply to mammograms? This is a very difficult question to answer. There is further question of how one should define sets of mammograms or regions of mammograms for statistical analysis and detection experiments. The present work was very carefully designed to avoid any biased sampling of breast structure. No special selection of background areas was attempted, other than the obvious one of restricting work to the constant thickness region. It is quite possible that there are defensible categories of breast tissue structure that ought to kept separate from one another. This is an entire avenue of investigation that remains to be explored.

Effect of power-law exponent variation: One simple way of classifying regions might be based on estimated local exponent of the power-law spectrum. Unfortunately, this type of measurement is not trivial, as work reported in two other papers[16,17] at this conference demonstrate. The spectral analysis results suggest that exponents, β, range from 2 to 4. This variation in power-law exponent has strong implications for variation of tumour detectability as a tumour grows. As was shown in figure 2, the range of CD diagram boundary line slopes is 0 -> 1 for the β range 2 -> 4. Consider detectability of a growing tumour in power-law structure, as shown in figure 6. As the tumour grows, its projected amplitude (contrast) will be determined by the local difference in x-ray attenuation and amplitude will increase linearly with size as long as the composition of the tumour and surrounding tissue do not change. The CD diagram line for a particular power-law exponent represents, for a given decision criterion, a boundary between detection and non-detection. For a given lesion, if its particular combination of size and amplitude places it above the appropriate CD diagram line then the lesion is detectable. Otherwise the lesion is not detectable. If the decision criterion for detection is changed, the CD diagram lines in figure 6 are shifted vertically (to new amplitudes for a given size) but their slopes remain the same.

Figure 6. CD diagram lines of constant decision accuracy for 5 power-law ($1/f^\beta$) noise exponents. For a given exponent, the lines represent boundaries between two regions. Above the line the signal is reliably detected for the selected decision accuracy (e.g. d' = 2). Below the line, the signal is not reliably detected. The contrast trajectory of a growing tumour (slope = +1) is also shown. The average mammogram structure power spectrum exponent is about 3 with a value range of 2 to 4.

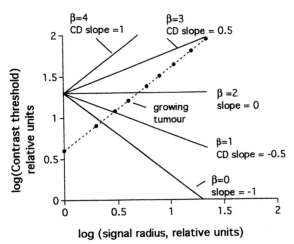

Now consider the consequences of a particular power-law ($1/f^\beta$) exponent. As the exponent, β, increases, the slope of the CD boundary line increases. This means that the rate of change of detectability with tumour size also decreases. The situation is particularly unfavourable for mammogram regions were the power-law exponent, β, is greater than or equal to 4. For β equal to 4 the slope of the detection threshold boundary line is unity and the detectability of the growing tumour in the mammogram will never increase due to contrast changes alone. Mammographic detection may occur either because the tumour eventually distorts organ morphology or because the tumour displaces normal structure and produces a large enough change in local statistical properties (architectural distortion) that it draws attention to itself. Obviously, there is also the possibility of detection by palpation.

ACKNOWLEDGEMENTS

We would like to thank a number of people who gave valuable advice or assistance during both planning and execution of this work. Larry Clarke and Maria Kallergi of University of South Florida provided the digitized mammograms and a variety of related information. John Heine and Robert Velthuizen of University of South Florida also gave valuable assistance. Jack Beutel, Sterling Diagnostic Imaging, kindly digitized the tumour specimen radiographs. He and David Richards, Sterling, provided Min-R/Microvision H&D curve data. Bijoy Misra of the Harvard-Smithsonian Institute of Astrophysics and Darrell Smith, Director of Breast Imaging in the BWH Radiology Dept., Harvard Medical School were party to many discussions on all aspects of the work. Kyle Myers and Robert Wagner of CDRH, US Food and Drug Administration made valuable comments on mathematical issues and took part in a number of helpful discussions. Ken Hanson, Los Alamos National Laboratories and Rodney Shaw, Hewlett-Packard Research Laboratories made helpful suggestions related to spectral analysis. Harold Kundel and Larry Toto, Univ. of Pennsylvania, made helpful suggestions about image display. This research was funded by grant R01-58302 from the US National Cancer Institute.

REFERENCES

1 H.R. Blackwell, "Contrast thresholds of the human eye," J. Opt. Soc. Am. **36**, 624-643 (1946).

2 A. Rose, "The sensitivity performance of the human eye on an absolute scale," J. Opt. Soc. Am. **38**, 196-208 (1948).

3 R.H. Morgan, "Screen intensification; A review of past and present research with an analysis of future development," Am. J. Roentgenol. **75**, 69-76 (1956).

4 R.F.Wagner, D.G. Brown, and M.S. Pastel, "Application of information theory to the assessment of computed tomography". *Med. Phys.* **6**, 83-94 (1979).

5 A.E. Burgess and K. Humphrey, "Visual Perception Limits in Angiography," in *Application of Optical Instrumentation in Medicine VI*, edited by J.E. Gray (Proceedings of the Society of Photo-optical Instrumentation Engineers, Boston. MA, 1977), Vol. 127, pp. 51-59.

6 S.E. Seltzer, P.F. Judy, R.G. Swensson, K.H. Chan and R.D. Nawfel, "Flattening of the contrast-detail curve for large lesions in CT liver images," Med. Phys. **21**, 1547-1555 (1994).

7 J. P. Rolland and H. H. Barrett, "Effect of random background inhomogeneity on observer detection performance," J. Opt. Soc. Am. **A 9**, 649-658 (1992).

8 A.E. Burgess, X. Li, and C.K. Abbey, "Nodule detection in two component noise: toward patient structure," in *Medical Imaging 1997: Image Perception*, edited by H.L. Kundel (Proc. Soc. of Photo-optical Instrumentation Engineers, Newport Beach, CA, 1997), Vol. 3036,2-13.

9 A.E. Burgess, "Prewhitening revisited," in *Medical Imaging 1998, Image Perception*, edited by H.L. Kundel (Proceedings of the Society of Photo-optical Instrumentation Engineers, San Diego, CA, 1998), Vol. 3340, pp. 55-64.

10 A.E. Burgess, "Visual signal detectability with two noise components: lowpass spectrum effects," J. Opt. Soc. Am. **A 16**, (in press, March issue) (1999).

11 D.O. North, "Analysis of the factors which determine signal-noise discrimination in pulsed carrier systems," RCA Tech. Rep. PTR6C (1943), reprinted in Proc. IRE **51**, 1016-1028 (1963).

12 A. Papoulis, *Probability, Random Variables, and Stochastic Processes. 3rd ed.* (McGraw-Hill, New York, 1991).

13 A.E. Burgess, X. Li, and C.K. Abbey, "Visual signal detectability with two noise components: anomalous masking effects," J. Opt. Soc. Am. **A14**, 2420-2442 (1997).

14 A.E. Burgess and B. Colbourne, "Visual signal detection IV: Observer inconsistency," J. Opt. Soc. Am. **A5**, 617-627 (1988).

15 A.Papoulis, *Systems and Transforms with Applications in Optics* (MacGraw-Hill, New York, 1968).

16 A.E. Burgess, "Bach, breasts and power law processes," in *Medical Imaging 1999, Image Perception*, edited by E. Krupinski (Proceedings of the Society of Photo-optical Instrumentation Engineers, San Diego, CA, 1999), Vol. 3663, to be published.

17 A.E. Burgess, "Mammographic structure: Data preparation and spatial statistics analysis," in *Medical Imaging 1999, Image Processing*, edited by K. Hanson (Proceedings of the Society of Photo-optical Instrumentation Engineers, San Diego, CA, 1999), Vol. 3661, to be published.

18 J. Beutel and D. Richards .Sterling Diagnostic Imaging (private communication)

19 P.F. Judy, "Detection of clusters of simulated calcifications in lumpy noise backgrounds," in *Medical Imaging 1997, Image Perception*, edited by H.L. Kundel (Proceedings of the Society of Photo-optical Instrumentation Engineers, Newport Beach, CA, 1996), Vol. 2712, pp. 36-49..

20 A.E. Burgess and S. Chakraborty, "Producing lesions for hybrid images: extracted tumours and simulated microcalcifications," in *Medical Imaging 1999, Image Perception*, edited by E. Krupinski (Proceedings of the Society of Photo-optical Instrumentation Engineers, San Diego, CA, 1999), Vol. 3663, to be published.

21 M24L monitor, "Image Systems Corporation," (11543 K-Tel Drive, Hopkins MN 55343, 1993).

22 IDL, Version 5.1 (Research Systems Inc., Boulder, CO, 1998).

23 A.B.Watson and D.Pelli, "QUEST: a Bayesian adaptive psychometric method," Percept. Psychophysics **33**, 113-120 (1983).

24 A.E. Burgess, "Comparison of receiver operating characteristic and forced choice observer performance measurement methods," Med. Phys. **22**, 643-655 (1995).

25 H.L. Kundel, C.F. Nodine, L. Toto, and S. Lauver, "A circle cue enhances detection of simulated masses on mammographic backgrounds," in *Medical Imaging 1997, Image Perception*, edited by H.L. Kundel (Proceedings of the Society of Photo-optical Instrumentation Engineers, Newport Beach, CA, 1997), Vol. 3032, pp. 81-84.

26 A. E. Burgess and H. Ghandeharian, "Visual signal detection II. Signal location identification," J. Opt. Soc. Am. **A1**, 906-910 (1984).

27 A. E. Burgess, "Visual signal detection III: On Bayesian use of prior knowledge and cross-correlation," J. Opt. Soc. Am. **A2**, 1498-1507 (1985).

28 M.P. Eckstein, A.J. Ahumada, and A.B. Watson, "Visual signal detection in structured backgrounds II: Effects of contrast gain control, background variations and white noise," J. Opt. Soc. Am. **A14**, 2406-2419 (1997).

Producing lesions for hybrid mammograms:
Extracted tumours and simulated microcalcifications

Arthur E. Burgess and Sankar Chakraborty,

Radiology Dept., Brigham & Women's Hospital,

Ha rvard Medical School, 75 Francis St., Boston, MA 02115

ABSTRACT

Experimental and theoretical investigations of signal detection in medical imaging have been increasingly based on realistic images. In this presentation, techniques for producing realistic breast tumour masses and microcalcifications will be described. The mass lesions were obtained from 24 specimen radiographs of surgically removed breast tissue destined for pathological evaluation. A variety of masses were represented including both lobular and spiculated ductal carcinomas as well as fibroadenomas. Mass sizes ranged from 4 to 18 mm. The specimens included only a small amount of attached normal tissue, so tumour boundaries could be identified subjectively. A simple, interactive quadratic surface generating method was used for background subtraction - yielding an isolated tumour image. Individual microcalcifications were generated using a 3D stochastic growth algorithm. Starting with a central seed cell, adjacent cells were randomly filled until the 3D object consisted of a randomly selected number of filled cells. The object was then projected to 2D, smoothed and sampled. It is possible to generate a large variety of realistic shapes for these individual microcalcifications by varying the rules used to control stochastic growth. MCCs can then randomly generated, based on the statistical properties of clusters described by LeFebvre et al.[1]

1. INTRODUCTION

Until recently, most signal detection experiments related to medical imaging have used mathematically generated lesions. Many experiments used simple smoothed 2D disc and 2D Gaussian signals, that are convenient for mathematical analysis but do not realistically represent lesions present in patients. One effort to produce realistic lung nodules signals was reported by Samei et al.[2]. They measured the profiles of a large number of nodules and gave a polynomial algorithm for generating profiles. Burgess et al.[3,4] gave a designer nodule equation that provided a convenient analytical function to their data. The radial amplitude equation is $a(\rho) = A \, \text{Rect}(2\,\rho)(1-\rho^2)^\mu$, where A is the peak amplitude, ρ is a normalized distance,(r/R), relative to the nodule radius, R, and the exponent, μ, is real and non-negative. The designer nodule equation, with exponent μ equal 1.5 gives an excellent fit to the average lung tumor profile reported by Samei et al. The range of nodule profiles that they described was fitted by exponents between 1 and 2. This generalized nodule function has a convenient analytic Hankel transform proportional to $J_{\mu+1}(2\pi Rf)/(2\pi Rf)^{\mu+1}$. There have also been realistic mathematical nodules[5,6], developed for liver CT. These simulated masses are mathematically convenience and, for some purposes, realistic enough. This is not the case for mammographic tumors. Tumors and microcalcifications are highly irregular in shape, so simple mathematical simulations are instantly recognized as artificial.

The topics of breast masses and microcalcifications have been the subject of innumerable research papers in the computer-aided diagnosis literature over the last 10 years. There is also a wealth of information about statistical distributions of tumor sizes and numbers and sizes of microcalcification in clusters. Two excellent reference books exist, one on breast imaging[7] that has several chapters dealing with masses, while the other book deals solely with microcalcifications[8]. There has been no attempt, to the best of our knowledge to create realistic breast tumor masses.

There has been several approachs used to simulating microcalcifications and microcalcification clusters

316

Part of the SPIE Conference on Image Perception and Performance
San Diego, California • February 1999
SPIE Vol. 3663 • 0277-786X/99/$10.00

(MCCs). LeFebvre et al.[1] used a database of 8611 binary microcalcification shapes extracted from 408 real clusters extracted from digitized mammograms. This binary database was used to generate artificial clusters based on a detailed list of statistical properties of both individual microcalcifications and clusters. The pertinent point with respect to this paper is that they did not generate completely synthetic microcalcifications. They used binary shapes selected from their database and then produced gray level variations using an *ad hoc* layering method. They evaluated their results by having two radiologists view 100 images, 49 had simulated clusters and 51 had real clusters. The radiologists did not know which were simulated and were asked for each example cluster 'Do you think you would see such a cluster in routine examination''. The result was that one radiologist stated that 86% of the real clusters and 79% of the simulated clusters seemed realistic. The other radiologist stated that 69% of the real clusters and 58% of the simulated clusters seemed realistic. The authors used a χ^2 test to conclude that the radiologists could not distinguish between real and simulated clusters. Lado et al.[9] created databases of real and simulated microcalcification clusters. It appears that the individual simulated microcalcifications were copied form real digitized microcalcifications. They reported ROC experiments using 74 real and 74 simulated clusters. Two radiologists and a physicist took part in the experiment, which gave an average area under the ROC of 0.54 ± 0.03, indicating that there was no significant difference in appearance. Kallergi et al.[10] also produced simulated clusters. Their individual simulated microcalcification were produced by manually drawing based on BIRADS morphological descriptions and published examples. They used Gaussian gray level distributions. They evaluated 30 real and 30 simulated clusters added to digitized mammograms shown on a high-resolution monitor. Three mammographers took part in the blind study of visual assessment. Responses were evaluated for agreement using the kappa statistic and for independence using the χ^2 test. They concluded that there were no significant differences between the real and simulated microcalcification clusters.

This paper describes a method of extracting real tumor images from specimen mammograms and also describes a method for generating individual microcalcifications using a stochastic growth method.

2. EXTRACTED TUMORS

The Brigham and Women's Hospital (BWH) does about 20,000 mammographic studies per year and has a high tumor surgery rate because most are referrals from clinics and small hospitals. On average, there are about 20 surgical tumor removals per week. The specimens are radiographed in the mammography division of the Radiology Dept. before being sent to the Pathology Dept. for examination. The purpose of the mammograms is to determine whether all of the tumour has been removed and document the result. The specimen mammograms are done in a conventional mammogram unit with the tissue compressed. The images are recorded using a mammographic screen-film system. Because there is no patient radiation risk, a number of mammograms are done at a number of orientations to ensure clear demonstration of the tumor. Many of the specimens include only a small amount of normal tissue so by careful search of departmental records it was possible to obtain 25 high quality tumor images.

The 25 tumor images used for this work were obtained in the following manner. A larger number of cases were selected from the mammography division record book using the following criteria: no microcalcifications present and a representative mix of lesion types. The mammograms of the surgical biopsy specimen tissues were then reviewed: In many cases, the guide wires overlapped the tumor and these cases were rejected In other cases, there was considerable overlapping parenchymal tissue and these cases were also rejected. The goal was to obtain a set of tumor images where the tumor and its speculations (if present) were clearly visible, a minimum of overlapping complex tissue and complete biopsy records in the film jacket. The ideal cases would have a nearly uniform background. After about 50 cases were selected, the films were reviewed with two radiologists and 25 examples were selected. The mammograms were digitized at 51 micron sampling (12 bits/pixel) by Dr. J. Beutel of Sterling Diagnostic imaging using a Lumisys digitizer with a 50 micron spot. The size of each raw image was 3937x3937 pixels. A square region surrounding the tumor was then selected to produce smaller image files (500x500 pixels, 25.5x25.5 mm). This image size was large enough to include all tumors plus some surrounding tissue.

Table I: The distribution of lesion types extracted from specimen mammograms. The carcinomas covered a range of Bloom-Richardson grades.

Lesion type	number	Size range (mm)
invasive ductal carcinoma	10	9 - 18
invasive lobular carcinoma	5	4 - 15
fibroadenoma	7	5 - 8
atypical hyperplasia	1	9
lobular carcinoma in situ	1	
complex sclerosing lesion	1	

The next step was to extract the tumor from its background. Since care had been taken to select cases without background complexity, the process was relatively straight forward. The background was estimated using a quadratic surface method as follows. A 3x3 square grid of points was centered on the tumor with the midpoints of the edges close to, but not overlapping, the nearest tumor point. The image data values for the 8 points on the boundary were recorded and the value of the central point that would be expected, if the tumor were not present, was then estimated by one of the authors. The 9 point values were then used to calculate a quadratic surface with 51 micron sampling. This surface was then subtracted from the specimen image and negative values were set to zero. The resulting first estimate of the tumor only image was compared to the specimen image. In every case, it was clear that this first estimate was a poor one because of the lack of agreement between apparent tumor boundaries. The visual disparity was used to estimate perturbations to the 9 grid values and the revised values were used to calculate a second quadratic surface. The boundary comparison was repeated and another set of perturbations to the 9 grid values were estimated to create a new quadratic surface. This interactive procedure was repeated a number of times until there was a satisfactory agreement between the appearance of the extracted tumor and the tumor in the specimen image.
The extracted and specimen tumor images were then compared by a radiologist and were considered to be realistic. The extracted tumors were then adjusted in amplitude (contrast) and digitally added to normal digitized mammograms for evaluation by radiologists.

Figure 1 shows an example image of a tumor, background and biopsy guide wire before extraction of the tumor. Figure 2 shows the four lesions used in the two-alternative forced-choice lesion detection experiment reported in another paper of this conference[11]. (A) Invasive ductal Ca, 18 mm B-R grade 2; (B) fibroadenoma, 12 mm; (c) Invasive ductal Ca, 8 mm, well differentiated, B-R grade 1; (D) Invasive lobular Ca (14 mm, well- differentiated, B-R grade 1. The abbreviation B-R indicates the modified Bloom-Richardson grade (3 levels). Note that the lesions are not shown in correct relative size. They were all rescaled after extraction to fit inside a 256x256 array.

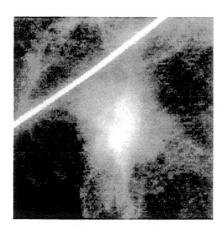

Figure 1. Example specimen mammogram

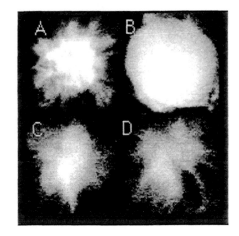

Figure 2; Four example lesions.

3. MICROCALCIFICATIONS

Our microcalcification simulation method is based on three-dimensional (3D) stochastic growth. A simple version of the method will be presented here. But it is easily varied to achieve increased complexity if desired. Some possibilities will be listed at the end of the section. It should be noted that the pixel and voxel dimensions used for growing the microcalcifications are arbitrary. Suppose one has digitized mammograms with 50 micron pixels, the stochastic growth can be done with smaller dimensions; voxels with 25 or 10 micron edges for example. The resulting 2D microcalcifications can then be rescaled to the desired pixel size and smoothed by the appropriate imaging system transfer functions for realism.

The basic idea is illustrated in figure 3, in two-dimensions for simplicity. The 2D array is labelled with left, right, top and bottom identified as (L, R, T, B). Each lattice point represents a pixel that may be filled (included in the calcification by setting its value to unity). A total number of calcification pixels is selected, N_p. The process starts with the center (seed) pixel filled. Then each step proceeds as follows. (1) One of the 4 edge views is random selected with equal probability. (2) The number of filled pixel edges that are visible from that view is determined and one of them is randomly selected to be the face to which the next pixel is added. (3) The appropriate pixel is filled. Then process is then repeated until all the available pixels have been used. So for figure 3, the sequence of steps will be described using the notation (view = T, fill #1 pixel of 1 choices). The resulting sequence is (L, #1 of 2), (R, #1 of 2), (B, #3 of 3), and finally (T, #2 of 3). This, of course, would be a silly procedure to use in 2D but is very convenient in 3D because the 'book-keeping' is straight forward.

The microcalcification growth occurs in a 3D array (64x64x64) with a center seed voxel filled. A total of N_v voxels will be filled. For the results presented here N_v had a fixed, selected value, but in practice N_v could be a random variable. There are now six possible views, the four listed above plus front and back (F, B). The steps are identical to the 2D example - (1) one of the six views is randomly selected, (2) one of the voxel faces visible from that view is randomly selected and (3) the adjacent empty voxel is filled. The process is repeated until all N_v voxels are filled. The 3D microcalcification is then projected to 2D to form the desired image. The amplitude of each pixel in the 2D image is determined by the number of filled voxels along the projection line associated with that pixel. During the procedure, the 3D data array serves as the complete memory of the process. The view and voxel face steps provide a simple and reliable way of ensuring that the next filled voxel is always attached to the face of an occupied voxel, ensures that every available voxel face has an equal probability of being selected as the point of growth and prevents voids.

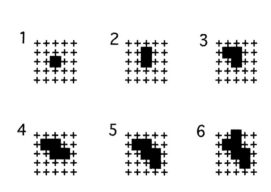

Figure 3. Two-dimensional illustration of the stochastic growth method. Described in the text

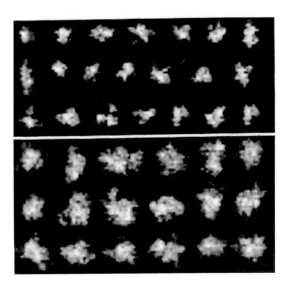

Figure 4. Example microcalcifications. The upper 3 rows were produced using 128 voxels. The lower 3 rows were produced using 512 voxels.

Example results are shown in figure 4. The upper 3 rows were produced using $N_v = 128$, while the lower 3 rows were done using $N_v = 512$. These examples were not specially selected, each set represents the sequential output of the algorithm (with a new random number seed for each realization).

Statistical properties:. The number of voxels filled is the main determinant of the microcalcification statistics. We investigated seven values of N_v: 64, 128,256,512,1024, and 2048. The mean area, A, of the resulting 2D images (in pixels) is related to N_v (in voxels) by $\log(A) = 0.71\log(N_v) + 0.159$. Lefebvre et al.[1] describe the statistical properties of their data base of 8611 microcalcifications and 408 clusters. Care must be taken in using their results because they are based on rectangular pixels (51x68 microns). This measurement asymmetric is very likely the source of such anomalies as a physically unreasonable height/width aspect ratio of 1.36 for both individual microcalcifications and clusters. Given random growth, one would be surprised by a value different from unity. Some of our results are presented in table II to allow comparison with the statistics of Lefebvre et al. . One might be trying to duplicate their individual microcalcification statistics, but then there are many reasons for using other possible size distributions. Lefebvre et al. also give an ad hoc algorithm for generating gray levels for the individual microcalcifications (which are binary shapes in their database). Their methods do deal very nicely with the realistic cluster generation problem, once one has obtained a collection of individual microcalcifications.

Table 2. Some statistical properties of the populations of microcalcifications generated with different starting numbers of voxels. These are provided to allow comparison with those obtained by LeFebvre et al. [1]. However, since no specific physical size is associated with a voxel, the user is free to select a size, use any appropriate growing lattice and then convert to the desired image pixel size, as well as include smoothing before or after scale change. The aspect ratio is the ratio of vertical/horizontal extent. The area/rect ratio refers to the microcalcification area as a fraction of the bounding rectangle area. The coefficient of variation for contrast (sd. dev./mean) is, of course, easily overridden by contrast scaling of the final microcalcification image.

N voxels	64	128	256	512	1024	2034
area mean (pixels)	27.2	45.7	74.2	123.7	196.4	321.8
area sd. dev.	4.9	6.5	10.3	15.2	20.7	33.2
aspect ratio sd. dev.	0.57	0.44	0.33	0.28	0.26	.23
Area/rect ratio.	0.80	0.74	0.70	0.68	.68	.67
Contrast sd. dev./mean	0.21	0.18	0.16	0.14	0.11	0.12

Possible growth variants. (1) The most obvious step is to make the number of voxels, N_v, a random variable. There is also the freedom to chose one of a number of probability distributions: uniform, Poisson, Gaussian, etc. and select the distribution parameters. This will have the effect of broadening the distributions of individual microcalcification statistical properties (2) It has been observed[8] that many microcalcifications appear to have lucent (lower physical density) cores. It would be straight forward to simulate any desired variation in layer density in the stochastic growth method. The above work was done with one density/attenuation value for all voxels. One could use a variety of densities or attenuation values. Consider two levels for example. The total number of voxels to be used could be divided so the first (central) N_1 voxels belong to the lower physical density class and the remainder (outer voxels) are of the higher physical density class. (3) Another possible variation could provide more needle-like microcalcifications of the type found in ducts. The above procedure did not have a preferred direction so any departure from spherical is due to statistical variation. A preferred direction, horizontal for example, can be obtained by modifying the view allocation probabilities from the current equality to 50% horizontal (L and R) and 25% for each of the other two directions. The choice is unimportant because one can then rotate the resulting microcalcifications to any angle one would like in the image.

4. SUMMARY

We have described a method for extracting real tumour images from specimen mammograms. The method requires interactive use of a quadratic surface background subtraction. This in turn requires that very little normal tissue be attached to the specimens and that the guide wire not overlap the tumour image. The quadratic surface subtraction success depends on good judgement of boundary comparisons, needs radiologist assistance and understanding of the anatomy. It, in principle, is possible to include full spiculations. We did not attempt this in the present work because the spiculations do not have enough contrast to be apparent at the low signal amplitudes used in 2AFC detection experiments.

Our 3D stochastic growth method for producing microcalcifications, even in its simplest from, produces very realistic lesions. The variants we have suggested have the potential to expand the range of possible shapes.

ACKNOWLEDGEMENTS

We would like to thank Jack Meyer MD, former Director of Breast Imaging in BWH Radiology for providing access to his personal biopsy records, which greatly facilitated the search for suitable cases. I would also like to thank Francine Jacobson MD, for considerable assistance in selecting cases and Darrell Smith MD, the current BWH Director of Breast Imaging for evaluating the final results. A special thanks to Jack Beutel of Sterling Diagnostic Imaging for digitizing the films. This research was funded by grant R01-58302 from the US National Cancer Institute.

REFERENCES

1 F. Lefebvre, H. Benali, R. Gilles *et al.*, "A simulation model of microcalcifications in digital mammograms," Med. Phys. 21, 1865-1874 (1994).

2 E. Samei, M.J. Flynn, G.H. Beue *et al.*, "Comparison of observer performance for real and simulated nodues in chest radiography,"in *Medical Imaging 1997: Image Perception*, edited by H.L. Kundel (Proceedings of the Society of Photo-optical Instrumentation Engineers, Newport Beach, CA, 1996), Vol. 2712, pp. 60-70

3 A.E. Burgess, X. Li, and C.K. Abbey, "Nodule detection in two component noise: toward patient structure," in *Medical Imaging 1997: Image Perception*, edited by H.L. Kundel (Proceedings of the Society of Photo-optical Instrumentation Engineers, Newport Beach, CA, 1997), Vol. 3036, pp. 2-13.

4 A.E. Burgess, "Visual signal detectability with two noise components: lowpass spectrum effects," J. Opt. Soc. Am. A16, (in press, March issue) (1999).

5 S.E. Seltzer, R.G. Swensson, R.D. Nawfel, J.F. Lentini, I. Kada and P.F. Judy, "Visualization and detection - localization on computed tomography images," Invest. Rad. 26, 285-294 (1991).

6 R.G. Swennson, P.F. Judy, C. Wester and S.E. Seltzer, "Nodule polarity effects on detection and localization performance in liver CT images," in *Medical Imaging 1997: Image Perception*, edited by H.L. Kundel (Proceedings of the Society of Photo-optical Instrumentation Engineers, Newport Beach, CA, 1997), Vol. 3036,pp. 85-17.

7 D. Kopans, *Breast Imaging, 2nd edition* (Lippincott-Raven Pub., Philadelphia, 1998).

8 M. Lanyi, *Diagnosis and differential diagnosis of breast calcifications* (Springer-Verlag, Berlin, 1986).

9 M.J. Lado, P.G. Tahoces, M. Souto *et al.*, "Real and simulated clustered microcalcifications in digital mammograms. ROC study of observer performance.," Med. Phys. 24, 1385-1394 (1997).

10 M. Kallergi, M.A. Gavrieldes, L. He *et al.*, "Simulation model of mammographic calcifications based on the ACR breast imaging reporting and data system, BIRADS," Acad. Radiol. 5, 670-679 (1998).

11 A.E. Burgess, "On the detection of lesions in mammographic structure," in *Medical Imaging 1999, Image Perception*, edited by E. Krupinski (Proceedings of the Society of Photo-optical Instrumentation Engineers, San Diego, CA, 1999), Vol. 3663, pp. to be published.

SESSION 9

Poster Session

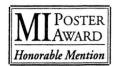

Appearance Matching of Radiographic Images
Using Lightness Index

Eiji Ogawa, Kazuo Shimura

Miyanodai Technology Development Center, Fuji Photo Film Co., LTD.

ABSTRACT

Appearances of images are closely related with the luminance dependence of human visual characteristics. Radiographic images are displayed on the CRTs with various luminance as well as on high luminance light-boxes. We studied a tone scale that can improve consistency in appearance among various devices with different luminance. It is likely that radiologists diagnose images based on the relation between the brightness of region of interest and that of surrounding area. Lightness is defined as a relative brightness of region of interest compared with the maximum luminance level of the image. We think the lightness index can be applied for realizing the appearance matching of radiographic images. Lightness matching can be realized by displaying images with the tone scale which gets agreement of the gradients of the display tone scale, on the logarithm of output luminance vs. input data level plane, among display systems. In this paper we call it a "lightness-equivalent" characteristic. We evaluated the appearance consistency of images displayed with the log-luminance linear tone scale, as realizing the lightness equivalent characteristic, compared with those displayed with the perceptual-linear tone scale. In evaluation the log-luminance linear tone scale gave almost the same appearance among devices with different luminance. On the other hand, the perceptual-linear tone scale gave lower visual contrast for images on the lower luminance device than the higher luminance device, which might have lead to observers perceiving as different appearances.

Keywords: Tone Scale, Appearance Matching, Lightness-Equivalent , Log-luminance Linear, Perceptual-Linear

1.INTRODUCTION

Digital imaging such as CT, MRI, and CR has been introduced in medical field for last three decades, and its popularity is significant now. With such digital acquisition, image can be handled as a soft copy. So it is now common that images are displayed on electronic devices such as CRT displays. Recently, filmless radiology has been in demand because of an economical matter. In the past, image quality on the CRT used to be much inferior to that on film, so hard copy film was used for diagnosis of radiographic images. However, as image quality of CRT is improved more recently, filmless diagnosis of image is in reality.

Digital images are likely to be reproduced and observed many times. As radiographic image display systems, there are a lot of CRTs and film/light-boxes with various image quality, such as the maximum luminance, MTF, and noise characteristic. When filmless radiology advances in the future, display systems with various specs will be used. It is important in terms of diagnosis to realize appearance matching of images presented on those display systems. Because the human visual perception is dependent on a luminance of a display system, differences in appearance may be mainly attributable to the maximum luminance, display tone scale of the system. As the maximum luminance has influence on an visual contrast sensitivity, we must realize appearance matching not with changing the maximum luminance but with modifying a display tone scale.

We studied a display tone scale that realizes appearance matching on display systems with various luminance. We also evaluated the level of appearance matching among images displayed with the tone scale.

Part of the SPIE Conference on Image Perception and Performance
San Diego, California • February 1999
SPIE Vol. 3663 • 0277-786X/99/$10.00

2. METHOD

2.1. Gradation Transformation Process

Digital Images are processed in several steps of gradation transformation process. For the computed radiography system(CR), an electrical signal read from an imaging plate is logarithmically converted and then normalized to a 10-bit signal. Next, gradation processing is performed on an image-by-image basis so that an optimal image for diagnosis is derived, and the resulting image is presented based on its display characteristic. This display characteristic means the relationship between an input signal level and an output luminance level of the system. The display characteristic is generally calibrated by performing tone correction on the system's intrinsic characteristic with a lookup table. [1] [2]

Usually data acquired by CT or MRI is processed by a console or modality workstation, so the resulting image is transferred, as data with window width and window level adjusted, to a hard copy output device or image viewing workstation. It is then presented with the display characteristic.

For medical imaging, gradation processing parameters are determined, on the assumption that an image is displayed with a certain display characteristic, and an image is processed with them to be used for diagnosis. That is, gradation processing which is optimized for that presumed display characteristic is performed. Thus, if an image is presented with a display characteristic other than the presumed characteristic, the resulting image may appear in an unexpected manner. In order to achieve reproduction of an image on various display systems in such a manner that the operator wants the image to appear, it is necessary to display an image with the display characteristic which gives appearance matching.

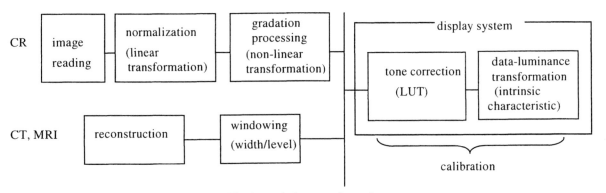

Fig. 1. gradation transformation process

2.2 Lightness equivalent characteristic

Appearance matching is to get appearance of whole image presented on a device with the same appearance of that on another device. Because there are a lot of devices with different luminance, and medical images are required to reproduce several times, we think it is valuable for diagnosis to realize appearance matching.

When considering appearance matching, we studied indexes of brightness perception. Several researches on brightness perception were done by Jameson, et al [3], Muka, et al [4]. They tested human contrast sensitivity by use of gray patches or sinusoidal patterns to derive rules and indexes, and suggested a relationship between contrast sensitivity and brightness.

However, it would be difficult to directly apply such indexes derived from the experiment as an index for representing the appearance matching of medical images. That is because radiographic images have complex patterns and are considered unlikely to be represented by an index that is determined from the contrast sensitivity experiment for a simple pattern.
When people observe medical images, it is likely that they judge information on a point of interest in terms of not only the brightness of that point but also the relative relationship with the brightness of its surrounding portions and the brightness of the entire image. We supposed that relative brightness might be applied as an index when considering appearance matching. As an index indicative of relative brightness, "lightness" that is generally used in the field of color imagery is

available. Lightness represents a brightness at a point of interest in terms of relative relationship with a brightness at the white point, and is given by the following equation [CIE 1976 psychometric lightness]:

$$116*(Y/Yn)^{1/3} - 16$$

We considered it possible to realize appearance matching by matching the levels of lightness for both images displayed on devices having different luminances. Lightness at a point of interest on an image may be represented by a relative relationship with the maximum luminance value. Assuming that observation point on an image is p, the maximum luminance values of devices A and B are L0_A and L0_B, and luminance values of p are Lp_A, Lp_B respectively, then the appearances at the observation points on the devices A and B can be described by:

$$116*(Lp\_A/L0\_A)^{1/3} - 16 \qquad\qquad 116*(Lp\_B/L0\_B)^{1/3} - 16$$

To give the same appearance to both of them, the ratios of the maximum luminance value to the luminance at the point p are required to be equal among the display devices having different luminance. This requirement is equivalent with the assumption that the gradients of tone scale curves of both systems are matched on the logarithm of luminance vs. input data level plane. We call this relationship the "lightness equivalent". The gradient means the level of Δ logarithm of luminance divided by Δ input data level. It is a common practice to put a hard copy film on light-box systems having different luminance for diagnostic observation. This means that films are observed with display characteristics having equal gradients among various luminance systems . Lightness equivalent is well accepted in hard copy film reading.

2.3 Experimental Method

We evaluated the lightness equivalent display characteristic from the standpoint of appearance matching. As a tone scale for realizing the lightness equivalent display characteristic, we employed a tone scale having a nearly linear characteristic on the logarithm of luminance vs. input data level plane, we call it "log-luminance linear tone scale" , that is currently used in many medical image printers as an output tone scale. For this study, we used a tone scale of Fuji-FL-IM-D (hereinafter referred to as "FI tone scale") as a typical example of the log-luminance linear tone scale. A main region of the FI tone scale is linear on the logarithm of luminance vs. input data level plane, however, gradients in the high luminance region are lower considering the fog characteristic of a film/light-box system, while in the low luminance region, gradients are higher considering the human low contrast sensitivity in the low luminance region.

As a tone scale for comparison, the perceptual linear tone scale that is currently part of the DICOM standard was used. [5] The perceptual linear tone scale is characterized by calibrating a display system to provide a perceptual linear characteristic. The log-luminance linear tone scale and the perceptual linear tone scale for the CRT with the maximum luminance of 300nit used for these evaluations are shown below. (Fig. 2)

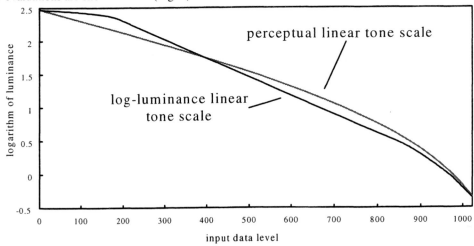

Fig. 2. Tone scales for CRT with the maximum luminance of 300nit

Evaluations were performed by determining which case provided more closely matched appearances among display systems: a case where high luminance and low luminance devices are calibrated to the perceptual linear tone scale and a case where they are calibrated to the log-luminance linear tone scale.

The display systems with different luminance used for these tests were a film/light-box system as a high luminance display system (laser printer film; the minimum and the maximum optical density of the system are 0.15, 3.0 respectively (Fuji-FL-IM-D)/light-box; the maximum luminance of 3000nit with no film); Fuji-HI-C655 with the maximum luminance of 300nit calibrated, as a standard-luminance CRT system; and Fuji HI-C655 with the maximum luminance of 100 nit calibrated, as a low-luminance CRT system.

The calibration of the CRT was implemented by measuring intrinsic characteristic of the CRT, creating a tone correction LUT that would eventually gives a target display characteristic with intrinsic characteristic, and transforming images by use of the LUT at the time of display. During evaluation, the dynamic range (the maximum luminance / the minimum luminance) of systems were matched.

Images used for evaluation included six CR images (two images of Chest, one image of Pelvis, Stomach, Leg, Mammography for each), three CT images (one image of Skull, Chest, and Abdomen for each), and three MRI images (one image of Abdomen, Skull, and Neck for each).

Evaluations were made regarding how appearances of images were matched, first between the film/light-box system and the standard-luminance CRT system, and then between the standard-luminance CRT system and low-luminance CRT system.

Fig. 3 shows the image presentation method of experiments. On the higher luminance device, a log-luminance linear optimized image (LOI) was presented. The log-luminance linear optimized image means an gradation processed image with optimal parameters to be displayed with the log-luminance linear tone scale. On the lower luminance device that was calibrated to the log-luminance linear tone scale, a log-luminance linear optimized image was presented, while a perceptual linear optimized image (POI) was presented on the lower luminance device that was calibrated to the perceptual linear tone scale.

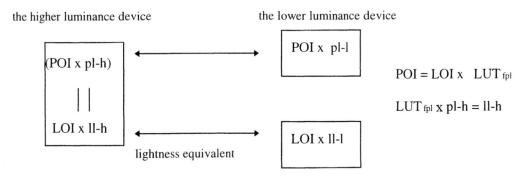

Fig. 3. image presentation method

In Fig. 3, "pl-h" and "pl-l" denote the tone scales of the higher luminance device and the lower luminance device that were calibrated to the perceptual linear tone scale, respectively. Meanwhile, "ll-h" and "ll-l" denote the tone scales of the higher luminance device and the lower luminance device that were calibrated to the log-luminance linear tone scale. X means an image transformation with display tone scale such as ll-l. A tone of the POI presented with pl-h is completely the same as that of the LOI presented with ll-h. The POI was created by processing the LOI with a lookup table (LUT_{fpl}) that would yield the tone scale, ll-h, when presented with pl-h.

With the higher luminance device and the lower luminance device arranged side by side, images optimized to the log-luminance linear tone scale were placed on the higher luminance device. Then, images optimized to the log-luminance linear tone scale and POI x pl-l simulated images are presented to the lower luminance device. The POI x pl-l simulated image means the image simulated so as to represent the same tone with POI x pl-l image when displayed on the ll-l calibrated device. Then, the image on the higher luminance device and the "LOI x ll-l" on the lower luminance device are images on the log-luminance linear calibrated device, and they have a lightness equivalent relationship, on the other hand, the image on the higher luminance device and the "POI x pl-l" on the lower luminance device are images on the perceptual linear calibrated device.

Evaluations were made through pair tests, whereby observers were instructed to choose one of the two images displayed on the lower that would appear more closely matched to the image presented on the higher luminance device.

The POI x pl-l simulated images and LOI x ll-l images were displayed in a CRT, and position of them were randomized. In order to reject the ambient light effect, tests were conducted in a darkroom, with a viewing distance of 50 cm, for an unlimited amount of observation time. The observer included 16 medical imaging scientists having more than five years of experience in this field, who evaluated appearance consistency for the film/light-box system and standard-luminance CRT system, while ten of those scientists evaluated appearance consistency for the standard-luminance and low-luminance CRT systems.

3. RESULTS AND DISCUSSION

The tone scales of the film/light-box system, standard-luminance CRT system, and low-luminance CRT system that were calibrated to the log-luminance tone scale, and those calibrated to the perceptual linear tone scale are shown below. (Fig. 4 and Fig. 5)
The relationship among log-luminance linear tone scales was the lightness equivalent. (Fig. 4)

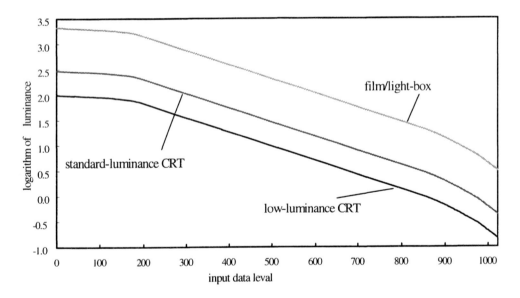

Fig. 4. log-luminance linear tone scale

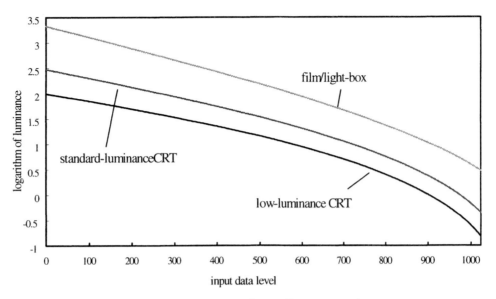

Fig.5. perceptual luminance linear tone scale

For the log-luminance linear tone scale, the gradients of curves in the entire data area are equal among the systems with different luminance. On the other hand, when calibrated to the perceptual linear tone scale, the lower the luminance of the system, the higher the gradients in the low luminance data area, while the gradients in the middle to high luminance area gets lower. The more different the luminance between devices is, the more significant the difference of gradients is.

Next, the results of evaluation on appearance matching for the film/light-box system and standard-luminance CRT system are shown in Fig. 6.

	CR Chest A	B	Pelvis	Stomach	Leg	Mammography
total number	16	16	16	16	16	16
LL>PL	16	16	16	16	16	16
p	0.1%	0.1%	0.1%	0.1%	0.1%	0.1%

	CT Skull	Chest	Abdomen	MRI Skull	Abdomen	neck
total number	16	16	16	16	16	16
LL>PL	8	16	9	16	15	14
p	*	0.1%	*	0.1%	0.1%	0.5%

LL: log-luminance linear tone scale   * over 50%
PL: perceptual linear tone scale

Fig. 6. appearance matching evaluation between film/light-box and standard luminance CRT

In Fig.6, LL>PL is the number of the observer who selected an image displayed with the log-luminance linear tone scale in terms of appearance matching.   For CR images, the results indicate that all of the images yielded better appearance matching when displayed with the log-luminance linear tone scale (p < 0.5%).   For CT and MRI images, the log-luminance linear tone scale gained better ratings in terms of appearance matching, excluding images of CT Skull and Abdomen.   After the evaluation, most of observers said that, the contrast of the image displayed with the log-luminance linear tone scale on the lower luminance device is more matched with that of the higher luminance device than that displayed with the perceptual linear tone scale.   The difference was significant in the contrast for the Lung of the Chest, tumor mass of the Mammography, the Lung of the CT Chest , and the internal organs of the MRI Abdomen.

Next, the mean value and the standard deviation of the image pixel for evaluations are shown in Fig. 7, while the gradient curves of the log-luminance linear tone scales and for the perceptual linear tone scales are shown in Fig. 8., Fig. 9. respectively.

	CR Chest			Pelvis	Stomach	Leg	Mammography
	A	B					
mean	454	520		612	472	403	480
σ	227	247		200	216	96	92

	CT Skull	Skull (brain)	Chest	Abdomen	Abdomen (liver)	MRI Skull	Abdomen	neck
mean	680	815	468	788	644	624	603	660
σ	336	92	412	236	72	288	336	352

Fig.7. mean value and σ of the input data level

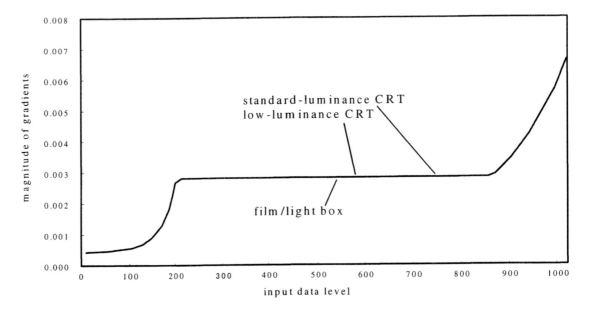

Fig.8. gradients of log-luminance linear tone scale

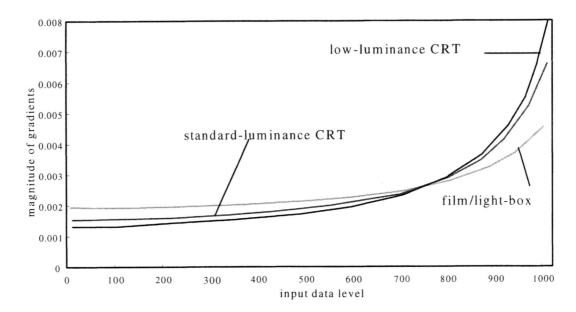

Fig.9. gradients of perceptual linear tone scale

Fig. 8 shows that the gradient curves of all the log-luminance linear tone scales are equal in the entire data range among the devices with different luminance. On the other hand, the gradient curves of the perceptual linear tone scales are different in most of data area among devices. (Fig. 9) It means the fact that the lightness of images are the same among devices calibrated to the log-luminance linear tone scale, while those are different among devices calibrated to the perceptual linear tone scale.

Fig. 7 shows the distribution of image pixel data used in the evaluation. The mean values of most images are in the middle portion of data range, and the standard deviations are around 100 to 400. This shows that the image pixel data exists over a wide range of the input data level. Because the log-luminance linear tone scales have the same gradients among devices in all region, appearance matching was achieved among images displayed with the log-luminance linear tone scales. On the other hand, in the perceptual linear tone scales, gradients of the tone scale of the lower luminance device is lower than the higher luminance device in most region of the input data level (up to about 800). Then contrasts in most of the image displayed on the lower luminance device are lower than those of the higher luminance device.

While, as shown in Fig.6, for the CT Skull and Abdomen images, about half of the observers chose the perceptual linear tone scale. In those images, Brain and Liver region occupy a large portion and the pixel data in those region distribute from 600 to 900. Around that input data level, the gradients of the perceptual linear tone scale of the higher luminance device and those of the lower luminance device are almost same, and the lightness equivalent relationship is locally exists in that data range. That is the reason why the perceptual linear tone scale gives as good appearance consistency as the log-luminance linear tone scale for those two images.

Next, Fig. 10 shows the result of appearance matching evaluation between standard-luminance CRT and low-luminance CRT .

	CR		Pelvis	Stomach	Leg	Mammography
	Chest A	B				
total number	10	10	10	10	10	10
LL>PL	9	10	10	8	8	10
p	3%	0.2%	0.2%	11%	11%	0.2%

	CT			MRI		
	Skull	Chest	Abdomen	Skull	Abdomen	neck
total number	10	10	10	10	10	10
LL>PL	7	10	8	9	9	9
p	35%	0.2%	11%	3%	3%	3%

Fig. 10. appearance matching evaluation between standard luminance CRT and low luminance CRT

For all the images, the log-luminance linear tone scale got better appearance consistency. Some observers chose the perceptual linear tone scale for images such as CR Stomach and Leg, while nobody chose the perceptual linear tone scale in evaluation between film/light-box and standard luminance CRT. It is probably because the difference of gradients between the standard luminance CRT and the low luminance CRT is smaller than that between film/light-box and standard luminance CRT. (Fig. 9)

4. CONCLUSION

We studied the lightness equivalent display characteristic to realize an appearance matching among devices having different luminances. And we evaluated the appearance consistency using the log-luminance linear tone scale, as the typical tone scale which realizes lightness equivalent characteristic, in comparison with the perceptual linear tone scale. The result shows that the log-luminance linear tone scale is obviously better than the perceptual linear tone scale in terms of realizing appearance matching.

Appearance matching was achieved among images displayed with the log-luminance linear tone scale regardless of the degree of difference in luminance between devices, while in most images displayed with the perceptual linear tone scale, contrasts of images on the lower luminance device were lower than those of the higher luminance device. The reason is supposed that the lightness of images are the same among devices calibrated to the log-luminance linear tone scale, while those are different among devices calibrated to the perceptual linear tone scale.

5. REFERENCES

[1] T. Tateno, T. Iinuma, M. Takano (Eds.): Computed Radiography, Springer-Verlag, Tokyo (1987)
[2] E. Ogawa, S. Arakawa et al: Quantitative analysis of imaging performance for computed radiography systems, Proc of SPIE, 2432-41(1995)
[3] D. Jameson & L.M. Hurvich: Theory of brightness and color contrast in human vision, Vision Res., 4 (1964)
[4] E. Muka, H. Blume, S. Daly: Display of medical images on CRT soft-copy displays: A tutorial, Proc of SPIE,2431-32(1995)
[5] DICOM: part 14 Grayscale Standard Display Function, NEMA, (1988)

Reconfigurable Parallel Processor for Noise Suppression

Michael Cuviello, Philip P. Dang, Paul M. Chau

Department of Electrical & Computer Engineering

University of California, San Diego

ABSTRACT

Digital images corrupted with noise regularly require different filtering techniques to optimally correct the image. Software provides convenience for implementing a variety of different filters, but suffers a speed penalty due to its serial nature of the filter calculations. In converse fashion, implementation using ASIC technology allows for a speed advantage due to parallel processing but at the cost of increased hardware overhead for implementing a variety of filters individually. Advances in Field Programmable Gate Array (FPGA) technology offers a middle ground in which the speed advantages of an ASIC and the reprogrammable aspect of a general purpose conventional CPU or DSP software approach are combined. In this paper, we present an FPGA-based, reconfigurable system, that can perform an assortment of noise filtering algorithms using the same hardware. Implementation of Gaussian and salt-and-pepper noise are evaluated for this system.

Keywords: Image, noise, suppression, median, average, filter, hardware, FPGA, reconfigure, reprogram

1 INTRODUCTION

In a system processing digital images, such as a communication channel, an assortment of sources inject a variety of noises with different characteristics into the image data. To correct for these, varied filtering techniques are applied to restore the corrupted images to an acceptable level. Gaussian noise for example, is commonly removed using low pass filter techniques. For other noises however, such as impulse noise, characterized by random white intensity values, and salt-and-pepper noise, characterized by random black and white intensity values, low pass filtering is insufficient, and thus, requires the utilization of other filters.[4]

For example, rank-ordered filters such as the median filter are widely used for cleaning impulsive noise without blurring sharp edges. Realizing median filters in general-purpose platforms is computationally costly because of the repeated data passing required to sort a large set of pixel values. Additionally, general-purpose platforms are overly complicated for the simple magnitude comparisons and selection operations that comprise the arithmetic of a median filter. Such a filter is most efficiently handled using array processing. This makes specific hardware implementation a better choice. In particular, the combinatorial cells, storage resources and interconnect of FPGAs are well suited for such a design.[5]

In this paper, we present a hardware architecture, realizable on a reprogrammable FPGA system, for noise suppression in digital images. The flexibility of this system allows for the development of new filters and for on-the-fly implementation of several different filters on the same hardware. Thus, not only do we achieve near ASIC parallel processing performance with the flexibility of reconfiguration, we demonstrate a system solution that also facilitates minimizing the overall system form-factor, weight, and power.

The remainder of the paper is organized as follows. In section 2 we present an overview of the reconfigurable system. In section 3, the architecture of the median filter and the average filter on the reconfigurable processor are discussed. Finally, the conclusion and a few remarks about our future works are provided.

2 SYSTEM OVERVIEW

2.1 RCP Description

The ReConfigurable Processor (RCP) board is a PC form-factor, FPGA based coprocessor designed by the VLSI-DSP Research Group at UCSD and L3 Communications, San Diego.[1] The RCP board consists of 6 Altera FLEX 10K70 FPGA

Part of the SPIE Conference on Image Perception and Performance
San Diego, California • February 1999
SPIE Vol. 3663 • 0277-786X/99/$10.00

processing elements, 4 ICube IQX160 PSID field programmable interconnect chips, two 4Kx18 FIFOs, 4 dual port 32Kx16 RAMs, an additional 1Mx32 single port RAM module, and a PCI interface. These components are interconnected to form a changeable pipelined data processing system. This flexibility enables the designer to have multiple degrees of freedom for architecture implementations that are not possible on other coprocessor boards. Data flow and functional control occur via the PCI bus and are managed with a custom software graphical user interface. This interface enables the user to build autonomous custom scripts that intermix the configuring of the board into various architectures with the actual use of those architectures for data processing. In this way, data sets, digital images for example, can be repeatedly processed several times through different hardware designs on one board. The RCP is shown in figure 1.

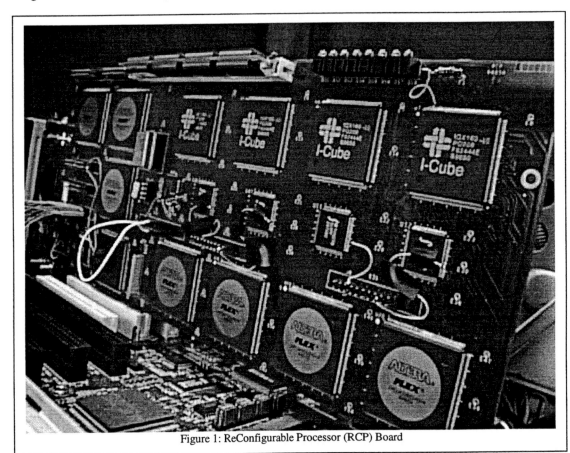

Figure 1: ReConfigurable Processor (RCP) Board

3 ARCHITECTURES

3.1 Case study: Median Filtering

3.1.1 Algorithm

Median filtering is a non-linear process that preserves the sharp edges in images. It effectively removes non-Gaussian and impulsive shaped noise.[2] Salt and pepper noise and impulse noise are examples of such noises. Figure 2 illustrates the median filter applied to a blood cell image.[10]

The filtering process is performed by taking a square window about a center pixel and ranking the pixels in the window in ascending order of intensity. A new value for the center pixel is set equal to the sample value in the window that is located in the middle of the list (figure 3). If the window size is 2n+1, the input values in the window, f(0, 0), f(0, 1), f(0,2n), f(1, 0), ... f(2n, 2n), are sorted into a magnitude ordered set, m(0), m(1), m(2), ... m($4n^2 + 4n$). The median value of this set is given by y(n)=m(2n(n + 1)).

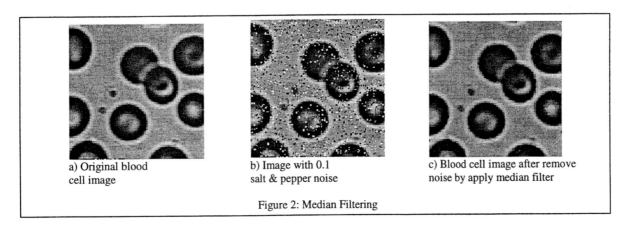

| a) Original blood cell image | b) Image with 0.1 salt & pepper noise | c) Blood cell image after remove noise by apply median filter |

Figure 2: Median Filtering

3.1.2 Hardware Architecture

For our system we implement a 3x3 window. Figure 4 depicts the exchange network required to sort the nine pixel-values of the window.[3.] The nine pixels are divided into three groups. Each group includes three pixels from the same column. The sorting process can be divided into three stages. In the first stage, the pixels in each group are compared to each other to determine the smallest, the median, and the largest pixel. This process takes 3 clock cycles. In the second stage, the smallest pixels from each group are compared for the largest value, the median pixels are compared for the median value, and the largest pixels are compared for the smallest value. These values are then compared in the third stage and the median value of this set is selected as the median value for the entire window.

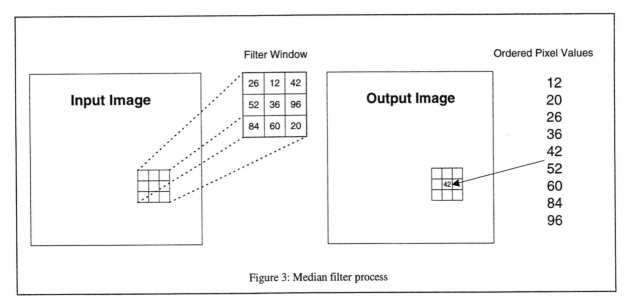

Figure 3: Median filter process

Slight modifications to this structure are required to handle pixels on the edge of the image. In which case, the window extends beyond the image. Window spaces beyond the edge are simply disregarded.

The complete sorting process in figure 4 requires 19 nodes and costs 9 clock cycles to determine the middle value. Each node is comprised of an 8-bit comparator requiring one clock cycle. At the output of the comparator, the lowest input goes to the left and the highest input goes to the right. A triangle group of nodes performs a full sort on three elements. Efficiency is achieved by having several (3) nodes operate simultaneously.

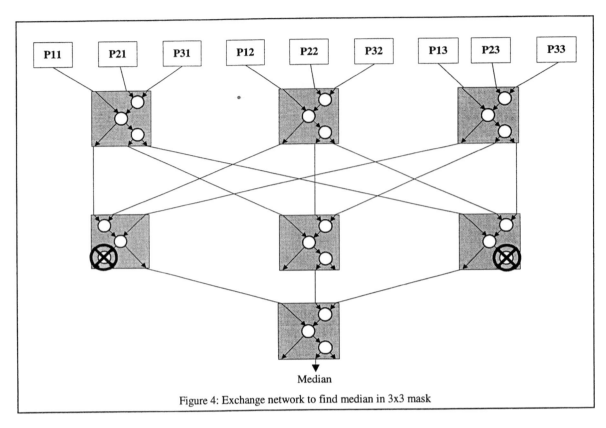

Figure 4: Exchange network to find median in 3x3 mask

3.2 Case study: Mean Filtering

3.2.1 Algorithm

The Mean filter, or average filter, is a simple linear spatial filter.[8.] It is a low pass filter that removes high spatial frequencies from an image. It is often applied for removing Gaussian noise from an image. Figure 5 shows the use of mean filtering.

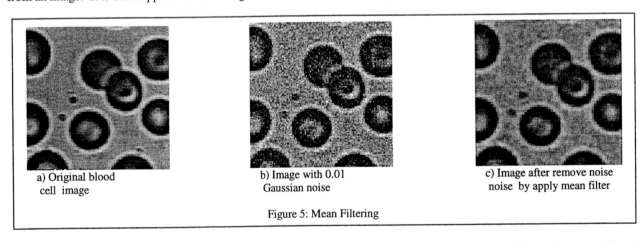

a) Original blood
cell image

b) Image with 0.01
Gaussian noise

c) Image after remove noise
noise by apply mean filter

Figure 5: Mean Filtering

The shortcoming of the average filter is that it reduces sharp edges located within the mask of the filter. The mean filter is implemented by a local averaging operation where the value of each pixel is replace by the average of all the values in the local neighborhood (figure 6).

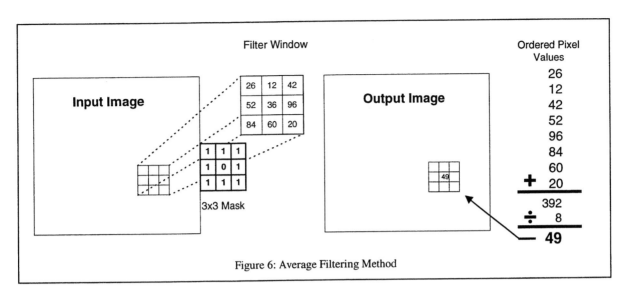

Figure 6: Average Filtering Method

3.2.2 Hardware Architecture

Typically, each value in the window is weighted the same, which means that the mean filter is spatially invariant, and can be implemented by using a convolution mask. However, in our implementation, to greatly simplify the hardware design, we set the weight of the center pixel in the window to zero and the rest to one. Therefore, the value of the output pixel will be the sum of the 8 surrounding pixels divided by 8. The divide by 8 operation is simply to drop the 3 lowest significant digits when the number is represented in binary. The architecture of mean filter is show below.

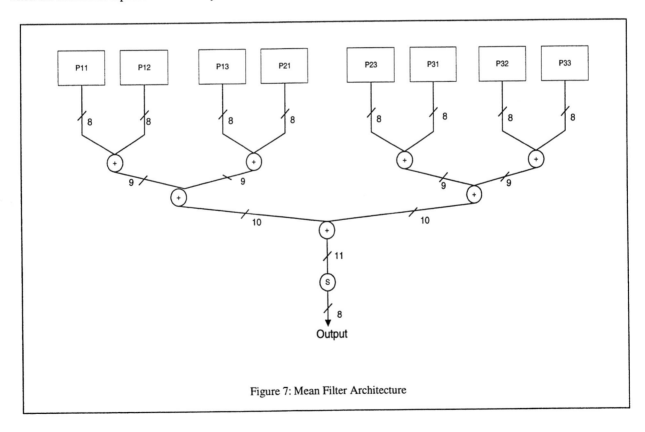

Figure 7: Mean Filter Architecture

The regular structure of this parallel architecture makes it easily implementable in an FPGA. The design requires four 8-bit adders, two 9-bit adders, and one 10-bit adder with a total latency of three clock cycles. To calculate the average values for the pixels on the edge of the image we assume that the values of pixels outside the image are zeros.

3.3 System Pipeline Architecture for Implementing Filters.

The images used in this study are grayscale with 8-bit pixel values stored sequentially from left to right and from top to bottom in a contiguous data block (figure 8). For both the median and mean filters and any filter that applies a local window, the calculations require simultaneous access to data in adjacent rows that are used in each window calculation. In our study we used a 512x512 image with a 3x3 filter window.

Since the data is read in sequential in order of byte number, processing a window requires the buffering of at least the first two rows used in the window. To handle this, our design uses a pipelined architecture as shown in figure 9. Data enters from the left side of the block diagram and is stored in a sequence of two dual port memories that are configured as FIFO buffers. Each are sized to store one row of pixels. The data bus on the RCP board is two bytes wide, allowing two pixels to be loaded with each memory cycle.

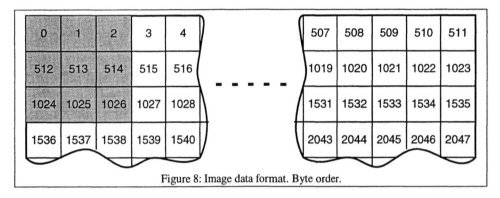

Figure 8: Image data format. Byte order.

Out of each memory and from the DATA IN bus, 3 adjacent rows of pixel data are simultaneously shifted left into a matrix of registers that comprise two sliding windows centered on registers (2,2) and (2,3). Because two pixels are read in at a time, processing of two windows simultaneously reduces control complexity and allows common calculations between two adjacent windows to be shared.

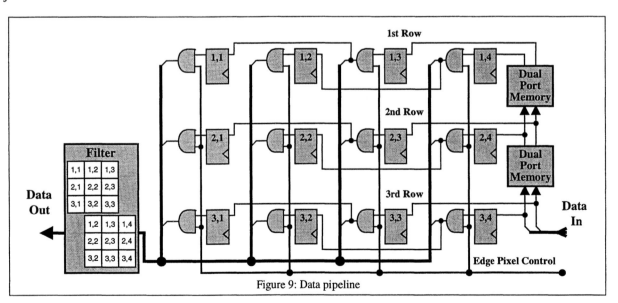

Figure 9: Data pipeline

For pixels on the edge of an image, gates are added to the outputs of each register to set window elements that lay outside the image to the appropriate value. For the mean filter, "AND" gates are sufficient to set these elements to 0 (as shown in figure 9). For the median filter, a mix of "AND" and "OR" gates would be used to set some of the values to 0 and some to the maximum value of 256.

One advantage of this architecture is that the entire image does not have to be stored in memory, as would a system that reads in 9 pixels of a window non-sequentially from random access memory. Storing only two rows at a time is sufficient. Additionally, since the data is stored sequentially, memory accesses can occur every clock cycle using burst reads and writes. Hence the architecture we have is amenable to real-time, in-line, image processing. This approach could be expanded upon to accommodate real-time in line video processing

Since data is processed as fast as the access time on the data bus, the processing time in cycles for an image is approximately equal to the number of pixels in the image. This estimate considers the latency of the filter and of 1 row of data to be stored before the first pixel can be calculated negligible.

3.4 Implementation

Figure 10 illustrates a simple block diagram of the RCP board with highlighted devices and data paths that are utilized in this design. Data enters from the PCI bus, through the PCI interface, through the input FIFO, through the PRE processing element, and into the programmable interconnect matrix, to the beginning of the design. This is the point labeled DATA IN on figure 9. The data path is then split in two. One path passes directly to processing element 0 (PE0) and the other passes through the 1st dual port memory and into (PE0). Both paths pass directly to PE1. The first path provides 3rd row data and the path through the dual port memory provides 2nd row data. In PE1, the 2nd row data is tapped out to the programmable interconnect and back through the 2nd dual port memory to provide the 1st row data. The window matrix and filters are implemented in PE1 with the output data passed out to the POST PE, through the output FIFO, and back to the PCI bus.

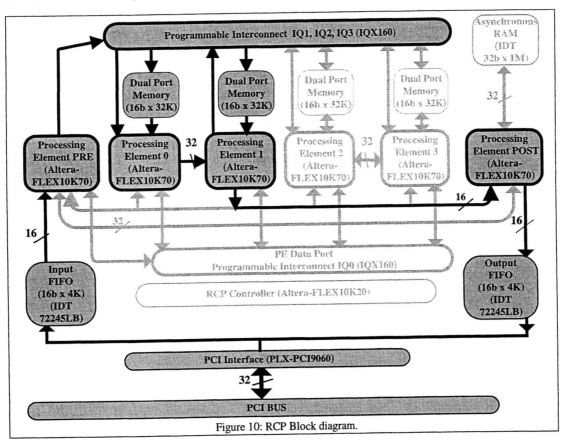

Figure 10: RCP Block diagram.

3.5 RCP Performance:

The maximum operating frequency for the RCP is 40MHz. This limit is a result of the maximum operating frequency of the FPGAs available when the RCP was built in 1997. For a 512x512 image, the processing time equates to 3.27mS to handle the entire 262Kbytes. More of a limiting factor in performance however is the I/O of the data bus that is shared for input and output data. Because of this, the data rate in and out of the board is cut in half, increasing the processing time to 6.55mS.

Image size is limited to the depth of the dual port memories that are required to hold one row. Each dual port memory holds up to 64Kbytes of data, making the image size effectively limitless.

3.6 Reconfiguration:

PE1 is large enough to implement several different simple filters, such as the median and mean, simultaneously. For more complicated algorithms however, the need may arise to change or modify filters programmed into the design. In our implementation, we need only to reconfigure the processing element PE1 to accomplish this. Copies of different designs for PE1 may be stored off-board or may be stored in the onboard 4Mbyte asynchronous RAM. Programming PE1 is done with a serial bit stream of configuration data that can be clocked into the device in approximately 100mS.[6.]

3.7 Summary

The table below lists some performance parameters of the RCP, the Texas Instruments TMS320C54x DSP, and the AMD-K6 RISC general-purpose processor for performing the median and mean filters. The Texas Instruments (TI) and AMD processors, with the speed grades used in these estimates, were introduced at roughly the same time as the FPGAs on the RCP and therefore provide a reasonable basis for comparing the RCP approach to the processor approaches.

Estimates for the TI and AMD processors are based on cycles per instruction obtained from their respective data books.[7,9] Calculations for the TI DSP are estimated using the formula, {(3 instructions / operation) x (1 cycle / instruction) x (# of operations / pixel) + (2 cycles store to memory / pixel)} x {# of pixels}. AMD calculations are calculated in a similar fashion but include penalties and benefits from additional load/store instructions and memory caching capabilities respectively. Adjustment to the number of operations required for each device was also considered. For the processors, reduced operations for the median filter take into account that calculations common to overlapping windows can be optimally shared. The average filter also uses shared operations but additionally includes the extra shift operation that is not necessary in the RCP.

Performance Comparison	Median Filter			Average Filter		
	RCP	'C54	AMD-K6	RCP	'C54	AMD-K6
Operations per pixel	19	12.5	12.5	7	7	7
Clock Cycles per pixel	1	~39.5	~29.5	1	~23	~23
Clock Latency (512x512) / (4096x4096)	267/4107	~0	~0	261/4101	~0	~0
Maximum operational clock frequency	40 MHz	40MHz	200MHz	40 MHz	40MHz	200MHz
Time per pixel	25ns	~988ns	~148ns	25ns	~575ns	~115ns
512x512 Processing Time	6.55ms	~259ms	~38.6ms	6.55ms	~151ms	~30.1ms
4096x4096 Processing Time	0.419s	~16.6s	~2.47s	0.419s	~9.66s	~1.93s
Reconfiguration Time	100ms	---	---	100ms	---	---
Speed Improvement	---	x39.5	x5.9	---	x23	x4.6

3.8 Conclusion

This paper presented a novel reprogrammable architecture to efficiently implement median and mean filters on a hardware reconfigurable processor. This architecture exploits the structure of digital image data that eliminates the requirement full image buffering. The comparisons of the embedding of our architecture on the RCP against two conventional software approaches provide a qualitative measure of speed advantage that can be obtained using our architecture while maintaining the same flexibility as software implementations. The TMS320C54 comparison provides a realistic comparison when considering the amount and speed of the hardware used for each implementation. The inclusion of the AMD-K6 comparison demonstrates that the RCP still performs favorably when hardware resources are not an issue.

Additionally, the pipeline system architecture developed for the two filters is applicable to real-time, in-line image processing and can be expanded upon to accommodate real-time, in-line, video processing. As the growth of the internet and wireless communications occur, we envision the emergence of increased remote site medical assistance. Hence efficient real-time in-line processing will be needed to achieve compact and portable medical imaging/video communications and processing. Since our architecture doesn't need full image buffering and is reconfigurable for implementing alternative filters, it facilitates the realization of such equipment.

The RCP board was designed and built in 1997 and is currently being used in several projects as a research development and demonstration tool for reconfigurable hardware. We are currently developing VHDL libraries to implement other filters and designs. Additionally we are developing a new reconfigurable platform that will be optimized for greater data throughput, have a wider flexibility in applications, and a faster reconfiguration scheme.

ACKNOWLEDGMENTS

We would like to thank the UCSD RCP team members, Mike Crawford and his staff of L3 Communications, and our undergraduate research assistants, Ted Barsenas and Victor Gallardo for their support of the RCP research. We would additionally like to thank the UCSD ICAS Center and the National Science Foundation for their partial support of our research in reconfigurable systems.

REFERENCES

1. K.J. Page, J. Arrigo, P. M. Chau , "ReConfigurable Hardware Based Digital Signal Processing for Wireless Communications." *Proceedings of the SPIE: Advanced Signal Processing Algorithms, Architectures and Implementation VIII, July 1997.*
2. R. Jain, R. Kasturi, B. Schunck, *Computer Vision,* McGraw Hill, Inc. New York, NY, 1995, pp:112-137.
3. J.L. Smith, "Implementing Median Filters in XC4000E FPGAs," *Xilinx XCELL Quarterly Journal, Q4 1996, pp16.*
4. R. Crane, *A Simple Approach To Image Processing,* Prentice Hall, Upper Saddle River, NJ, 1997, pp:95-96.
5. S.M. Trimberger (Editor*), Field Programmable Gate Array Technology,* Kluwer, Boston, MA. 1994.
6. Altera, *Altera Data Book.* 1998.
7. Texas Instruments, *TMS320C54x DSP Reference Set, Volume 3: Algebraic Instruction Set.,* Oct. 1996.
8. K.R. Castleman, *Digital Image Processing,* Prentice-Hall, Englewood Cliffs, NJ, 1996. pp208.
9. H.Kalish (Editor), J.Isaac (Editor), *The AMD-K6 3D Processor,* Abacus, Grand Rapids, MI, 1998, pp.465.
10. MathWorks, "blood1.tif", *Matlab Image Processing Toolbox, Version 1.3,* 1997.

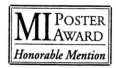

Image compression and feature stabilization of dynamically displayed coronary angiograms

Jay L. Bartroff[1], Craig A. Morioka, James S. Whiting, Miguel P. Eckstein

Department of Medical Physics and Imaging, Cedars-Sinai Medical Center, 8700 Beverly Blvd., Davis 6065, Los Angeles, CA 90048-1865

ABSTRACT

Eigler et al (1994) proposed an optimized display for coronary angiograms where each image of the sequence is digitally shifted so that the feature of interest within an artery remains fixed at the center of the screen and the background moves (stabilized display). We measure the effect of JPEG and CREW (a wavelet-based software) image compression on the detectability of a simulated morphological feature (filling defect) for the stabilized display and compare it to the conventional moving artery display. Our results show that 15:1 compressed JPEG for the stabilized display and the moving artery display does not significantly degrade human performance but a 19:1 CREW did. The stabilized display significantly improved performance with respect to the conventional moving artery display for the uncompressed and the 15:1 JPEG but not for the 19:1 CREW.

Keywords: Image compression, visual detection, feature motion, image quality, x-ray angiography

1. INTRODUCTION

Digital catheterization laboratories are quickly becoming the norm in cardiology [1]. Among the benefits of the digital system are the availability of enhancement and filtering techniques that improve image quality, manipulation of variable display options by the cardiologist, and the ability to copy the original data for availability to multiple physicians. Storage of digital catheterization procedures is expensive however (~ 1 Gigabyte per individual procedure) and lossy image compression is a possible solution. The amount of compression then becomes critical and must be tempered by its affect on the cardiologist's visual detection, classification, and/or estimation of a lesion. A small number of studies have investigated the impact of lossy compression on diagnosis in coronary angiograms [2-4]. Baker et al [2] found that 15:1 JPEG compression did not significantly degrade the detection of morphological features while Rigolin et al [3] similarly concluded that stenosis measurement precision was not significantly affected.

Eigler et al [5] proposed an optimized display for coronary angiograms where each image of the sequence is digitally shifted so that the feature of interest within an artery remains fixed at the center of the screen while the background moves (see figure 1). This stabilized display (S.D.) allows the observer to scrutinize the feature of interest without having to eye-track its sometimes abrupt motion. Previous results using computer simulated arterial motion showed that the S.D. improves feature detectability over the standard display where the artery is moving (M.A.). The purpose of this paper is to investigate the interaction between image compression and method of display (S.D. vs. M.A.). It is unknown whether a 15:1 compression ratio will not degrade lesion detectability for the feature-stabilized display.

---

[1] Correspondence: Email: miguel@medphysics.csmc.edu WWW: http://www.csmc.edu/medphys; Telephone: 310 855 7770; Fax: 310 652 8338

Part of the SPIE Conference on Image Perception and Performance
San Diego, California • February 1999
SPIE Vol. 3663 • 0277-786X/99/$10.00

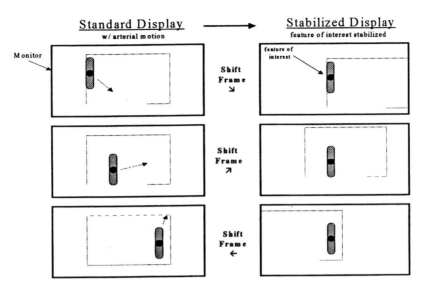

Standard Display ⟶ Stabilized Display
w/ arterial motion   feature of interest stabilized

Monitor

feature of interest

Shift Frame ↘

Shift Frame ↗

Shift Frame ←

Figure 1. The standard moving-artery display (M.A.) and the stabilized display (S.D.). The stabilized display is obtained by digitally shifting each frame of the standard moving-artery display so that the feature of interest remains in the center of the screen throught the sequence.

The Baker et al. [2] study relied on consensus committees to determine the gold-standard in the observed images. Images in which no consensus was reached were discarded from the study. One potential limitation of this methodology is that most of the difficult cases with subtle lesions may not result in consensus and thus might be discarded from the study. In addition, recent results with computer simulated lesions suggest that relying on a consensus committee to establish a gold standard can lead to a "false gold standard" [6]. In order to avoid the shortcomings of establishing a gold standard, the present paper uses simulated lesions embedded in patient coronary angiograms. In addition, the Baker study used fixed quality levels in the compressions so we do not know which compression level or levels were actually being studied[2]. The present paper uses a program to iteratively compress the images at different quality levels to try to achieve a fixed compression for all images. Finally, the majority of available image compression software can be categorized as either cosine-transform or wavelet-based by their basis of choice for image decomposition. JPEG is the forerunner of the cosine class yet the more recent wavelet algorithms have not been evaluated for coronary angiograms. We test JPEG as well as the wavelet-based CREW software.

2. METHODS

2.1 Acquisition of x-ray coronary angiograms and generation of simulated arteries and lesions

Clinical angiograms were acquired at 30 frames/sec using a 7-in. image intensifier (Advantx/DXC, General Electric Medical Systems). The images were digitized to 512 x 512 pixel matrices with resolution of .3 mm/pixel and 256 gray levels.

Normal arteries and arteries with lesions (filling defects) were simulated on individual frames of the acquired clinical sequences. The simulation algorithm, described extensively by Eckstein et al [7], takes into account scattering, veiling glare, and focal spot blur, generating arteries as 3-D right circular cylinders with a diameter of 12 pixels (3.6 mm) and a narrowing at the center (minimum diameter of 8 pixels). Four arteries were generated on each frame of the test sequences and one out of these four would contain the filling defect target, a hemi-ellipsoidal shape (diameter of 6 pixels) located at the vertical and horizontal center of the artery.

---

[2] A quick test compressing 25 x-ray angiograms using JPEG and a fixed quality factor of 50 yielded a mean compression ratio 20.9 with a standard deviation of 4.4 and a range of 14 to 30.

The arterial motion was achieved using data from 40 different manually tracked clinical angiogram sequences as positions for the simulated arteries. The feature-stabilized display was achieved by digitally shifting the images by these same displacements.

2.2 Compression of images

Copies of the images were compressed and decompressed with the fifth public release of the Independent JPEG Group's free JPEG software [8] and the RICOH corporation's CREW code, a wavelet based software (RICOH Company Ltd., Menlo Park, CA) [9]. We chose these software packages because they were easily available and well-documented. Neither the JPEG nor the CREW codes allow the user to specify a desired compression ratio; instead, both take a quality factor (or level) parameter which influences the compression ratio. In JPEG, the quality factor varies between 1 and 100; entering 100 will return a high quality, but uncompressed image while 1 returns a poor quality, but highly compressed image. CREW's quality factor, on the other hand, varies between 1 and 75; entering 1 results in a virtually-uncompressed image while 75 returns a highly compressed image. Furthermore, a fixed quality factor will compress different images at different compression ratios[2]. Thus, to compare the different algorithms at a specified compression ratio we used a computer program that iteratively adjusts the quality factor at each image to get as close as possible to the desired ratio. Figure 2 shows the JPEG and CREW codes' relationships between quality factor and compression ratio for a single coronary angiogram with simulated arteries. With JPEG it is possible to get almost arbitrarily close to any value in its near-continuity of compression ratios. But the CREW code's response is highly discontinuous and the available compression ratios are limited.

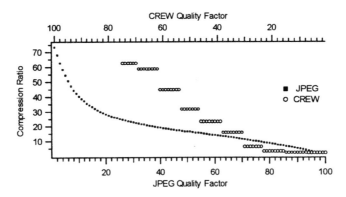

Figure 2. Compression ratio (size of original file / size of compressed file) of a single frame of x-ray cine-angiogram with simulated arteries at various JPEG and CREW quality factors. JPEG quality factors can vary between 1 and 100 while CREW quality factors range between 1 and 75.

With a target ratio of 15:1 the JPEG achieved (average ratio $\pm$ standard deviation) 14.9:1 $\pm$ 0.2 while CREW achieved 19.2:1 $\pm$ 5.5. The CREW code's inability to compress at or near the target ratio is due to this descretized characteristic of the algorithm.

2.3 Psychophysical studies

Two naïve observers (GR, CH) and one radiologist (DV) participated in the study. The naïve observers both had extended training visually detecting simulated lesions in medical images and the radiologist had previous experience reading x-ray coronary angiograms. The task was to detect the simulated filling defect in one of the four simulated arteries in each sequence (4 alternative forced choice). Each sequence consisted of 32 frames with simulated arteries with real coronary motion and was displayed at 32 frames/s. Three compression conditions (uncompressed, 15:1 JPEG, and 19:1 CREW) and two display types (M.A. and S.D) gave a total of six conditions and observers ran five sessions of 100 trials (sequences) for each, in a randomized order. The 100 available sequences for each compression modality and were viewed in a randomized order for each session.

2.4 Data analysis

The accuracy for a given session of 100 trials was recorded as the percent correct (Pc), the proportion of trials in which the observer correctly identified the artery containing the lesion. Pc was then transformed to index of detectability (d_a) for an M-alternative forced choice, given by [10]:

$$Pc(d_a, M) = \int_{\Re} g(z - d_a)[G(z)]^{M-1} dz \qquad (1)$$

where $g(z) = \frac{1}{\sqrt{2\pi}} e^{-z^2/2}$, $G(z) = \int_{-\infty}^{z} g(z')dz'$, and M is the number of alternatives (4 in this case).

The index of detectability has been shown to be approximately constant with the number of alternatives in the task and linear with signal contrast in white noise [11] and x-ray coronary angiograms [12, 13].

3. RESULTS AND DISCUSSION

Figure 3 shows each observer's performance as well as an average across observers, measured by index of detectability, for both display methods (M.A. and S.D.) in the uncompressed, JPEG, and CREW compression methods. Given that the three observers displayed very similar patterns of results we performed statistical comparisons on performance averaged across the observers' data. T-tests with Bonferroni corrections for multiple tests resulted in non-significant differences ($p > .005$) between human performance in the uncompressed and the 15:1 JPEG compression for either display type (S.D. or M.A.). On the other hand, the CREW compression caused a significant drop in performance ($p < .005$) from the uncompressed condition for both display types.

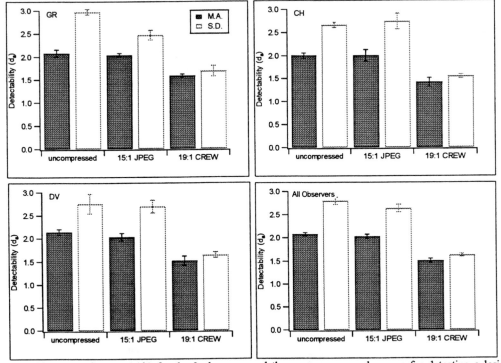

Figure 3. Human performance (d_a) for the 3 observers and the average across observers for detecting a lesion in simulated arteries for M.A. and S.D. display types and the uncompressed, 15:1 JPEG, and 19:1 CREW compression conditions.

The stabilized display resulted in a significant increase in performance ($p < .005$) over the M.A. display for the uncompressed and JPEG-compressed images. Furthermore, this S.D. effect caused performance on the

15: 1 JPEG images to be significantly higher (p < .005) than M.A.-displayed images, even at the uncompressed level. On the other hand, although the stabilized display did cause an increase in performance over the M.A. display for the CREW-compressed images, the small increase was not statistically significant (p > .005).

4. CONCLUSIONS

Our results suggest that 15:1 JPEG compression does not significantly degrade human visual detection of a morphological feature for either the conventional moving artery display or the motion stabilized x-ray coronary angiograms. In contrast, the 19:1 CREW compression does. The stabilized display significantly improves lesion detectability for uncompressed and JPEG-compressed images over the conventional moving artery display, but not significantly for the CREW images. Finally, our findings suggest that for the present task, 15:1 JPEG-compressed angiograms with the stabilized display result in higher performance than the uncompressed images with the conventional moving artery display.

ACKNOWLEDGMENTS

The authors would like to thank Darko Vodopich, Cedric Heath, and George Ruan for their participation as observers in the study. This research was supported by NIH-HL 53455.

REFERENCES

1. S. E. Nissen et al., "Cardiac angiography without cine film: Erecting a 'tower of babel' in the cardiac catheterization laboratory", Journal of the American College of Cardiology, 24, 834-837, 1994.
2. W. A. Baker et al., "Lossy (15:1) JPEG compression of digital coronary angiograms does not limit detection of subtle morphological features", Circ., 96, 1157-1164, 1997.
3. V. H. Rigolin, P. A. Robiolio, L. A. Spero, B. P. Harrawood, K. G. Morris, D. F. Fortin, W. A. Baker, T. M. Bashore, and J. T. Cusma, "Compression of digital coronary angiograms does not affect visual or quantitative assessment of coronary artery stenosis severity." American Journal of Cardiology, 78, 131-135, 1996.
4. J. S. Whiting, M. P. Eckstein, C. A. D. Honig, S. Gu, S. Einav, N.L. Eigler, "Effect of lossy image compression on observer performance in dynamically displayed digital coronary angiograms, Circ., 86 (Suppl.) I-444, Abs., 1993.
5. N. L. Eigler, M. P. Eckstein, K. Maher, D. Honig and J. S. Whiting, "Effect of a stenosis stabilized display on morphological feature detection", Circ., 89, 2700-2709, 1994.
6. M. P. Eckstein, T. D. Wickens, G Aharanov, G. Ruan, C. Morioka, and J. S. Whiting, "Quantifying the limitations of the use of consensus expert committees in ROC studies", Proceedings of the SPIE Medical Imaging Conference of the Society of Photo-Optical and Instrumentation Engineers, 3340-12, 128-134, 1998.
7. M. P. Eckstein, J. L. Bartroff, C. A. Morioka, D. Vodopich, and J. S. Whiting, "Feature stabilized digital x-ray coronary amgiograms improve human visual detection in JPEG compressed images", Opt. Exp., submitted.
8. W. B. Pennebaker and J. L. Mitchell, JPEG Still Image Data Compression Standard, Van Nostrand Reinhold, New York, 1992.
9. M. Boliek, M. J. Gormish, E. L. Schwartz, and A. Keith, "Next generation image compression and manipulation using CREW", International Conference on Image Processing, 1997.
10. D. M. Green and J. A. Swets, Signal Detection Theory and Psychophysics, Wiley, New York, 1966.
11. A. E. Burgess and H. Ghandeharian, "Visual signal detection II: Signal-location identification|", J. of the Opt. Soc. Am. A, 1, 906-910, 1984.
12. M. P. Eckstein and J.S. Whiting, "Visual signal detection in structured backgrounds I: Effect of number of possible locations and signal contrast", J. of the Opt. Soc. of Am. A, 13, 1777-1787, 1996.
13. J. S. Whiting, M. P. Eckstein, C. A. Morioka, and N. Eigler, "Effect of additive noise, signal contrast and feature motion on signal detection in structured noise in Medical Imaging", Proc. SPIE, Ed. Harold L. Kundel, 2712, 39-47, 1996.

Addendum

The following papers were announced for publication in this proceedings but have been withdrawn or are unavailable.

[3663-28]   **Real-time registration of video images and volumetric patient data during stereotactic surgery**
R. Shahidi, B. Wang, M. Epitaux, E. Wilkinson, J. Alder, Stanford Univ. School of Medicine

[3663-39]   **Bach, breasts, and power law processes**
A. E. Burgess, Brigham and Women's Hospital/Harvard Medical School

Author Index

Abbey, Craig K., 243, 273, 284
Alder, John, Addendum
Andrew, Rex K., 225
Barrett, Harrison H., 264
Bartroff, Jay L., 243, 342
Baysinger, Andrew, 253
Berbaum, Kevin S., 91
Bochud, François O., 243, 273, 284
Bruijns, Tom J., 170
Burgess, Arthur E., Addendum, 304, 316
Chakraborty, Dev P., 82
Chakraborty, Sankar, 316
Chamberlain, Charles C., 44, 180
Chau, Paul M., 333
Chen, Yeh-Fong, 91
Conetta, Donald A., 24
Cowen, Arnold R., 170
Cowley, Helen C., 157
Cuviello, Michael, 333
Dang, Philip P., 333
Davies, Andrew G., 170
Davis, Scott D., 14
Dorfman, Donald D., 91
Duerk, Jeffrey L., 232
Eckstein, Miguel P., 243, 273, 284, 342
Ellsworth, Lansing G., 199
Epitaux, Marc, Addendum
Foos, David H., 108
Friedman, Paul J., 2
Gagne, George M., 180
Gale, Alastair G., 157
Gallas, Brandon D., 264
Geiser, Edward A., 24
Gennari, Rose C., 8
Gerritsen, Frans A., 34
Gifford, Howard C., 187
Good, Walter F., 8, 100
Gur, David, 8, 74, 100
Hanlon, William B., 14
Hansen, Ronald C., 199
Hendrickson, Dan, 108
Hite, Pamela, 199
Howard, Nelson Scott, 82
Huda, Walter, 44
Jabri, Kadri N., 296
Jacobson, Francine L., 14, 207, 304
Jiang, Yulei, 56
Jiang, Zhiming, 180
Johnson, Jeffrey P., 253
Judy, Philip F., 14, 207, 304
Kieffer, Jean-Claude, 180
Kim, Hyae Young, 212

King, Jill L., 8, 74, 100
King, Michael A., 187
Kohm, Kevin S., 108
Krol, Andrzej, 180
Krupinski, Elizabeth A., 151, 199, 217, 253
Kundel, Harold L., 82, 122, 146
Langer, Steven G., 225
Lee, Elisa T., 61
Lee, Jin Seong, 212
Lee, Samuel C., 61
Lenth, Russell V., 91
LeSueur, Behjamin W., 199
Levine, Norman, 199
Lim, Tae-Hwan, 212
Lopez, Ana Maria, 199
Lubin, Jeffrey, 253
Maeder, Anthony J., 129
Maitz, Glenn S., 8, 74
Mello-Thoms, Claudia, 146
Misra, Bijoy M., 14
Morioka, Craig A., 342
Muka, Edward, 108
Nawfel, Richard, 207
Nishikawa, Robert M., 56
Nodine, Calvin F., 122, 146
Ogawa, Eiji, 324
Peterson, Heidi A., 253
Phillips-Hughes, Jane, 136
Renvyle, Ted T., 180
Roberts, Geraint M., 136
Roehrig, Hans, 151, 217, 253
Salem, Kyle A., 232
Sarantopoulos, Peter, 199
Scalzetti, Ernest M., 180
Seltzer, Steven E., 207
Shahidi, Ramin, Addendum
Shimura, Kazuo, 324
Silvis, Nancy, 199
Sivarudrappa, Mahesh, 217
Slone, Richard M., 108
Smith, Darrel N., 207
Song, Koun-Sik, 212
Stewart, Brent K., 225
Strasters, Karel C., 34
Swensson, Richard G., 74, 100
Toto, Lawrence C., 122
Verdonck, Bert, 34
Wang, Bai, Addendum
Wang, Yiming, 61
Weinstein, Ronald S., 199
Wells, R. Glenn, 187
Wendt, Michael, 232

Whiting, Bruce R., 108
Whiting, James S., 243, 342
Wilkinson, Eric, Addendum
Wilson, David L., 232, 296
Wojtowycz, Andrij R., 44
Wooding, David S., 136
Wurzel, James P., 199
Young, Susan S., 108
Yu, Jianfan, 180
Zong, Xuli, 24